Clinical and Diagnostic Pathology

Editor

ALESSANDRO MELILLO

VETERINARY CLINICS
OF NORTH AMERICA:
EXOTIC ANIMAL PRACTICE

www.vetexotic.theclinics.com

Consulting Editor
AGNES E. RUPLEY

January 2013 • Volume 16 • Number 1

ELSEVIER

1600 John F. Kennedy Boulevard • Suite 1800 • Philadelphia, Pennsylvania, 19103-2899
http://www.theclinics.com

VETERINARY CLINICS OF NORTH AMERICA: EXOTIC ANIMAL PRACTICE Volume 16, Number 1
January 2013 ISSN 1094-9194, ISBN-13: 978-1-4557-7347-3

Editor: John Vassallo; j.vassallo@elsevier.com
Development Editor: Teia Stone

Veterinary Clinics of North America: Exotic Animal Practice (ISSN 1094-9194) is published in January, May, and September by Elsevier, Inc., 360 Park Avenue South, New York, NY 10010-1710. Subscription prices are $243.00 per year for US individuals, $389.00 per year for US institutions, $124.00 per year for US students and residents, $289.00 per year for Canadian individuals, $457.00 per year for Canadian institutions, $326.00 per year for international individuals, $457.00 per year for international institutions and $159.00 per year for Canadian and foreign students/residents. To receive student/resident rate, orders must be accompanied by name of affiliated institution, date of term, and the *signature* of program/residency coordinator on institution letterhead. Orders will be billed at individual rate until proof of status is received. Foreign air speed delivery is included in all *Clinics* subscription prices. All prices are subject to change without notice. **POSTMASTER:** Send address changes to *Veterinary Clinics of North America: Exotic Animal Practice*, Elsevier Health Sciences Division, Subscription Customer Service, 3251 Riverport Lane, Maryland Heights, MO 63043. **Customer Service: Telephone: 1-800-654-2452** (U.S. and Canada); **1-314-447-8871** (outside U.S. and Canada). **Fax: 1-314-447-8029. E-mail:journalscustomerservice-usa@elsevier.com** (for print support); **journalsonlinesupport-usa@elsevier.com** (for online support).

Reprints. For copies of 100 or more of articles in this publication, please contact the Commercial Reprints Department, Elsevier Inc., 360 Park Avenue South, New York, New York 10010-1710. Tel.: (212)-633-3813; Fax: (212)-633-1935; E-mail: reprints@elsevier.com.

Veterinary Clinics of North America: Exotic Animal Practice is covered in *MEDLINE/PubMed (Index Medicus)*.

Printed and bound by CPI Group (UK) Ltd, Croydon, CR0 4YY

Transferred to digital print 2012

Contributors

CONSULTING EDITOR

AGNES E. RUPLEY, DVM
Diplomate, American Board of Veterinary Practitioners–Avian Practice; Director and Chief Veterinarian, All Pets Medical & Laser Surgical Center, College Station, Texas

EDITOR

ALESSANDRO MELILLO, DVM
Clinica Veterinaria OMNIAVET, Roma; Department of Veterinary Clinical Sciences, University of Teramo, Italy

AUTHORS

MARÍA ARDIACA, LV (Veterinarian)
Centro Veterinario Los Sauces, Madrid, Spain

ERIKA AZZARA, DVM
San Donà, Veneto, Italy

MATTIA BIELLI, DVM
Ambulatorio Veterinario Dott. Mattia Bielli, Novara, Italy

CRISTINA BONVEHÍ, LV (Veterinarian)
Centro Veterinario Los Sauces, Madrid, Spain

RAFFAELLA CAPITELLI, Dr Med Vet
CSV-Labvet Missaglia, Lecco, Italy

AUGUSTO CARLUCCIO, DVM, PhD
Department of Veterinary Clinical Sciences, University of Teramo, Italy

SALVATORE CATANIA, DVM, PhD
Istituto Zooprofilattico Sperimentale delle Venezie, Legnaro, Padua, Italy

DIEGO CATTAROSSI, DVM, PhD
Treviso, Italy

SIMONE CELIBERTI, DVM
Clinica Veterinaria OMNIAVET, Roma, Italy

ALBERTO CONTRI, DVM, PhD
Department of Veterinary Clinical Sciences, University of Teramo, Italy

LORENZO CROSTA, Dr Med Vet, PhD
Clinica Veterinaria Valcurone Missaglia, Lecco, Italy

ALESSIA GLORIA, DVM, PhD
Department of Veterinary Clinical Sciences, University of Teramo, Italy

FRANCES MARGARET HARCOURT-BROWN, BVSc, FRCVS, RCVS
Diplomate, European College of Zoological Medicine; Recognised Specialist in Rabbit Medicine and Surgery, Crab Lane Veterinary Surgery, Bilton, Harrogate, North Yorkshire, United Kingdom

MINH HUYNH, DVM
Exotic Department, Centre Hospitalier Vétérinaire Fregis, Arcueil, France

FLORA LALOI, DVM
Exotic Department, Centre Hospitalier Vétérinaire Fregis, Arcueil, France

STEFANIA LEOPARDI, DVM
Exotic Animal Department, Clinica Veterinaria Modena Sud, Spilamberto, Modena, Italy

ALESSANDRO MELILLO, DVM
Clinica Veterinaria OMNIAVET, Roma; Department of Veterinary Clinical Sciences, University of Teramo, Italy

ANDRÉS MONTESINOS, LV (Veterinarian)
Centro Veterinario Los Sauces, Madrid, Spain

GIORDANO NARDINI, DVM
Medical Director of the Exotic Animal Department, Clinica Veterinaria Modena Sud, Spilamberto, Modena; Lecturer, Faculty of Veterinary Medicine, University of Teramo, Teramo; PhD Student, Faculty of Veterinary Medicine, University of Bologna, Italy

TANJA PERIC, DScA
Department of Food Sciences, University of Udine, Udine, Italy

DOMENICO ROBBE, DVM, PhD
Department of Veterinary Clinical Sciences, University of Teramo, Italy

Contents

The presence of nucleated erythrocytes and thrombocytes in reptile blood limits the use of electronic cell-counting devices for leukocytes so that manual counting techniques and evaluation of blood smears are necessary, resulting in time-consuming procedures requiring good training and experience. The evaluation of most hematologic values is complicated by the many physiologic adaptations occurring in reptiles, making references values very difficult to interpret. This article brings together most of the bibliography about hemochrome evaluation in reptiles, with schematic instruction about sample collection, handling, and evaluation. Information about evaluation of both qualitative and quantitative aspects of reptile hematology are also given.

The canary (*Serinus canaria*) is a highly popular bird with families as a companion animal and among breeders for competitive purposes. The mortality rate in these animals is very high at the onset of an epidemic, and the technical times of a laboratory often necessitate starting treatment before having completed the diagnostic procedure. This article describes a practical approach that deals with the first things to do in the clinic as soon as the animal arrives or the breeder asks for advice and explains the procedure in a specialist laboratory for processing samples and completing the diagnosis.

The i-STAT PCA can be used as a blood analyzer in critical avian patients, although single values must be interpreted carefully. The study of the acid-base status in companion birds is still in its infancy. Further research is needed to establish normal reference values in arterial blood gases, compare them with venous blood gas, and to determine if the formulas that deviate from small animal medicine are or are not applicable.

Part 1 presents a comprehensive overview of the differences between mammals on sampling methods, processing, testing, and interpretation of data, with special attention to the meaning of pathologic and normal, and the differences among species and diseases. Part 2 critically analyzes 150 different hematologic and biochemical profiles obtained over 5 years from 150 psittacine birds belonging to 29 different species, brought to our clinic and/or examined in other locations, with confirmed or strongly suspected diseases. The results are grouped according to the various pathologies observed with respect to species and the degree of variation from the reference range of each species.

Liver disease in ferrets is often subclinical and underdiagnosed. Clinical pathology and diagnostic imaging are needed to guide clinicians but definite diagnosis is based on histopathologic lesions. Inflammatory digestive conditions can lead to ascending tract infection and hepatobiliary inflammation. Ferrets have a specific sensitivity to hepatic lipidosis. Incidence of hepatic neoplasia is high in ferrets. After a summary of anatomy and physiology of the ferret liver, hepatic diseases known in ferret species are reviewed with their subsequent diagnostic procedures.

There are differences in renal anatomy and physiology between rabbits and other domestic species. Neurogenic renal ischemia occurs readily. Reversible prerenal azotemia may be seen in conjunction with gut stasis. Potentially fatal acute renal failure may be due to structural kidney damage or post-renal disease. Chronic renal failure is often associated with encephalitozoonosis. Affected rabbits cannot vomit and often eat well. Weight loss, lethargy, and cachexia are common clinical signs. Polydypsia/polyuria may be present. Derangements in calcium and phosphorus metabolism are features of renal disease. Radiography is always indicated. Urolithiasis, osteosclerosis, aortic and renal calcification are easily seen on radiographs.

This article outlines a practical approach for the use of blood-gas analysis in pet rabbits using the I-STAT analyzer. Sampling techniques and a theoretic approach to diagnosis are described. The following 95% RI were obtained from venous samples of 45 healthy rabbits: pH (7.245–7.533), PCO_2 (28.9–52.9 mm Hg), HCO_3 (17.0–32.5 mmol/L), total CO_2 (18–34 mmol/L), BE_{ecf} (−10–8 mmol/L), AnGap (11–26 mmol/L), Na (136–147 mmol/L), K (3.4–5.7 mmol/L), Cl (93–113 mmol/L), Glu (93–245 mg/dL), BUN (9–33 mg/dL). Results from 20 arterial samples were pH (7.358–7.502), PCO_2 (29.1–36.8 mm Hg), HCO_3 (17.5–27.6 mmol/L), BE_{ecf} (−7–5 mmol/L), PO_2 (75–101 mm Hg), iCa (1.67–1.85). The article also includes some conclusions obtained comparing results from healthy and ill rabbits over an 18-month period.

Simone Celiberti, Alessia Gloria, Alberto Contri, Augusto Carluccio,
Tanja Peric, Alessandro Melillo, and Domenico Robbe

> The data about chinchilla (*Chinchilla laniger*) reproduction are limited and
> in some cases discordant. The aim of this study was to monitor the sexual
> hormone fluctuation by fecal progesterone level and colpocytology analy-
> sis by vaginal smears in order to evaluate the different phases of the oes-
> trus cycle. Twenty-four non pregnant chinchillas aged from 1 to 4 years old
> and subdivided in three groups were monitored. In contrast with findings
> reported in other study, the high values of progesterone recorded in
> autumn suggested the presence of a ciclicity also in this period. The
> data indicate that chinchilla presents a continuous cycle.

Alessandro Melillo

> Serum Protein Electrophoresis (SPE) is a useful diagnostic and prognostic
> tool in human and companion animals medicine: several experiences
> show that it can be useful in exotic practice as well. The fundamentals
> of SPE interpretation as well as some normal and pathological patterns
> for the species most commonly seen in practice are provided.

VETERINARY CLINICS OF NORTH AMERICA: EXOTIC ANIMAL PRACTICE

THE CLINICS ARE NOW AVAILABLE ONLINE!
Access your subscription at:
www.theclinics.com

Preface

Clinical and Diagnostic Pathology

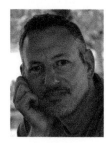

Alessandro Melillo, DVM
Editor

Since the first tentative steps in the field of exotic animal medicine, I have always been frustrated by the lack of information about laboratory medicine of less conventional or common species, and I have looked with envy at the flights of fancy of my colleagues, who reflected, discussed, and extrapolated information from complete blood cell counts and biochemical profiles of dogs and cats.

The small size of the patients, the difficulty in collecting representative samples, and, especially, the lack of reference values and statistical studies available for most species seemed to make every attempt to do so in exotic pets only a futile exercise of skill that produced useless or misleading results.

Luckily, over the years, the situation has changed as we have learned techniques for handling and safer sedation that allow us to take samples safely for us and patients; we use machines that work with small volumes of blood, and, especially, we continue to accumulate data.

Laboratory medicine is based on statistical studies: for many exotic animals, the amount of data available doesn't yet allow one to make an accurate assessment of the health of an individual from just a few drops of blood, but only through gradually collecting data and documenting our experiences will new connections be made and new uses for laboratory analysis tested.

The goal is to be able to reach, whenever possible, a precise diagnosis and useful targeted therapies in the least invasive and respectful animal welfare way. The commitment of all our colleagues who have contributed, sacrificing their precious little free time to bring their experience to us, is deeply appreciated.

My thanks go to all of them and to Elsevier, which has allowed the publication of these experiences, reflections, and notes in the hope that they will be helpful in

Vet Clin Exot Anim 16 (2013) ix–x
http://dx.doi.org/10.1016/j.cvex.2012.11.003
1094-9194/13/$ – see front matter © 2013 Published by Elsevier Inc.

vetexotic.theclinics.com

developing an exotic animal medicine that is more efficient and useful to the difficult task of protecting the welfare of these animals in captivity.

Alessandro Melillo, DVM
Clinica Veterinaria OMNIAVET
Piazza G. Omiccioli 5
00125 Roma, Italy

E-mail address:
birdalec@gmail.com

Clinical Hematology in Reptilian Species

Giordano Nardini, DVM[a,b,c,]*, Stefania Leopardi, DVM[a],
Mattia Bielli, DVM[d]

KEYWORDS

- Blood • Clinical pathology • Erythrocytes • Hematology • Leukocyte • Reptile

KEY POINTS

- The interpretation of hematologic data is still challenging in reptiles in comparison with small animals, because of the lower number of studies and the lack of reference values for the majority of species.
- The presence of nucleated erythrocytes and thrombocytes in reptile blood limits the use of electronic cell-counting devices for leukocytes, so that manual counting techniques and evaluation of blood smears are necessary.
- Despite problems in interpretation, hematology should always be done, thus giving the veterinarians the opportunity to increase knowledge in this field.
- Other than a good differential count, the evaluation of cellular morphology is essential while reading a blood smear, to detect signs of regeneration, inflammatory responses, toxicosis, and the presence of parasites or inclusions.
- As great variability exists in reptilian hematologic parameters in response to many intrinsic and environmental situations, serial sampling is always preferred to single results, as they may be useful in monitoring the progress of the disease.

INTRODUCTION

In reptile medicine very few pathognomonic indicators are known, so the diagnosis often requires a combination of diagnostic tests, including hematology, biochemistry, cytology, histopathology, microbiology, clinical pathology, and serology. Hematology is commonly used in mammals to investigate conditions that may affect the blood cells, such as anemia, inflammatory diseases, hematopoietic disorders, hemostatic

This work was not supported by any funding.
The authors have nothing to disclose.
[a] Exotic Animal Department, Clinica Veterinaria Modena Sud, Piazza dei Tintori 1, Spilamberto 41057, Modena, Italy; [b] University of Teramo, Piazza Aldo Moro, 45, Teramo 64100, Italy; [c] University of Bologna, Via Tolara di Sopra, 50, Ozzano dell'Emilia 40064, Bologna, Italy; [d] Ambulatorio Veterinario Dr Mattia Bielli, Viale Buonarroti 20/a, Novara 28100, Italy
* Corresponding author.
E-mail address: giordano.nardini@gmail.com

alterations, and parasitemia. Nevertheless, the interpretation of hematologic data is still challenging in reptiles in comparison with small animals, because of the lower number of studies and the lack of reference values for certain species. Furthermore, different physiologic conditions and adaptations to the environment in reptiles may consistently vary these parameters, making it difficult to establish the clinical significance of variations from the reference values.

SAMPLE COLLECTION

Besides proper testing and interpretation, obtaining reliable results starts with a proper collection and handling of the sample. Poor sample collection and handling produce poor-quality blood data, which can be useless or can even mislead the clinician. Other than a clean blood sample, every diagnostic procedure requires an appropriate volume of blood and an appropriate anticoagulant. Furthermore, it is always important to keep in mind that blood collection represents an invasive procedure, thus pain and risk of infection may be considered.[1] To minimize this collateral effect, the asepsis of the technique must be always guaranteed, and the least traumatic site that leads to the most diagnostic sample should be always chosen. Sedation or anesthesia may be necessary for the safety of the animal and/or the clinician. For this purpose many protocols are adequate, but only ketamine alone or combined with xylazine or midazolam has been proved not to affect hematologic parameters.[2]

The total blood volume of reptiles varies between species; the range is estimated at between 5% and 8% of the body weight. Before collecting blood it is important, especially for small animals, to accurately calculate the maximum safe volume of the sample. Because most healthy reptiles can tolerate an acute loss of up to 10% of the total blood volume, most investigators agree that an amount of blood of up to 0.5% to 0.8% of body weight in grams can be collected safely.[3–6] According to some investigators,[2] the withdrawal can reach 1% of the body weight. Usually lower volumes are sufficient for complete biochemistry and hematology, so the smallest useful volume should be collected (usually 1.5–2 mL/kg). If trials or monitoring of animals requires serial blood collections over an extended period of time, the total amount of withdrawal increases, as much larger blood loss can be tolerated chronically, also depending on the health of the animal and its environmental and nutritional management. Nevertheless, further studies are necessary to estimate a safe volume and safe intervals between samples.

The use of anticoagulant is necessary when collecting blood for hematologic evaluation. Whereas in mammals ethylenediaminetetraacetic acid (EDTA) is the anticoagulant of choice for such evaluations, it has been found to cause hemolysis in reptile blood samples, especially in chelonians.[2,7] Thus, lithium heparin (LiHe) is widely used for reptile hematology in many reptilians. However, LiHe can cause clumping of leukocytes and thrombocytes and creates a blue tinge to blood films, resulting in difficulties in the evaluation of cell morphology.[2] To minimize these effects, it is wise that blood samples are processed as soon as possible after collection. However, EDTA can be used in most lizards, and is considered the anticoagulant of choice in some species such as the green iguana (*Iguana iguana*) and the Chinese water dragon (*Physignathus cocincinus*).[2] According to these investigators, in the aforementioned species EDTA allows for better staining of the cells and therefore makes cells' identification easier than for cells exposed to heparin. Also, in chelonians some clinicians use a combination of EDTA and LiHe to preserve samples for hematology.[7] Once again, samples need to be processed soon after collection. Other investigators suggest citrated blood samples to be also suitable for hematology.[7] Thus, it is clear that there is no single preferred anticoagulant for hematology in reptiles, because cells' reaction to anticoagulant may be taxa specific.[3]

For a complete diagnostic panel, blood samples should be always accompanied by blood smears, used for differential white blood cell (WBC) count, for the evaluation of cell morphology and to assess toxic changes, the presence of blood parasites, and bacterial and viral inclusions. To avoid any interference during staining, blood film slides should be quickly prepared following collection from a drop of blood containing no anticoagulant.

Many sites are available for blood collection in reptiles. Details about the venipuncture sites mostly used for blood collection from reptiles are summarized in **Table 1**. Usually the site that allows the safest and least traumatic withdrawal both for the animal and the clinician should be used. Many parameters need to be borne in mind while choosing the venipuncture site:

- Species
- Size
- Volume of blood needed
- Physical condition of the patient
- Temperament of the patient
- Clinician confidence: venipuncture in reptiles is often a blind technique, so anatomic knowledge about position of vessels is essential
- Considerations about hemodilution

In reptiles, lymphatic vessels often accompany blood vessels, so the collection of a mixture of blood and lymph may occur. This mixture will lead to a dilution of blood resulting in lower packed cell volume (PCV), hemoglobin concentration (Hb), erythrocyte count (TRBC), and leukocyte count (TWBC).[2] Some biochemical parameters seem to be also influenced by lymphodilution with a reduction of lactate dehydrogenase, uric acid, alkaline phosphatase, albumins, globulins, and alanine aminotransferase.[7] Furthermore, lymphodilution leads to an abnormally stained background of smears, similar to the blue tinge typical of heparinized samples. This risk varies from site to site depending on vessel anatomy and, according to the evidence of a different composition of the lymph depending on location, the effect is often unpredictable. Investigators generally agree that lymphodilution is least likely to occur during collections from the jugular veins and the heart, so this site should be always preferred whenever possible. Nevertheless, it is important to consider also the parameters previously described before attempting venipuncture. For example, the collection from the heart is only suggested in snakes and neonatal turtles, usually under general anesthesia, to prevent cardiac laceration and excessive hemorrhage. Furthermore, it is possible to dilute cardiac samples with pericardial fluid. Moreover, although conventional wisdom dictates that jugular samples should be taken as a gold standard, no definitive studies prove this. Jugular samples from chelonians have been compared with tail samples and with subvertebral venous sinus samples.[7] Although samples from the subvertebral venous sinus have been considered less reliable, in 20% of animals the PCV measured was actually higher in the tail sample compared with the jugular ones. This fact raises the possibility that lymphodilution may also occur in jugular blood samples. More studies are needed to better estimate the reliability of each venipuncture site.

Because lymphatic vessels are usually more superficial compared with blood vessels, lymph appears as a transparent fluid often entering the syringe immediately before the appearance of the blood. When this occurs, the sample collection needs to be attempted again with new materials.

Table 1
Venipuncture sites used in reptiles

	First Choice		Jugular Vein	Venous Sinuses
Chelonians	Jugular vein		According to the species: Internal and external Ventral and dorsal The right may be larger	Supravertebral: Dorsal, mainly sea turtles Postoccipital, mainly freshwater turtles Subcarapacial Dorsal tail Easily approachable
		Pro	Lymphodilution less frequent; may be visualized especially in tortoises	Possible lymphodilution; Caution not to damage the spinal cord (postoccipital sinus)
		Con	Requires head restraint: may be dangerous or impossible without sedation in big or feisty animals	
Snakes	Heart	Pro	—	—
		Con		
Lizards	Ventral tail vein (ventral and lateral approach)	Con	Right one usually bigger	—
Crocodilians	Supravertebral vein. for bigger ones; Ventral tail vein for smaller ones	Con	—	Supravertebral Possible lymphodilution; caution to avoid spinal trauma

	Coccigeal Vein	Heart	Other (Less Frequent)
Chelonians	Dorsal Useful site for dangerous animals not approachable from the front Possible lymphodilution. Risk of damage to the central nervous system and of contamination of renal tubules	Only site for very small individuals with soft plastron Require a drill to pass the plastron unless cases of soft plastron (physiologic or pathologic)	Veins of the limbs (brachial plexus, femoral plexus) Difficult Small samples often obtained
Snakes	Ventral Possible lymphodilution. Well developed only in some species (eg, rattlesnake); pay attention to hemipenes (males) and musk glands (females)	Safe if the heart is stabilized Harder in small individuals (<300 g); may require sedation if restraint is difficult	Palatine-pterygoid vein Well visualized in big snakes Very fragile, easy formation of big hematomas
Lizards	Ventral Possible lymphodilution (lateral approach). Attention to hemipenes in males (ventral approach). Not possible in some lizards with semicalcified scales	Dangerous because the heart cannot be stabilized	Ventral abdominal vein High risk of uncontrollable hemorrhage
Crocodilians	Ventral	Dangerous because the heart cannot be stabilized	

HEMATOLOGIC METHODS

Hematology is used to evaluate blood cell number and morphology, hematocrit, hemoglobin concentration, and erythrocytic indices. Erythrocyte counts can be performed with automatic counting machines, and the same systems can be used to determine hematocrit and hemoglobin.[1,8,9] On the other hand, the presence of nucleated erythrocytes and thrombocytes in reptile blood precludes the use of electronic cell-counting devices for WBC count, so that manual counting methods are necessary. For a thorough examination, the hemogram should always be accompanied by the evaluation of blood smears, which requires special training to obtain reliable and consistent results. **Tables 2** and **3** summarize all the parameters that must be considered for a complete hematologic investigation, and the methods commonly used for the evaluation of every parameter.

Other secondary parameters can be obtained using published references.[2]

$$MCV = \frac{PCV(\%)}{TRBC} \times 10 \qquad MCH = \frac{Hb}{TRBC} \times 10 \qquad MCHC = \frac{Hb}{PCV(\%)} \times 100$$

Microhematocrit Centrifugation

This technique, described in **Fig. 1**, is used to assess the PCV, which provides the percentage of whole blood that is composed mainly of erythrocytes. As in mammals, in reptiles this is considered the quickest and most practical method; furthermore, it is thought to be the most reproducible technique.[10]

Table 2
Hematologic parameters considered in the reptile hemogram and relative methods

Quantitative Parameter		Method
Erythron	Packed cell volume (PCV)	Microhematocrit
	Total erythrocyte count (TRBC)	Erythrocyte Unopette system (manual) (Unopette, Becton Dickinson) (no longer available[a]) Natt and Herrick solution (manual) (Natt and Herrick, 1952) Electronic cell counter
	Hemoglobin concentration (Hb)	Cyan methemoglobin method
	Reticulocyte number	Slide stained with new methylene blue
Leukogram	Total leukocyte count (TWBC)	Semidirect Phloxine B method (manual) Direct Natt and Herrick method (manual)
	Differential leukocyte count	Slides evaluation
Thrombocytes	Total thrombocyte count (TTC)	Natt and Herrick solution (manual)
	Subjective thrombocyte count	Slides evaluation

Qualitative Parameter	Method
Cell morphology Presence of inclusions Presence of parasites	Slides evaluation

[a] In 2007, the Unopette system (Becton Dickinson) was replaced by the Avian Leukopette kit. This method is only recommended for birds.

Data from Pendl H. Avian and reptilian hematology. In: Proceedings of 11th European AAV conference, 1st Scientific ECZM Meeting. EAAV: Madrid; 2011. p. 550–64.

Table 3
Application, advantages, and disadvantages of Natt and Herrick solution versus Phloxine B solution for the leukocyte count

Natt and Herrick			Phloxine B
Can be used to count erythrocytes, leukocytes, and thrombocytes	Pro	Con	Only used for heterophils and eosinophils
Best in species with higher number of circulating lymphocytes and low heterophil count (eg, pythons)	Pro	Con	Increased errors in samples with low heterophil count
Difficulty in the differentiation between lymphocytes, thrombocytes, and immature erythrocytes	Con	Pro	Best in species with higher number of circulating heterophils and eosinophils (eg, iguanas, some tortoises)
Requires preparation of the diluent/stain and the use of manual diluting pipettes	Con	Pro	Mixing vials and pipettes commercially available
Short shelf life of the staining solution	Con	Pro	Stability of the staining solution

It is always imperative to keep in mind that results from different manual counting techniques may not be correlated with each other. Furthermore, because manual methods are not as precise as automated ones, counts need to be validated by an estimation on the blood slide.

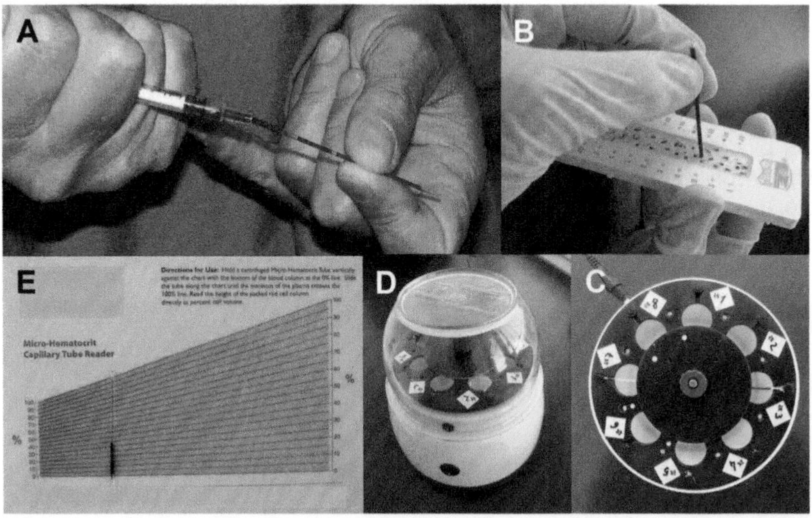

Fig. 1. Microhematocrit centrifugation technique. (*A*) Fill the microhematocrit tube (75 × 1.5 mm tubes) via capillary action to about 70% to 90% of its capacity directly from the syringe. (*B*) Seal with clay at one end by pressing the tube once or twice into the tube sealant while keeping it horizontally to prevent blood from dripping. (*C*) Position the tubes on a microhematocrit centrifuge with the clay-sealed end positioned toward the outside. (*D*) Centrifuge in the microhematocrit centrifuge at 12,000 × *g* for 5 minutes. (*E*) Use the tube-reading card to assess the packed cell volume (PCV) by comparing the percentage of erythrocytes packed in the bottom of the tube with the total volume of the tube. On aligning the erythrocyte-clay interface with the 0 line and the top of the plasma column with the 100 line in the card, the value indicated on the scale at the top of the erythrocytes column is the PCV%.

Manual Cell-Counting Methods

Different methods are available for red blood cell (RBC) and WBC counts in reptiles; whereas some are translated by mammal hematology (erythrocyte Unopette system [Unopette, Becton Dickinson], Phloxine B method), the Natt and Herrick solution has been developed specifically for avian and reptile blood cell count. Whatever method is used to dilute the blood, cells are always counted using a hemocytometer chamber. The procedure is based on the count of the number of cells in a determined volume. Specific formulae depending on the starting dilution and the volume of the hemocytometer used allow the determination of the total number per microliter of blood. In the Neubauer hemocytometer, the grid is composed of 9 major squares, which clearly appear on observing the slide under the microscope at 40× magnification (**Fig. 2**). Cells are included in the count according to their position in the grid, with different methods depending on the counted cells, explained in **Table 4**. It has been determined that any of these manual counting methods may have an inherent error of 10%.[2] It may be very useful to always count and compare both sides of the chamber[2]: when the difference between the counts obtained from each chamber exceeds 10%, the procedure should be repeated.

Blood Smear Preparation

As already mentioned, the evaluation of blood slides is an essential part of the hemogram assessment. Blood smears are used for the differential leukocyte count but are also important for the evaluation of cell morphology and the presence of blood parasites. To avoid anticoagulants artifacts, smears have to be prepared with fresh blood immediately after collection without anticoagulants.[1]

The aim of any blood slide technique is either to create a monolayer of individually dispersed cells and a minimal disturbance of the relative cell distribution that reflect the cell concentration in the mixed blood.[11] The visible result should be a uniform film of blood that gets progressively thinner. Because big cells such as monocytes and heterophils are concentrated at the margin of the smear, its edges must be examinable. It is always wise to prepare at least 3 good smears. To prepare a blood smear

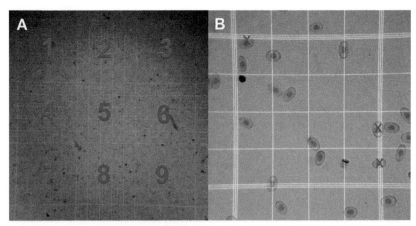

Fig. 2. Neubauer hemocytometer chamber. (*A*) Nine major squares, × 100 magnification. (*B*) Conventionally, cells touching the left and lower lines are always included in the count, whereas cells touching the right and upper lines are not, × 400 magnification.

Table 4 Manual cell-counting techniques		
	Squares in Which Cells are Counted[a]	Equation to Obtain Total Number per Microliter of Blood
Erythrocytes (either method)	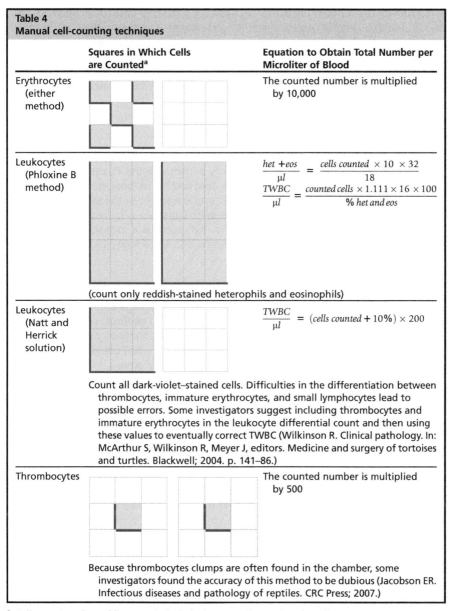	The counted number is multiplied by 10,000
Leukocytes (Phloxine B method)		$\dfrac{het + eos}{\mu l} = \dfrac{cells\ counted \times 10 \times 32}{18}$ $\dfrac{TWBC}{\mu l} = \dfrac{counted\ cells \times 1.111 \times 16 \times 100}{\%\ het\ and\ eos}$
	(count only reddish-stained heterophils and eosinophils)	
Leukocytes (Natt and Herrick solution)		$\dfrac{TWBC}{\mu l} = (cells\ counted + 10\%) \times 200$
	Count all dark-violet–stained cells. Difficulties in the differentiation between thrombocytes, immature erythrocytes, and small lymphocytes lead to possible errors. Some investigators suggest including thrombocytes and immature erythrocytes in the leukocyte differential count and then using these values to eventually correct TWBC (Wilkinson R. Clinical pathology. In: McArthur S, Wilkinson R, Meyer J, editors. Medicine and surgery of tortoises and turtles. Blackwell; 2004. p. 141–86.)	
Thrombocytes		The counted number is multiplied by 500
	Because thrombocytes clumps are often found in the chamber, some investigators found the accuracy of this method to be dubious (Jacobson ER. Infectious diseases and pathology of reptiles. CRC Press; 2007.)	

[a] Cells crossing the red lines are included whereas cells crossing the others are not.

2 main procedures are known: the slide-to-slide technique, also called the wedge technique, and the coverslip method.

After being rapidly air-dried, these smears can be also stained later. McArthur and colleagues[7] recommend gentle use of a hair dryer to achieve rapid drying with good cell preservation.

Slides are commonly stained with Romanowsky-type stains such as Giemsa, Wright, or Wright/Giemsa, as they allow the best differentiation of cells, especially between leukocytes and thrombocytes, of which cytoplasm remains translucent.

Romanowsky quick stains such as Diff-Quick are less likely to be used because they tend to damage lymphocytes and lead to underestimation of immature erythrocytes and lymphocytes.[10] Furthermore, quick stains determine a more evident coalescence of heterophil granules compared with other stains, making the evaluation of these cells difficult. On the other hand, rapid stains have obvious advantages; some investigators[12] consider them to be adequate. May-Grunwald Giemsa is especially good for marine turtles, as it is the best to differentiate basophils.[12]

SAMPLE EVALUATION: QUALITATIVE ASPECTS
Microhematocrit Tube Evaluation

After centrifugation, the blood's components separate in the microhematocrit tube (**Fig. 3**). Other than the presence of the buffy coat and the percentage of RBC (hematocrit), the microhematocrit centrifugation technique also allows the technician to evaluate the color of plasma, which should be clear to light yellow. In herbivorous reptiles an orange-yellow plasma can be due to the diet, such as a greenish-yellow one in snakes[4]; otherwise a green coloration of plasma should be related to a high concentration of biliverdina.[2]

Cell Evaluation

The evaluation of reptile blood cells requires a good knowledge and a lot of practice, as differentiation between cellular types is not always so obvious, even for experts. Furthermore, discussions are still ongoing about the significance of certain cellular types, such as azurophil cells. Other than a good differential count, the evaluation of cellular morphology is essential while reading a blood smear, to detect signs of regeneration, inflammatory responses, toxicosis, and the presence of parasites or inclusions. As some of these cellular alterations have no pathologic significance, a good knowledge is once again essential for a good diagnosis.

Red blood cells
The functions of a reptile RBC is similar to that of mammals. The main difference is the presence of the nucleus, which reptiles have in common with birds, bony fish, and amphibians. Just as in the other animals, reptile RBC contain hemoglobin tetramers that carry oxygen and carbon dioxide to and from the tissues, respectively. The structure of the hemoglobin seems to be similar across the different species of reptiles; however, small changes in the molecular structure result in significant variation of the oxygen affinity among different species and individuals. The highest affinity is reported in lizards, whereas the lowest one is reported in chelonians. Differences in the oxygen affinity are also related to the age of some species (eg, turtles) whereby 2 functionally different hemoglobin tetramers can be found in the same RBC.[4]

Reptile RBC are mostly produced in the extravascular space in the bone marrow, although erythroid precursors may also replicate in the peripheral blood. In neonates and up to the first year the yolk sac is the primary site of erythropoiesis. Old RBC undergo programmed cell death and are removed from the blood by phagocytes

A   B   C

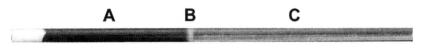

Fig. 3. Microhematocrit tube. (A) Sedimented red blood cells (RBC). (B) Buffy coat, corresponding to white blood cells (WBC) and considered as an evidence of leukocytosis. (C) Plasma.

present in the splenic tissue. The reptile RBC life span is much higher than that of mammals (2–5 months) and birds, lasting up to 600 to 800 days.[4]

Unlike in mammals, reptilian, amphibian, avian, and piscine RBC are nucleated. The nucleus is irregularly round to oval with irregular nuclear margins, oriented along the cell's long axis, centrally positioned, with dense purple chromatin. RBC without nuclei (erythroplastids) are occasionally seen as well as bare nuclei named hematogones.[13] Reptilian RBCs are elliptical and large, ranging in length from 14 to 23 μm and in width from 8 to 14 μm[14]; only amphibians' RBC are larger. Both the general and the nuclear shape are slightly variable among different species (**Fig. 4**). Poikilocytes are RBC of irregular shape. Their presence could be due to diseases (anemia, toxicosis) or to improper sampling or blood smear preparation (graphic A in **Table 5**).

No unequivocal classification exists for early stages of erythrocytes. Frye[13] talks about proerythroblast, erythroblast, and early and late polychromatophil. Early stages are bigger and rounder than mature RBC and are characterized by a round, large nucleus and a scant amount of dark blue cytoplasm; they are capable of replication, thus their increased number, binucleated cells, and cells containing mitotic figures are an appropriate physiologic response to anemia and do not have to be associated with neoplastic processes.[4,5] The normal maturation process provides an increase in cytoplasm, which progressively loses its blue stain, an elongation of the shape, and a condensation of the nuclear chromatin. The latest precursors of reptile RBC directly identifiable using Romanowsky-type stains are the polychromatophilic erythrocytes. These cells are yet rounder in shape with more basophilic cytoplasm compared with RBC, and have a larger nucleus with a disperse chromatin with obvious pale

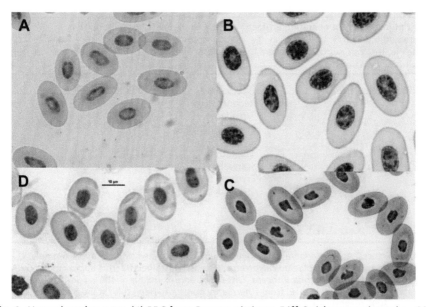

Fig. 4. Normal erythrocytes. (*A*) RBC from *Pogona vitticeps*, Diff-Quick; approximately × 800 magnification. (*B*) RBC from *Testudo hermanni boettgeri*, Hemacolor stained (Merck, Darmstadt, Germany); approximately × 1000 magnification. (*C*) RBC from *Boa constrictor*, Hemacolor stained (Merck); approximately × 800 magnification. (*D*) RBC from *Emys orbicularis*, Giemsa; approximately × 800 magnification. Rounder cells are likely to occur in chelonians and some snakes. Nuclei are particularly round in shape in chelonians. (*Courtesy of* M.L. Fioravanti DVM, Bologna, Italy).

Table 5
Morphologic alteration of erythrocytes

Erythroplastids
Anucleated erythrocytes
Incidental finding
Especially in snakes

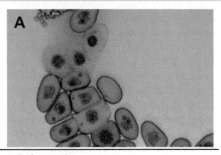

Poikilocytosis	Polychromasia
Irregular-shaped erythrocytes (arrow)	Presence of polychromatophils

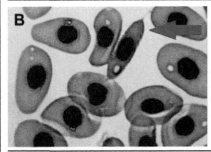 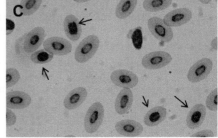

Low number: Slide preparation artifact	Low number (<1% RBC): normal
Increased number:	Increased number:
Anemia, toxicosis, septicemia, severe chronic infections	Regenerative response in moderately to severely anemic reptiles

Anisocytosis	Erythrocyte Mitosis

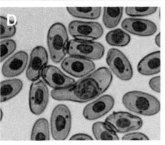

Regenerative response
Severe inflammatory disease
Malnutrition
Starvation
Erythrocyte disorders (rare)

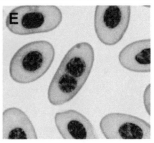

Original pictures: A: from *Vipera ammodytes,* Hemacolor stained (Merck) approximately × 1000 magnification; B: from *Chamaeleo calyptratus,* Hemacolor stained (Merck) approximately × 1000 magnification; C: from *Pogona vitticeps,* Diff-Quick approximately × 400 magnification, arrows indicate polychromatophils; D, E: from *T hermanni boettgeri,* Hemacolor stained (Merck); approximately × 1000 magnification.

euchromatin (indicating the active hemoglobin production).[4] These cells are normally found in reptilian blood, usually representing 1% of total RBC in healthy animals. This number is low in comparison with mammals and birds, probably because of the slow turnover rate of reptilian erythrocytes, the large erythrocyte life span (600–800 days in some species),[13] and the relatively low metabolic rate of reptiles. Campbell and Ellis[2] report how young reptiles tend to have a greater degree of polychromasia than adults. Different stages of RBC maturation are presented in **Fig. 5**. The erythrocyte's aging is characterized first by a progressive cytoplasmic swelling, then by the rounding of the nuclei up to perfect spheres, and finally pyknosis (evident dark, dense chromatin). These old cells are normally seen in low number (**Fig. 6**). Large evanescent cells with similar aspect to old RBC but with an intact nucleus may be found on the blood slide. These cells, named ghosts, correspond to damaged RBC in which the membrane rupture has caused the loss of chromatin (**Fig. 7**).

Morphologic alterations of RBC, including some of the more common cytoplasmic inclusions, are shown in **Tables 5** and **6**. A description of hemoparasites infecting RBC is not included in this section.

White blood cells

Reptilian WBC are commonly divided into granulocytes and mononuclear cells. Among granulocytes, eosinophils and heterophils are characterized by acidophilic granules, whereas basophils have basophilic granules. The presence of eosinophils is still controversial in snakes and in some lizards, but are present and well differentiated in chelonians and crocodilians.[15] Mononuclear cells are lymphocytes, plasma cells, and monocytes. There is still much confusion about the correct classification of azurophils; they may be considered immature forms of monocytes, because they are ultrastructurally and cytochemically similar.[16] Azurophils are typical of snakes but may also be found in low numbers in the other groups. However, some investigators highlight the little clinical advantage in separating azurophils from monocytes in the differential count.[2] The basic morphologic description of different cells is reported in **Tables 7 and 8**. Every group of cells is thus characterized by species-specific peculiarities.

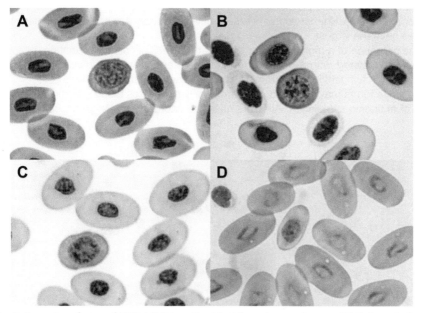

Fig. 5. Immature forms of RBC. (*A*) Proerythroblast from *Iguana iguana*. (*B*) Rubrocyte from *T hermanni boettgeri*. (*C*) Proerythrocyte from *T hermanni*. (*D*) Polychromatophil from *T hermanni*. All Hemacolor stained (Merck). Approximately × 1000 magnification.

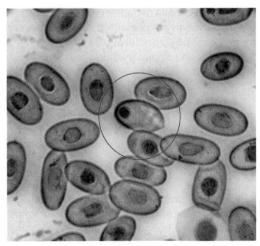

Fig. 6. Old erythrocyte (circled cell) from *Testudo graeca*, Hemacolor stained (Merck); approximately × 100 magnification.

The size of heterophils varies depending on the species, even if cells of different diameters may be seen in one blood smear from the same animal. Otherwise, shape and number of granules are characteristic of each species (**Fig. 8**).

Eosinophils granules from some species (eg, green iguanas, tegus, and rainbow lizards) stain blue-green with Romanowsky-type stains. These cells, referred to as green eosinophils, also differ from normal eosinophils because they are not known to stain with any cytochemical stains used thus far,[4] whereas the "normal" ones stain positive with benzidine peroxidase.

Regarding size, lizards also show the smallest basophils, whereas crocodiles and turtles have the largest.

The presence of a higher number of immature WBC is called left shifting, which is usually associated with severe inflammation (heterophils) or in infectious diseases that result in antigenic stimulation (lymphocytes and plasma cells).

Reactive forms may be found, with reactive lymphocytes being a particular indication of antigenic stimulation. All WBC have the capability to phagocytose infectious

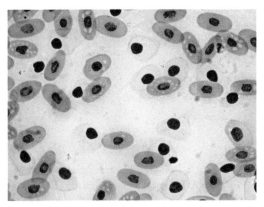

Fig. 7. Ghosts from *I iguana*, Diff-Quick; approximately × 400 magnification.

Table 6
Cytoplasmic inclusions of erythrocytes

Squared to Rectangular Clear Crystalline Inclusion	Single Round to Irregular Basophilic Inclusion	Cytoplasmic Vacuoles
Alteration; unknown significance Associated in the iguana with the common hemoglobin crystals also observed in mammals by using electron microscopy in 2001 by Harr et al	One: slide preparation artifacts especially chelonians More than one (basophilic stippling) coupled with Regenerative response Iron deposition/iron deficiency Lead toxicosis Septicemia (mainly alligators)	Slide preparation artifacts often a result of slow drying of the blood film

Small Eosinophilic Punctate Inclusion (Lizards and Snakes)	Crystalline Hexagonal Inclusion with Unknown Protein (Snakes)
Iridovirus inclusions	
May be oval in lizards identified as viral particles by using electron microscopy in 1993 by Telford and Jacobson	Increasing in size with the infection progression; viral origin confirmed in 1994 by Smith et al

Original pictures: A–C: from *I iguana*, Diff-Quick; B: from *T hermanni boettgeri*, Hemacolor stained (Merck). Approximately × 400 magnification.

agents, cells, and debris. Finding many WBC engulfed with bacteria or debris in circulating blood indicates inflammation and/or infection. Some examples of reactive WBC are illustrated in **Fig. 9**. Toxic changes of heterophils are the main morphological alterations of WBC: they are shown in **Table 9.**

Thrombocytes
Reptilian thrombocytes play a significant role in thrombus formation, assuming basically the same function of avian thrombocytes and mammalian platelets. Their primary role is the formation of the initial hemostatic plug through adhesion and aggregation, so they tend to clump or form aggregates in blood films. Furthermore, they secrete thromboplastin, which is involved in the polymerization of fibrinogen in the formation of clots.[2]

Normal thrombocytes (**Fig. 10A**) are smaller than erythrocytes, elliptical to fusiform in shape, with a round and small nucleus with dense purple chromatin, centrally placed. Thrombocytes are characterized by a small quantity of colorless to pale blue cytoplasm, which may contain a few azurophilic granules or clear vacuoles (glycogen stores). It can be challenging to distinguish some thrombocytes from small lymphocytes, which may lead to errors in the total and differential WBC count, eventually misleading the diagnosis. Differences include a rounder shape of lymphocytes and their darker cytoplasm. Differences between similar cells are shown in **Fig. 11**. Differentiation is easier with Romanowsky-type stains, in which thrombocyte cytoplasm tends to remain colorless. A definitive differentiation is made on the positivity

Table 7
Normal morphology of reptile white blood cells and granulocytes

	Granulocytes		
	Acidophils Heterophils	Eosinophils	Basophils
Shape	Round. Margins may be irregular, pseudopodia may be present	Round	Round
Range size	10–23 μm	9–20 μm	7–20 μm
Cytoplasm	Colorless	Light blue	Clear, packed with granules
Cytoplasmic granules	Eosinophilic (bright orange), shape and number varies among species	Eosinophilic, spherical, numerous, staining blue-green in some species (green eosinophils)	Basophilic (dark blue to purple), metachromatic, round, variable in number
Nucleus	Eccentric, round to oval; densely clumped chromatin. Lobed in some lizards May be partially obscured by the granules	Central or slightly eccentric, round to oval May be lobed in some species of lizards (eg, I iguana)	Slightly eccentric, round, and monolobed Often obscured by the granules
Cytochemical stain reaction	Peroxidase negative except for few species of snakes and lizards (green iguana)	Peroxidase positive except for green eosinophils (lizards)	Not reported
Function	Phagocytosis and microbicidal activity	Participation in the immune response; phagocytosis of immune complexes	Processed surface immunoglobulins and release of histamine

Original pictures: A: from *Trachemys scripta*; B: from *T hermanni boettgeri*; C: from *Vipera ammodytes*, all Hemacolor stained (Merck). Approximately × 1000 magnification.

Table 8
Normal morphology of reptilian white blood cells, mononuclear

	Mononuclear			
	Lymphocytes	Plasma Cells	Monocytes	Azurophils
	A	B	C	D
Shape	Round to oval, may be irregular	Round to oval, distinct borders	Round to amoeboid	Irregular, possible pseudopodia
Range size	Small (5–10 μm); large (15 μm or larger)	Slightly larger than lymphocytes	8–25 μm (the largest cells)	Slightly smaller than monocytes
Cytoplasm	Scant amount (more in large lizards), slightly basophilic (pale blue). Homogeneous, generally lacks vacuoles and granules	Intensely basophilic (deep blue) with a perinuclear halo (Golgi)	Abundant, pale blue-gray, may be slightly opaque or foamy. Phagocytized material and vacuoles can be found	Darker than monocytes Vacuolation and phagocytized material may be present within the cytoplasm
Cytoplasmic granules	Not present	Not present	Fine eosinophilic or azurophilic granules may be present	Small number of fine, dustlike, azurophilic granules
Nucleus	Central or slightly eccentric, large, round to oval. Dark chromatin heavily clumped. Large nucleus/ cytoplasm ratio	Eccentric, round/oval; clumped chromatin. Lower nucleus: cytoplasm compared with unstimulated lymphocytes	Variably shaped (round, oval, or lobed). Chromatin less condensed and paler staining compared with lymphocytes	Irregularly round to oval to lobed. Coarse chromatin
Function	Immune response	Stimulated lymphocytes	Granuloma and giant cell formation	Not defined

Original pictures: A, B, D: from *B constrictor*, Diff-Quick; C: from *T hermanni boettgeri*, Hemacolor stained (Merck). Approximately × 1000 magnification.

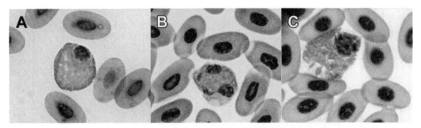

Fig. 8. Heterophils from different species. (*A*) Snake heterophils have eosinophilic granules, pleomorphic and elongated in shape, and are so abundant that they may obscure the nucleus, so the whole cell appears as heterogeneous eosinophilic material (*Phyton molurus*, Diff-Quick). (*B*) Lizard heterophils have many small eosinophilic granules, angular or pleomorphic in shape. Bilobed nuclei are frequent (especially in green iguana) (*I iguana*, Hemacolor stained [Merck]). (*C*) Chelonian heterophils have eosinophilic granules, fusiform in shape (*T hermanni boettgeri*, Hemacolor stained [Merck]). Approximately × 1000 magnification.

to the PAS stain (thrombocytes usually stain PAS positive, whereas lymphocytes stain PAS negative). Because a manual count of blood cells is time consuming, thrombocytes are rarely counted; therefore, thrombocytosis and thrombocytopenia need further investigations in reptile medicine. The activated form usually appears as aggregated clusters of cells with cytoplasm decreased in volume, with irregular margins and presence of vacuoles and fine granular material. Usually many fibrin-like filaments radiate between and around the cells (see **Fig. 10**B). Morphologic alterations observed include the presence of polymorphic nuclei, mitosis, and double nuclei (see **Fig. 10**C), and cytoplasmic projections. Polymorphic nuclei are rare and are usually associated with severe inflammatory diseases.[2]

Hemoparasites

The evidence of blood parasites in the slides is usually an incidental finding, as most of them are considered not to be pathogenic, differently than in mammals and birds. Nevertheless, some investigators highlight how some of these parasites have the potential to cause diseases such as hemolytic anemia and inanition, especially in geriatric and young individuals.[16] All reptilian hemoparasites have indirect life cycles; the main vectors for terrestrial species are arthropods, whereas leeches are commonly

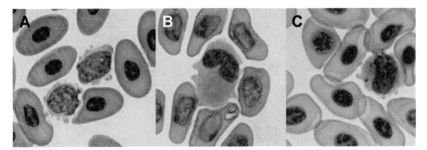

Fig. 9. Reactive forms of WBC. (*A*) Reactive lymphocytes: larger than small lymph, larger nucleus with evident nucleoli and cytoplasmic projections. (*B*) Reactive monocytes: cytoplasmic projection and evident Golgi area. (*C*) Monocytes with phagocytic bacteria. (*A*) From *I iguana*, (*B*) from *Chamaeleo calyptratus*, (*C*) from *T hermanni boettgeri*. All Hemacolor stained (Merck). Approximately × 1000 magnification.

Table 9
Morphologic alteration of white blood cells

Heterophils		
Toxic changes		
Occur in the bone marrow before the release of WBC in the peripheral blood. Associated with severe inflammatory/infective diseases		

Increased cytoplasmic basophilia	Degranulation	Vacuolation
Mild disease ⟶	Sample handling, prolonged storage in anticoagulant, inadequate fixation. If nuclear pyknosis is also present, this appearance may be part of the normal in vivo aging	

Excessive nuclear lobation	Abnormal cytoplasmic granules (color, size, or shape)	
The nucleus is normally lobated in some species		⟶ Severe disease (frequently from bacterial toxins)

Original pictures: A: from *I iguana*, Diff-Quick; B: from *T hermanni boettgeri*, Hemacolor stained (Merck); C: from *I iguana*, Hemacolor stained (Merck); D: from *C calyptratus*, Hemacolor stained (Merck); E: from *T hermanni*, Hemacolor stained (Merck); F: from *I iguana*, Diff-Quick. Approximately × 1000 magnification.

involved in aquatic species. Classification, life cycles, and pathology of different hemoparasites are explained in the following paragraphs, and a morphologic description is reported in **Table 10**.

Apicomplexa, subclass Coccidiasina

Parasites in the phylum Apicomplexa and subclass Coccidiasina are the most commonly found.[16] This large group of protozoa includes unicellular, spore-forming, and exclusively parasites of animals such as coccidians, gregarines, piroplasms, haemogregarines, and plasmodia.

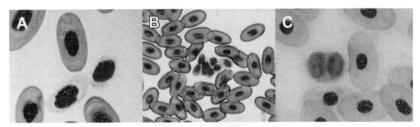

Fig. 10. Thrombocytes. All Hemacolor stained (Merck). (*A*) Normal thrombocytes from *T hermanni boettgeri*. Approximately × 1000 magnification. (*B*) Cluster of activated thrombocytes from *I iguana*. Approximately × 400 magnification. (*C*) Binucleated thrombocyte from *Testudo marginata*. Approximately × 1000 magnification.

Reptiles represent the intermediate host for these parasites, whereas the invertebrate vector is the final host. Life cycles are similar and all are heteroxenous, schematically shown in **Fig. 12.**

Hemogregarines Phylum Apicomplexa subclass Coccidiasina, suborder Adeleorina, family Haemogregarinidae.

This group includes the 4 genera most commonly found in reptiles: *Haemogregarina, Haemolivia, Hepatozoon*, and *Karyolysus*. As appropriate classification can be only accomplished based on the appearance of the oocytes in the invertebrate host, the evidence of such parasites in blood films is usually attributed to haemogregarines in general. Indeed, different parasites are differently spread among reptilian groups, and each species within these genera only infects its specific reptile and vector.[17] In particular, *Haemogregarina* are spread among freshwater turtles (*Haemogregarina stepanovi* is a common parasite of *Emys orbicularis*) (**Fig. 13**),[18] tortoises of genera *Geoemyda* and *Testudo*, the tuatara, some lizards, and most snakes and crocodilians.[16] *Haemolivia* are encountered in turtles, with *Haemolivia mauritanica*

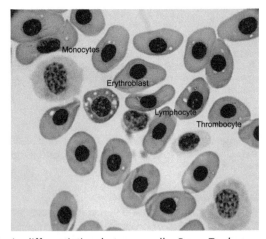

Fig. 11. Morphologic differentiation between cells. From *Trachemys scripta*, Hemacolor stained (Merck). Approximately × 1000 magnification.

Table 10	
Morphologic description and localization of reptilian hemoparasites	
Plasmodium's Pigments May Help the Distinction Between These 2 Groups of Parasites	
Plasmodiidae	Haemogregarines
RBC	RBC
Gametocytes: round oval or elongated shape, pale eosinophilic cytoplasm with deep pink or bluish structure containing many refractile pigments; trophozoites appear as focal packets or signet-ring structures Saurocytozoon is the only Plasmodiidae that lacks pigment granules. It can be found in immature erythrocytes	Sausage-shaped parasites with pale to purple cytoplasm and one central to slightly eccentric darker nucleus. Both the host cell shape and nucleus may appear altered. One or more organisms may be found in the same cell
Piroplasmida	Lainsonia and Schellackia (lizards)— haemococcidia
RBC	RBC and mononuclear leukocytes
Rare. Granular basophilic inclusions, usually in small aggregates, surrounded by clear vacuoles	Sporozoites: small, round to oval, pale staining, nonpigmented inclusions that deform the host cell nucleus into a crescent shape
Microfilaria	Sauroleishmania (lizards)
Free in the bloodstream	Mononuclear leukocytes
	Rare Singular to numerous basophilic inclusion Tend to condense in round aggregates with a central hollow

having as its own intermediate host *Testudo graeca* and rarely *Testudo marginata*, and the turtle tick *Hyalomma aegypticum* as its own final host. *Testudo hermanni* can be infected experimentally but natural infections have not been found.[17] *Hepatozoon* are found primarily in snakes, and *Karyolysus* primarily in old-world lizards and tree snakes.[16] No cases of haemogregarines have been reported in sea turtles.[16]

Even if it is assumed that many cells may be damaged during the asexual reproduction (spleen, lung, liver, kidney), these parasites are well adapted to their natural hosts and are considered not to cause disease. Clinical signs including lethargy, open-mouth breathing, weight loss and dehydration may be seen in unnatural or aberrant host species, or in immune-compromised patients. Most commonly, newly imported wild caught animals may be affected.[17]

Plasmodiid parasites Phylum Apicomplexa, subclass Coccidiasina, order Haemosporideae.

This order includes *Plasmodium*, *Haemoproteus*, and *Saurocytozoon* species. The peculiarity of Saurocytozoon species is the absence of refractile pigments typical of other species.

Over 60 species of *Plasmodium* have been described, mostly in lizards and rarely in snakes.[2] Even if rarely reported, these parasites are potentially dangerous for reptiles, and may cause severe hemolytic anemia or splenomegaly.[2] Owing to the peculiarity of possible schizogony in blood cells, both trophozoites and merozoites may be identified in the blood films in erythrocytes.[2]

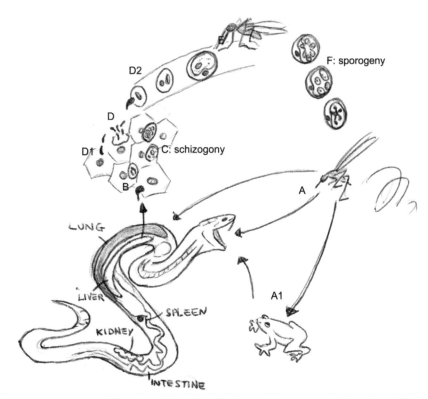

Fig. 12. Heteroxenous life cycle of Coccidia. (A) Transmission occurs via ingestion of the infected invertebrate vector (mites, ticks, bugs, biting flies, mosquitoes, and leeches) or of an infected vertebrate prey (A1): secondary transmission). (B) Sporozoites penetrate cells of liver, lungs, spleen, kidneys, and other organs, and grow to be trophozoites. (C) Schizogony. Trophozoites replicate asexually, developing schizonts containing merozoites. Schizogony may occur in blood cells in some families, including *Plasmodium* spp. (D) Merozoites are released after cell rupture, and may repeat the asexual multiplication (D1) or may infect RBC and develop into gametocytes (D2). (E) The final host is the invertebrate vector, which sucks parasite gametocytes together with the blood when feeding in the reptile. (F) Sporogeny. Sexual reproduction takes place in the invertebrate vector. The final infectious stage is the sporozoite, ready to infect another reptile.

Even if the primary hosts of *Haemoproteus* are considered to be birds, this parasite is reported in lizards, turtles, and snakes.[16] Vectors include sandflies, mosquitoes, gnats, and perhaps mites. It is generally considered nonpathogenic, but may cause hemolytic anemia.

Saurocytozoon is reported in lizards and is usually transmitted by mosquitoes; it is considered harmless for the reptilian host.

Piroplasmids Phylum Apicomplexa, subclass Coccidiasina, suborder Piroplasmorina.
These parasites are reported in lizards, chelonians, and snakes, and are called *Sauroplasma* in chameleons and lizards, and *Serpentoplasma* in snakes.

Lainsonia and Schellackia (Haemococcidia) Phylum Apicomplexa, subclass Coccidiasina, suborder Eimeriorina.

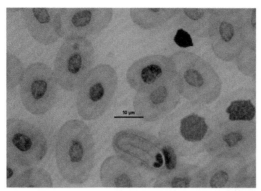

Fig. 13. Haemogregarina. From *Emys orbicularis*, Giemsa; approximately × 1000 magnification. (*Courtesy of* M.L. Fioravanti DVM, Bologna, Italy.)

Most of the other species included in this same suborder (*Cryptosporidium*, *Eimeria*, *Isospora*, *Sarcocystis*, and *Toxoplasma*) inhabit the intestinal epithelium of reptiles and may be detected by a fecal examination. On the other hand, only the schizogonic stage of these parasites takes place in the intestine, whereas sporozoites are found

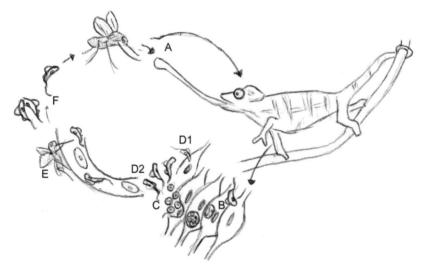

Fig. 14. Heteroxenous life cycle of Trypanosomatidae. (A) The infective form (metacyclic trypomastigote) is transmitted by blood-sucking arthropods (biting flies such as phlebotomine sandflies or leeches in aquatic species) by biting or ingestion. (B) The infective form turns into the amastigote form in the vertebrate host. (C) Asexual reproduction occurs by binary fission in cells of different tissues until cell rupture. New trypomastigotes can infect new cells (D1) or enter the bloodstream (D2). Differently from the other hemoparasites, trypanosomes are found extracellularly in the peripheral blood. (E) The vector is infected during the blood meal. (F) In the invertebrate host the parasite turns into the epimastigote stage, which multiplies in the insect's midgut. The infective form develops in the hindgut, ready to infect another reptile.

in the cytoplasm of erythrocytes and mononuclear leukocytes, so that a blood smear is necessary to point out the infection. These parasites have been reported mostly in lizards and they seem not to be associated with clinical disease.[2]

Flagellates, family Trypanosomatidae

Many members of the family have an heteroxenous life cycle (**Fig. 14**).

Trypanosomas class Zoomastigophorea, order Kinetoplastida, family Trypanosomatidae.

These flagellate protozoa closely resemble trypanosome species found in mammals and birds, with the presence of a single flagellum and a prominent undulating membrane (trypomastigote). There are at least 58 species spread in all orders of reptiles.[18]

Even if all species of *Trypanosoma* can cause severe parasitemia, infection is often subclinical and lifelong.[2]

Leishmania These parasites rarely infect reptiles. Parasites from the subgenera *Sauroleishmania* may be found in thrombocytes and mononuclear leukocytes of reptiles, primarily in lizards, transmitted by the sandflies *Sergentomyia* spp.[2]

Microfilaria Different genera of *filaridae* parasites can be detected in reptiles, usually as an incidental finding (**Fig. 15**). In fact, no clinical signs are associated with the infection. As for the other hemoparasites, these worms are transmitted by blood-sucking arthropods or insects.

SAMPLE EVALUATION: QUANTITATIVE ASPECTS

As in other ectotherms, profound physiologic adaptation may occur in reptiles in response to many intrinsic and environmental situations. Thus, because of the great variety of different factors influencing them, the evaluation of hematologic parameters is challenging. To not consider all these variations may lead to erroneous considerations or a failure to reach a diagnosis. Intrinsic factors to be considered are species, age, gender, nutrition, physiologic status, hibernation, stress, and disease status; extrinsic factors include environmental conditions such as the season, the temperature, and the habitat. As published hematologic reference values often fail to include information about testing conditions, these ranges should be used with caution. In fact it can be difficult to assess the clinical relevance of a variation from these references,

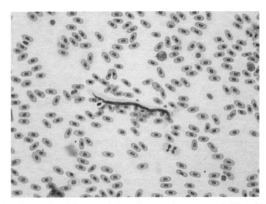

Fig. 15. Microfilaria. From *Furcifer pardalis*, Hemacolor stained (Merck). Approximately × 100 magnification.

and more reliance should be placed on previous testing of the same individual. Serial sampling is always preferred to single results, as they may be useful in monitoring the progress of the disease. Otherwise, it has been suggested that only counts at least double those of normal values should be considered significant.[4]

As blood collection (venipuncture site, use of manual or chemical restraint) and sampling technique may be an influence as well as hematology results, a standardization of the technique may help in achieving comparable results. Care should be taken not to evaluate hemodiluted samples. This goal may be achieved by avoiding venipuncture sites where lymphodilution is considered to occur more often, or by attempting collection again if dilution is supposed. Sykes and Klaphake[19] suggest immediately measuring the PCV and discarding the sample if less than 10%, unless severe anemia is clinically feasible.

Information about intrinsic and extrinsic influences are reported in **Table 11**.

RBC

Anemia

Anemia is to be considered a clinical sign rather than a disease. Typical clinical signs are weakness, exercise intolerance, reluctance to walk, tachycardia, and dyspnea; mucosa can be moderately to severely pale.[20] The diagnosis of anemia in reptiles should always follow consideration about artifactual (eg, due to hemodilution) or physiologic low PCV values (eg, the range in ball phytons [*Python regius*] is 16%–21%). It is also important to consider other physiologic adaptations that may influence hematologic values: for example, starvation results in decreased RBC, PCV, and hemoglobin in some elapid snakes[4]; a statistically significant decrease in the PCV and hemoglobin have been documented in a laboratory setting in the Cunningham skink (*Egernia cunninghami*) when exposed to low temperatures.[21]

Different pathologic conditions may lead to a decrease in RBC and PCV values:

- Blood loss (hemorrhagic anemia; regenerative anemia)
  - Associated with traumas, both internal and external, gastric ulcers, neoplasia rupture or other causes of internal hemorrhage, blood-sucking parasites.
    - Internal hemorrhages may be related to traumas, foreign-body ingestion, or ulcers. The rupture of a high vascularized neoplastic mass may cause regenerative anemia, whereas most neoplastic conditions are accompanied by nonregenerative forms of anemia. Hemorrhages caused by the ingestion of rodents exposed to anticoagulant rodenticides may occur in free-ranging snakes.[20] Other coagulopathies are very rare in reptiles.[20]
    - Blood-sucking parasites include flies (Ixodidae and Argasidae), mites (*Ophionyssus natricis*, the snake mite), leeches in aquatic wild reptiles. Juveniles are more susceptible to developing anemia from these infestations.[20]
- Increased RBC destruction (hemolytic anemia; regenerative anemia)
  - Seen in course of septicemia, parasitemia, toxemia.
    - Parasitemia: Usually hemoparasites are considered apathogenic. Nevertheless, anemia is reported in severe infestation by the malarial hemoparasites (*Plasmodium*), *Haemoproteus*, and *Saurocytozoon*.[20]
    - Lead toxicosis and zinc toxicosis can induce hemolytic anemia. Furthermore, the use of calcium EDTA as anticoagulant has been reported to cause hemolysis in some chelonians.[20]
    - Inherited hemolytic anemia has not been reported so far.[20]
- Decreased RBC production (nonregenerative anemia)

Table 11
Intrinsic and extrinsic factors influencing the reptilian leukogram

	Species Dependence	Sex Dependence	Age Dependence	Hibernation Dependence	Seasonal Variation
PCV %		Generally higher in males			
RBC (10^6/μL)	Highest number in lizards; lowest in chelonians	Generally higher in males	Higher in adult marsh crocodiles	Decrease	Highest in summer
MCV (fL)	Higher number in chelonians; lowest in lizards				
WBC (10^3/μL)		Higher in male crocodiles			
Heterophils %	Predominant cell type in chelonians and crocodilians	Higher in male crocodiles; higher during gravidity		Decrease	Highest in summer
Lymphocytes %	Predominant cell type in iguanas and some snakes	Higher in females	Higher in young crocodiles	Decrease	Highest in summer
Monocytes %					Minimal dependence
Azurophils %	Typical of snakes				
Eosinophils %	Highest number in turtles, lowest in lizards			Increase	Lowest in summer
Basophils %	Predominant cell type in freshwater turtles			Decrease in desert tortoises	Minimal dependence

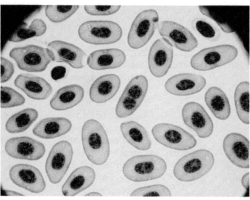

Fig. 16. Anisocytes and presence of binucleated RBC are signs of regeneration. From *T hermanni boettgeri*, Hemacolor stained (Merck) Approximately × 1000 magnification.

- o Seen in course of many chronic inflammatory diseases, especially associated with infectious agents, liver and renal failure, neoplasia, chemical or drug reaction, hypothyroidism.
    - ■ Viral infection, for example from herpesvirus, may cause moderate to severe nonregenerative anemia. Other hematologic signs associated with this pathology are a decrease of total protein and WBCs (lymphocytes, basophils, and eosinophils), probably as a consequence of bone marrow dysfunction.[4] Tortoise erythrocytes may show eccentric, pale blue, long intracytoplasmic inclusions.[2]
    - ■ Other systemic chronic infectious diseases commonly associated with anemia are mycobacteriosis, mycoplasmosis, chlamydiosis, salmonellosis, iridovirosis, coccidiomycosis, and aspergillosis, attributable to serious damage in the liver, kidneys, spleen, bone marrow, and/or lungs.
    - ■ Renal disorders, including nephritis, nephrosis, amyloidosis, and nephrocalcinosis, may cause nonregenerative anemia.[20]
    - ■ Liver disorders may cause a nonregenerative anemia, including hepatic lipidosis (commonly found in captive lizards), hepatitis, and tumors.[20]

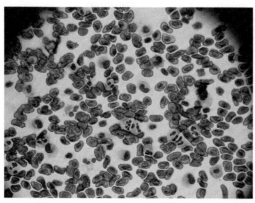

Fig. 17. Leukocytosis, mostly heterophilic, with degranulation and nuclear degeneration. From *Chamaeleo calyptratus*, Hemacolor stained (Merck) Approximately × 1000 magnification.

Table 12 Causes of altered WBC count			Increased Values	Decreased Values
Granulocytes	Acidophils	Heterophils	Infective inflammation, tissue injuries, tissue necrosis, neoplasia, granulocytic leukemia, stress, glucocorticoid administration	Overwhelming infection, resulting in excessive tissue demand for heterophils
		Eosinophils	Parasitic infection, immune response	Unknown
	Basophils		Blood parasites, viral infection	Unknown
Mononuclear	Lymphocytes		Wound healing, chronic infectious/ inflammatory disease, viral disease, parasitic disease (anisakiasis, spirorchidiasis, hematozoa) Lymphoid leukemia, inclusion body disease (IBD) of boid snakes (total WBC higher than 100,000 in early stage, with most being lymphocytes; IBD intracytoplasmic inclusions may be noted)	Malnutrition, immunosuppression, stress, corticosteroid administration
	Plasma cells		Severe infection or inflammatory disease	
	Monocytes		Chronic infectious processes, granulomatous response to bacteria and spirorchid trematodes	
	Azurophils		Acute inflammatory/ infectious disease	

Signs of a regenerative response should be detected in the blood smears to differentiate a regenerative anemia from a nonregenerative one. Typical signs of regeneration are polychromasia, erythrocytic mitosis, anisocytosis, and the presence of immature erythrocytes such as rubriblasts. **Fig. 16** shows a blood smear with some characteristics of regeneration. Furthermore, regenerative anemia is characterized by a reduction in mean corpuscular hemoglobin concentration and MCV, owing to a decreased quantity of hemoglobin in polychromatophils where it is actively produced, and to the smaller size of these cells. This situation is in contrast to the increased MCV seen in mammals during regeneration, associated with the larger size of reticulocytes.[4] Nevertheless, the chronicity of anemia should be considered if no signs are visible, as the reptilian response is particularly slow compared with mammals, requiring up to 30 days to be visible and up to 8 weeks before the maximal regeneration.[4] This delay may be related to a long development time for rubriblasts in the bone marrow and the long life span of reptilian red blood cells.[2,14] Usually an anemic process is considered nonregenerative if no signs of response are seen before 1 month.[4]

Polycythemia

A reptile is considered polycythemic when the PCV is higher than 40%.[19] Dehydration is a common consequence of hibernation and dry periods, when a reptile may not drink for weeks to months; this results in increasing PCV and RBC. Both hemoglobin and PCV are also susceptible to annual and seasonal changes.[4]

WBC

Leukogram pattern

Leukocytosis is often associated with infection. Nevertheless, unlike in mammals, this diagnosis in reptiles should not be only based on the leukogram evaluation, as leuko-penia, leukocytosis, and even a normal leukogram can all be recorded.[19] Furthermore, as already mentioned, definitive and reliable references are not always present. Thus to reach a diagnosis, it is essential to associate the study of leukocyte values, the eval-uation of cell morphology, and the clinical presentation of the patient. An example of a leukocytic blood smear is shown in **Fig. 17**.

Neoplastic leukemia is rare in reptiles, mainly being reported in lizards and snakes.[19] The main causes of leukogram variations are summarized in **Table 12**.

Thrombocytes

Thrombocytopenia

Thrombocytopenia is most likely to occur as a result of excessive peripheral use or a decrease in production in pathologic conditions such as severe septicemia or disseminated intravascular coagulation.

SUMMARY

In reptiles, hematology is a good instrument for investigation of conditions that may affect the blood cells, but it requires extensive knowledge, training, and experience for it not to be misleading. Indeed, not only reference values are sometimes absent or incomplete, but hematologic parameters are also strongly influenced by many intrinsic and extrinsic factors, including sample collection and processing. Thus, serial sampling is more useful than single results, as it allows monitoring of the progress of the disease. More indicative of pathologic situations is the observation of alteration in the morphology of blood cells, so that a good blood smear always has to accompany any hematologic examination. Once again, serial evaluation of slides is an efficient prognostic device.

REFERENCES

1. Strik NI, Alleman RA, Harr KE. Circulating inflammatory cells. In: Jacobson ER, editor. Infectious disease and pathology of reptiles. Boca Raton: CRC Press; 2007. p. 167–218.
2. Campbell TW, Ellis CK. Avian and exotic animal hematology and cytology. Yowa State Press: Blackwell; 2007.
3. Martinez-Jimenez D, Hernandez-Divers SJ. Emergency care of reptiles. Vet Clin North Am Exot Anim Pract 2007;10:557–85.

4. Jacobson ER. Infectious diseases and pathology of reptiles. Boca Raton: CRC Press; 2007.
5. Girling SJ, Raiti P. BSAVA manual of reptiles. Gloucester (England): BSAVA; 2004.
6. Pendl H. Avian and reptilian hematology for practitioners basic and advanced lab. SIVAE hematology course. Edizioni Veterinarie: Cremona (Italy); 2004.
7. McArthur S, Wilkinson R, Meyer J. Medicine and surgery of tortoises and turtles. Oxford: Blackwell Publishing Ltd; 2004.
8. Bielli M, Nardini G. Hematological values for Boettger tortoise (*Testudo hermanni boettgeri*). In: Proceedings of International Conference on Reptile and Amphibian Medicine. Edizioni Veterinarie: Cremona (Italy); 2012. p. 81–4.
9. Raskin RE. Reptilian complete blood count. In: Fudge AM, editor. Laboratory medicine avian and exotic pets. Philadelphia: WB Saunders; 2000. p. 193–7.
10. Mader DR. Reptile medicine and surgery. St Louis (MO): Saunders Elsevier; 2006.
11. Thrall MA. Veterinary hematology and clinical chemistry. Oxford: Blackwell Publishing Ltd; 2006. Accessed at: http://www.sciencedirect.com/science/article/pii/S1557506309000421.
12. Wiliknson R. Clinical pathology. In: McArthur S, Wilkinson R, Meyer J, editors. Medicine and surgery of tortoises and turtles. Oxford: Blackwell Publishing Ltd; 2004. p. 141–86.
13. Frye FL. Hematology as applied to clinical reptile medicine. In: Frye FL, editor. Biomedical and surgical aspects of captive reptile husbandry. Malabar: Krieger Publishing Co; 1991.
14. Campbell TW. Clinical pathology of reptiles. In: Mader DR, editor. Reptile medicine and surgery. St Louis (MO): Saunders Elsevier; 2006. p. 453–70.
15. Montali RJ. Comparative pathology of inflammation in the higher vertebrates (reptiles, birds and mammals). J Comp Pathol 1988;99:1–26.
16. Campbell TW. Hemoparasites. In: Mader DR, editor. Reptile medicine and surgery. St Louis (MO): Saunders Elsevier; 2006. p. 801–6.
17. Schneller P, Pantchev N. Parasitology in snakes, lizards and chelonians. Frankfurt (Germany): Chimaira; 2008.
18. Hnìzdo J, Pantchev N. Medical care of turtles and tortoises. Frankfurt am Main: Chimaira; 2011.
19. Sykes JM, Klaphake E. Reptile hematology. Vet Clin North Am Exot Anim Pract 2008;11:481–500.
20. Saggese MD. Clinical approach to the anemic reptile. J Exot Pet Med 2009;18: 98–111.
21. Maclean G, Lee A, Wuthers P. Hematological adjustments with diurnal changes in body temperature in a lizard and a mouse. Comp Biochem Physiol 1975;53: 15–29.

Clinical and Laboratory Practice for Canaries and True Finches

Diego Cattarossi, DVM, PhD[a],*, Erika Azzara, DVM[b],
Salvatore Catania, DVM, PhD[c]

KEYWORDS

- Canaries • True finches • Laboratory • Cytology • Diagnostic procedure
- Treatment

KEY POINTS

- The canaries and true finches are highly popular birds with families as a companion animal and among breeders for competitive purposes.
- Practicing vets must have everything in their clinic that could be needed for the correct collection of biological samples, be able to perform a first screening, and also be in contact with a laboratory for the more specialist diagnostic examinations that require specific skills and equipment.
- The postmortem examination, imprint cytology, and examination of the animal excrements are most commonly performed in the clinic.
- Cytology can be a considerable help in diagnosing various pathologies in almost all animal species, including the pet canary and all small cage and aviary passerines.
- In the last few years the diagnostic avian laboratory has developed several new tests to detect specific avian pathogens.

INTRODUCTION

The canary (*Serinus canaria*) is a highly popular bird with families as a companion animal and among breeders for competitive purposes. Domestic canaries fall into 3 groups based on 3 basic characteristics: song, color, and conformation-shape. Each group is made up of many distinctive races and varieties.

The canary is the most common finch among the small cage and aviary passerines although many other species are pure bred and crossbred to produce hybrids.

Clinical vets must be sure of the diagnostic possibilities and the protocol to follow to apply effective and well-targeted treatment for a problem in canaries and passerines.

The authors have nothing to disclose.
[a] Treviso, Italy; [b] San Donà, Veneto, Italy; [c] Istituto Zooprofilattico Sperimentale delle Venezie, Legnaro, Padua, Italy
* Corresponding author.
E-mail address: diegocattarossi@gmail.com

Vet Clin Exot Anim 16 (2013) 31–46
http://dx.doi.org/10.1016/j.cvex.2012.09.002

Practicing vets must have everything in their clinic that could be needed for the correct collection of biological samples, be able to perform a first screening, and also be in contact with a laboratory for the more specialist diagnostic examinations that require specific skills and equipment.

Examinations in the clinic allow practitioners to narrow the range of differential diagnoses, to refer their diagnostic suspicion to the laboratory (given in the accompanying letter), and, in particular, to prescribe a therapy immediately. The mortality rate in these animals is very high at the onset of an epidemic, and the technical times of a laboratory often necessitate starting treatment before having completed the diagnostic procedure. Emergency treatment is corrected or supplemented by the final therapy once the laboratory tests have been finished. Samples to the laboratory should always be collected before starting the emergency treatment so as not to affect results.

This article describes a practical approach that deals with the first things to do in the clinic as soon as the animal arrives or the breeder asks for advice and explains the procedure in a specialist laboratory for processing samples and completing the diagnosis.

Examinations in the Clinic

When one or more canaries arrive at the clinic, a physical examination is performed as for any other animal. All our observations are entered on a chart that has been specially studied for small passerines and will include the most important information given by the owner/breeder, for example, cage structure; feed at different times of the year; climatic conditions of the environment where the animals are housed with particular reference to temperature, humidity, and photoperiod; vaccinations, such as poxvirus; remote history; onset and progress of the problem; therapies already tried out; and so forth. This chart becomes extremely useful both for prescribing the treatment and as a clinical chart of the livestock if the breeder comes back to the clinic in subsequent years.

The postmortem examination, imprint cytology, and examination of the animal excrements are most commonly performed in the clinic.

There are 2 techniques for examining excrements in the clinic: fresh or through concentration and flotation with 1030 solution (**Fig. 1**). Examining fresh specimens is extremely useful for detecting moving protozoa, such as *Cochlosoma*, *Giardia*, and *Trichomonas*. Examination after flotation reveals parasites such as *coccidia* (eg, *Isospora* and *Atoxoplasma*), helminths (very rare in canaries), or protozoan cysts (**Figs. 2–4**).

An examination of a swab of the crop and cloaca is easy to perform (**Fig. 5**). Because the animals are small, a turkey endotracheal or human urethral swab is used for taking samples. After smearing the swab on the glass slide and staining it, the microbial flora of the gastrointestinal tract can be assessed. It is advisable to prepare at least 3 slides, one of which stained with Diff Quick and another with Gram, while one is left in reserve for any special stains that may prove necessary (eg, for acid-fast bacilli). The more easily identifiable microorganisms are yeasts (*Candida spp.*), *Macrorhabdus ornithogaster* (**Fig. 6**) and bacteria in various shapes (cocci, bacilli, spores, and so forth). Distinguishing between the gram-positive and gram-negative bacteria is an important first step for deciding on the correct emergency antibiotic treatment in the event of an existing high mortality rate.

An autopsy is always extremely useful for correct diagnosis (**Fig. 7**). If there is more than one carcass, some autopsies can be performed in the clinic and some animals kept for the laboratory. Biological samples as well as organs may be removed during the autopsy for histologic examination.

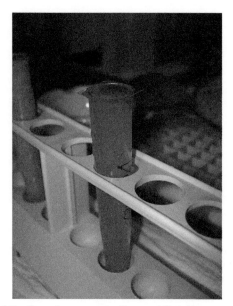

Fig. 1. Examination of the feces by concentration and flotation.

Observing damaged feathers under the microscope allows parasites, such as lice, to be detected (**Figs. 8** and **9**).

Blood samples are rarely taken in clinical practice, but a certain amount of blood can be taken from the jugular vein, taking care not to exceed 1% of the canary's total weight (**Fig. 10**). The blood can be used for a biochemical profile, a blood smear with assessment of the leukocyte formula or for serologic tests to search for example for *Paramyxovirus* or *Chlamydophila spp*.

Imaging

Radiography is extremely useful in the diagnostic procedure of a single canary bred as a pet bird, but rarely used in breeding diagnostics.

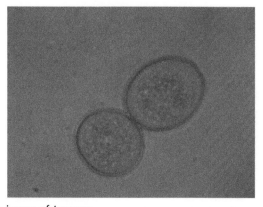

Fig. 2. Microscopic image of *Isospora*.

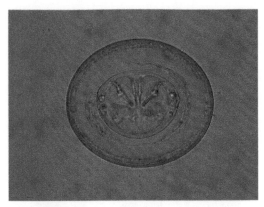

Fig. 3. Microscopic image of *Taenia*.

A radiograph can provide a great deal of information on the shape and size of the various organs in the coelomic cavity. At least 2 whole body images must be taken with both ventrodorsal and laterolateral views, extending the wings and feet well. During imaging the animal is often anesthetized with fast-acting isoflurane or sevoflurane gas anesthesia.

Ultrasonography is not much used in clinical practice. The best acoustic window is the ventromedial area with the ultrasound probe placed under the sternum, after having separated the feathers and applied the gel, and moving it in a cranial direction. The high-frequency micro convex probes are the best. Ultrasonography is most frequently used for the diagnosis of coelomic masses, coelomic effusions, and ultrasound-guided centesis, diagnosis of egg binding, and relative ovocentesis.

Computed tomography and magnetic resonance imaging are used rarely because of the high costs and because agreed well-tested implementing protocols are not available. In the not too distant future they will surely be of great help in managing pet canaries (**Fig. 11**).

Cytology in the Canary

Cytology can be of considerable help in diagnosing various pathologies in almost all animal species, including the pet canary and all small cage and aviary passerines.

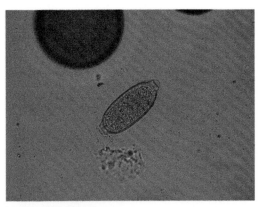

Fig. 4. Microscopic image of *Capillaria*.

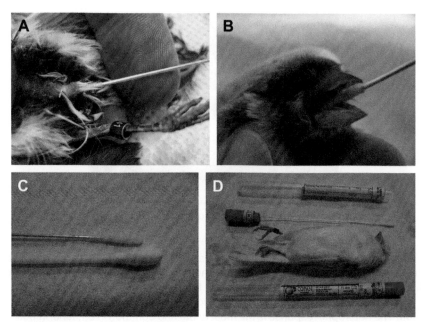

Fig. 5. (*A*) Cloacal swab sampling. (*B*) Crop swab sampling. (*C*) Real size of turkey endotracheal swab. (*D*) Size of classic swab compared with turkey endotracheal swab.

Cytology is used to study cells from tumefactions and other surface lesions, cavitary liquids, and internal organs that are usually taken from dead animals requiring an autopsy. Masses and surface lesions are evaluated cytologically using apposition, capillary-action, fine-needle aspiration, or scrape techniques that are quick, easy, and economic to perform and often require only a short confinement period, without needing to anesthetize the animal.

Cytology differentiates between inflammation and tumors, and frequently detects the pathogen, enabling a diagnosis to be made.

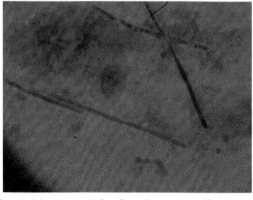

Fig. 6. *Macrorhabdus ornithogaster* under the microscope with quick stain.

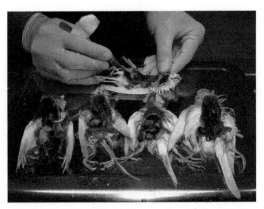

Fig. 7. Multiple postmortem examination with opening of the carcasses.

The same cytologic principles as for the cat and the dog are applied to unconventional companion animals. The main differences are in recognizing the inflammatory cell types and the unusual infectious agents that can affect these animal species.

Heterophils, macrophages, eosinophils, and lymphocytes can be found in an *inflammation*. The heterophil response is the most acute and common in bacterial infections. Heterophils in birds are easy to recognize because they contain numerous bright orange-pink granules with segmented nuclei, and they have functions that include phagocytic and microbicidal activity. There is a mixed cell reaction when macrophages are also present, which in birds are similar to those in mammals; a peculiarity found in birds is that within just a few hours giant cells can appear created by macrophages grouping together. The presence of giant cells does not indicate chronicity as in mammals.

To understand the effectiveness of cytology in diagnosing pathologies that affect the canary, *egg yolk peritonitis* is taken as an example.If a turbid coelomic effusion is found in a bird that in the smear background under the microscope has the appearance of an amorphous (protein) basophilic material, suggests the presence of egg yolk due to the breaking of the actual egg inside the body cavity. Again, in peritonitis there is a mixed type inflammatory response with heterophils and macrophages englobing

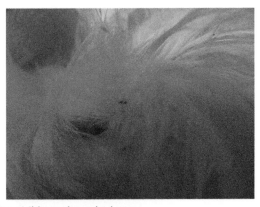

Fig. 8. Mites and lice visible to the naked eye.

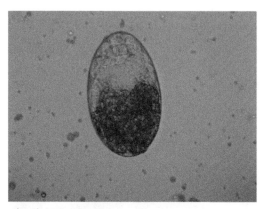

Fig. 9. Louse egg under the microscope.

cell debris in the cytoplasm. No bacteria will be found, however, which would be immediately recognizable under the microscope.[1]

In *bacterial infections,* rod-shaped or spherical-shaped bacteria can be found within the cytoplasm of heterophils and macrophages. This finding distinguishes abscesses caused by microtraumas, in which inflammatory cells and bacteria can be detected, from other frequent pathologies in canaries, such as lumps of the feathers, pox lesions, or neoplasms.

With Canary candidiasis, intense proliferation of a single-cell yeast is seen, which is considered an opportunistic pathogen of the gastrointestinal tract, frequent in canaries subject to stress, malnutrition, or prolonged antibiotic treatment. Symptoms are regurgitation, anorexia, diarrhea, and undigested seeds in the feces. An autopsy usually reveals whitish oropharyngeal plaques.[2–8] The disease can also be caused by the frequent and prolonged use of antibiotics, and because candidiasis is recognizable under the microscope, cytology can avoid prolonging unsuitable therapy that encourages rather than counteracts this pathology.

Amorphous debris, horny scales, and cholesterol crystals are cytologic features of *feather cysts (hypopteronosis cystica)* (**Figs. 12** and **13**).[9]

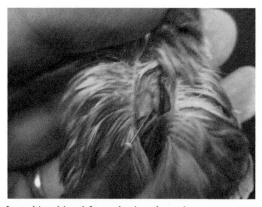

Fig. 10. Technique for taking blood from the jugular vein.

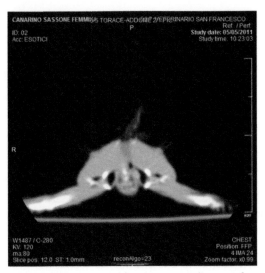

Fig. 11. Computed tomographic image with contrast medium performed on a canary at Ospedale Veterinario San Francesco Treviso (Italy).

Pox in the canary is caused by poxvirus and its clinical presentation can take various forms. In the skin form the lesions involve feet, eyelids, and areas around the eyes and nostrils. The cutaneous form differs from the forms of bacterial or mycotic dermatitis or conjunctivitis. Antemortem cytology followed by postmortem histopathology can reveal intracytoplasmic inclusions in the epithelial cells during poxvirus infection.[2]

The canary has *neoplasms*, such as tumorlike pox lesion and leukosis.[2] Apart from abscesses, the uropygial gland can also have neoplastic pathologies.

Tumors of this gland in avian species include squamous cell carcinoma, adenoma, adenocarcinoma, and fibrosarcoma (the latter seemingly the most common). Adenomas and adenocarcinomas are commonly found in the canary.[10]

Based on cytology, neoplasia is distinguished as benign neoplasia (recognizable cytologically by the presence of cells similar to the tissue of origin) from malignant

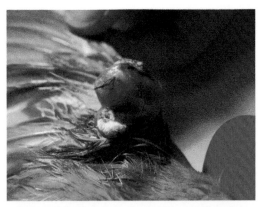

Fig. 12. Classic presentation of feather cysts (lumps) in pterylae of the wing.

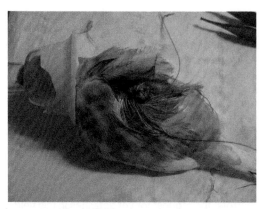

Fig. 13. Canary under gas anesthesia for lump removal.

neoplasia (consisting of cells that are atypical and always revealed by the cytologic test).

Epithelial tumors (also of glandular origin) can also be distinguished from mesenchymal tumors (with spindle cells, such as fibromas and fibrosarcomas) and lastly round-cell tumors (eg, lymphoma and plasmocytoma), (**Fig. 14**).

Summing up, cytology is indispensable for distinguishing inflammations from infections, neoplasms from cystic neoformations. Cytology sometimes reveals a precise pathogen and, points the clinical vet toward the most suitable therapy.

LABORATORY PROCEDURE

Canary or finch breeding is common in Italy, with a large number of breeders. The estimated production is around 2 million ornamental birds a year although this is probably an underestimate.

Finch breeding focuses on the selection of a specific livery variety, in particular, for the canary that can have almost 400 different color combinations.

This kind of breeding is susceptible to several types of health problems. High density husbandry, high selection rates, variability of nutrition standards, no specific

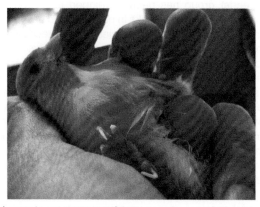

Fig. 14. Abdominal mass in a canary, xanthoma.

standards regarding the production site, and the absence of precise health protocols focused on limiting or eradicating disease could be the most important predisposing factors that contribute to the spread or development of specific health problems.

Vets must remember that each breeder manages his farm with individual knowledge that often has no scientific basis but relies only on empiric activities.

Given the specialized nature of the ornamental bird field, it is hard to define a relevant general laboratory approach although the clinical vet could be the key figure to achieving diagnosis.

In the last few years, the diagnostic avian laboratory has developed several new tests to detect specific avian pathogens and, apart from the poultry areas, the most important goals have been in the parrot sector, which is of most interest for practitioners.

Even if the number of canaries and finches in Italy and probably the world is higher than the number of parrots, the request for vet activities in this field is scarce: therefore specific laboratory methods are lesser in number and investigations are limited.

We perform about 1000 gross pathologic examinations on finches in our laboratory each year as well as other types of test, such as bacteriologic (about 1500 per year) and virological tests, and various polymerase chain reactions (PCRs) for specific pathogens, for a total of 3500 tests per year. For this bird species, the samples come mostly from aviaries or farms whereas very few samples are a companion bird. This is probably because in the case of a single sick canary, current laboratory tests are not helpful or are not specialized enough.

Hence in our laboratory we prefer to consider the finch sector as more similar to industrial poultry production than the parrot or other ornamental bird sectors in which each patient is treated as an individual. From our viewpoint, in the finch sector, the group of birds should be considered as the main goal for practitioners and accordingly we try to set specific laboratory tests to help indicate, evaluate, and analyze the general state of health of the finch stock.

Based on these considerations, our diagnostic approach to the group is very similar to that applied to the poultry sector, trying to adapt the very few specimens that we collect from a finch farm.

The most common specimens are excrements from live birds, but a carcass can be had during a disease outbreak.

In the finch sector, excrement can provide a good indication of the health status of the group and over the years, we have developed and applied a scheme of sampling and a set of laboratory tests that allow the vet to evaluate the group's well-being. This approach to the breeder group has been developed based on the main bacterial species involved during mortality outbreaks in nestlings and has focused on assessing the presence of these specific bacterial species in the breeders and then applying corrective measures to limit them before the breeding season.

The scheme proposed by the authors, called prebreeding check,[11,12] is based on previously obtained data in which aerobic bacterial flora in the gut of the canaries is considered to be scarce, meaning that the isolation of any bacteria belonging to the Enterobacteriaceae family can normally be correlated to a disease status.[13,14] The presence of potential pathogens, such as bacteria and parasites can have an adverse impact on breeding performance. Bacterial diseases are widely discussed as the cause of embryo and nestling mortality in canaries.

Our laboratory has been applying this scheme for about 6 years and has a good feedback from the owners and vets involved. The scheme performs particularly well when there is no viral infection in the aviaries, and earlier problems were instead due mainly to bacterial species, poor management activities, and feed deficiencies.

This scheme is based on the random collection of droppings in the aviary. We particularly recommend collecting the excrement for the parasitologic test in a different cage to where the birds are present to obtain a representative specimen. For the bacteriologic test, we advise collecting fresh droppings by swabs with Amies agar to keep the bacteria viable. Collection should be focused on all cages containing females (during the breeding phase they are usually kept in cages housing at least 15 females), touching at least 20 fresh droppings with one swab, while a collection is taken from only a part of the males (50%) including the new arrivals. After the collections, which provide a picture of the health status of the stock, the owner is forbidden to introduce new birds because they could be asymptomatic carriers of some pathogens. In the laboratory, the specimens are inoculated into blood agar, MacConkey agar, and b*rain-heart infusion* broth and incubated at 37°C in an aerobic environment. After 24 hours, the plates are read as described in our previous article.[15] The scheme of reading the plates is based on identifying the 2 most prevalent bacterial colonies and if other types of colonies are noticed, polymicrobism is confirmed and are added to the list. After the 2 most prevalent types of colonies are identified, we perform the Kirby Bauer (KB) test so that the drug susceptibility data can be given to the practitioners. The selection criterion for application of the KB test is based on the pathogenic impact of the bacterial species.[11] We consider species such as *Salmonella, Escherichia coli, Klebsiella spp, Listeria spp, Enterobacter sakazakii, Staphylococcus spp,* and *Pseudomonas* important because of their presence during mortality outbreaks in nestlings. *Pseudomonas* is often associated with poor quality drinking water or inadequate hygiene during the preparation of soft food by the owners. We advise an improvement in management practices to eliminate the primary source of *Pseudomonas*. Based on the results we discuss with the practitioners the best way to reduce the presence of the bacterial species in question in the flocks, basing the therapy on the KB test and the parasitologic test. We also advice regarding the critical points of the breeding phase, with a great deal of attention paid to the preparation of soft food with a large quantity of free water, very often used by owners to stimulate or increase feeding activities in the nestlings.

To evaluate our procedure, we decided to establish how correct application of the prebreeding check can improve the parent health status and consequently, the reproductive performance in canary husbandry.

On this basis, we decided to monitor the farms 1 month before the beginning of the breeding season through the clinical examinations of the bird group and microbiological and parasitologic examinations of the excrement.[12]

During the experiment, the owner was instructed to fill out a datasheet containing all the reproductive parameters of each examined couple of canaries. These data included several reproductive indices, such as fertility (%), hatchability (%), and neonatal mortality (%).

To assess the feasibility of our proposal a pilot experiment was started in 8 canary husbandries, where the prebreeding check was applied to evaluate the health status of the parents. The farms were divided into 2 groups: Group 1, where slight modification of management and a specific drug therapy were applied based on laboratory results; Group 2, no management or drug measures were applied based on laboratory results. At the end of the breeding season, we analyzed and compared the productive data between groups and our results showed better reproductive performance in husbandries belonging to group 1 (**Fig. 15**).

Based on our activities in the field and on these results, we can say that the veterinarian and the laboratory could play an important role in canary husbandry, and the

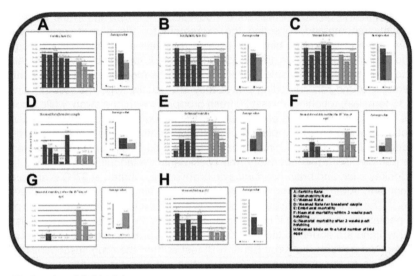

Fig. 15. Results of field trial.

prebreeding check should be considered a helpful tool in managing the reproductive season of the canary.

In our diagnostic laboratory, we also applied 2 main protocols during the gross pathologic examinations. Because health problems are common during finch breeding and are usually related to the age of bird or the reproductive period, we consequently used one protocol for nestlings up to the third week of age and another one for adult birds (after the third week of age).

The nestlings protocol included a bacteriologic test on tissue from the brain, lung, and gut to detect the pathogen bacterial species involved in infectious diseases and to determine if it was able to invade other organs such as the brain and lung. We usually performed the bacteriologic test on the 2 most interesting nestlings in terms of the gross pathologic findings. We also performed electron microscopy on a pool of gut samples to detect any virus and then we performed a specific PCR for circovirus, even if the role of this virus remains unclear because the presence of PCR positivities is not always related to disease. We performed a parasitologic test of the gut, which is very important in the Carduelius species, where we have found the presence of coccidia at 10 days of age. A mucosal scraping of the proventriculus was observed under the microscope to detect the presence of *Macrorhabdus ornithogaster*, even if we were only able to find it after 20 days of age using the microscope and PCR methods.[16] Infestation by cryptosporidium species in the proventriculus in a few clinical cases is interesting.

The adult protocol included an important necropsy procedure in which we checked all the organs, using a scheme designed to focus our attention on certain possible causes of disease only. To explain all the steps would require more space and so we will define the most important activities performed in these cases.

Our adult protocol included a scraping of proventriculus and gut for each carcass to reveal any parasitic infestation.

Regarding the most common diseases, during the first 4 months of age, we noticed a high incidence of atoxoplasmosis with associated spleen and liver enlargement. In this case we used a Diff Quick stain on a lung smear if the carcass was fresh, whereas

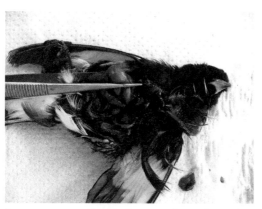

Fig. 16. Enlarged spleen, a common finding in atoxoplasmosis or plasmodiosis infestation.

a PCR method when the carcass was frozen; the PCR test is also best for examining excrements.[17] We have noticed the presence of atoxoplasmosis during the breeding phase and, in particular, that the dead birds are usually females that died during the laying of eggs. The 2 above-mentioned tests are used to obtain the diagnosis.

Another common disease is avian pox, which can cause several types of lesion. When we suspected poxvirus, a histopathological test on fresh samples was performed and, in other cases, electron microscopy was used to confirm our diagnostic suspicion.

A high-mortality rate can be frequent in the summer in birds (especially canaries) kept outdoors, and gross pathologic findings of the carcasses showed a noticeably enlarged spleen (**Fig. 16**) and liver, for which we prepared a lung smear to test for plasmodium (**Fig. 17**) or atoxoplasma (**Fig. 18**).[18]

In the last few years we have noticed the comeback of clinical cases of salmonellosis. In some aviaries the clinical symptoms are atypical, with increase in the mortality of adult birds and a very high rate in nestlings. Birds show anorexia and sometimes, hemorrhagic diarrhea, enlarged spleen, and liver, while some necrotic foci can be detected (**Fig. 19**). Diagnosis is based on the isolation of bacteria using microbiology techniques. In this case the serotype involved is typhimurium. Similar gross pathologic features can be found in listeriosis and yersiniosis, even if the presence of necrotic foci is more frequent and evident (**Fig. 20**), and the disease seems to be mild with a long

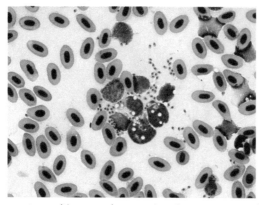

Fig. 17. Plasmodium mature schizont and merozoites, in canary smear (Diff Quick stain).

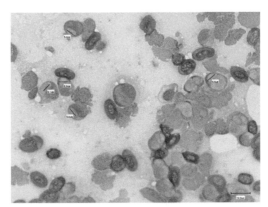

Fig. 18. Atoxoplasma in canary smear (Diff Quick stain).

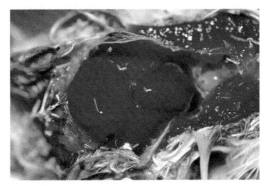

Fig. 19. Enlarged of the liver with evident necrotic areas caused by *Salmonella* infection.

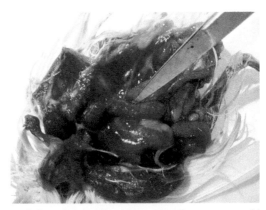

Fig. 20. Enlargement of the spleen with evident necrotic areas caused by *Listeria* infection.

period of lethargy in the affected birds. A bacteriologic test allows the bacteria to be isolated and the identification procedure to reach a diagnosis.

Chlamydophila is present in the finch, even though few data are available regarding the pathologic effects. In our laboratory we have noticed the presence of Chlamydophila in some aviaries in which a decrease in hatchability was the only symptom. A long period of treatment with doxycycline lasting at least 6 weeks is recommended, and an interesting improvement in the hatchability rate is noticed in this case. If chlamydia is suspected, liver or spleen samples are taken from the affected birds, whereas the best way to monitor dead-in-the-shell embryos is to collect excrements for at least one week and then perform a PCR for Chlamydophila. The collection of excrement for a whole week is necessary because of the intermittent shedding of this pathogen.

If viral disease is suspected, we prefer to use the specific PCR based on its availability. In other cases with no clear suspicion or the unavailability of PCR, electron microscopy on the affected organs can be a good solution, even if isolation in the eggs or cell culture can be a valid tool. In this instance, however, it is truly important to contact the diagnostic laboratory to decide on the best solution and the best sampling protocol.

REFERENCES

1. Raskin RE. congresso "International Congress of the Italian Association of Companion Animal Veterinarians". Rimini, May 19–21, 2006.
2. Harrison GJ, Lightfoot TL. Clinical avian medicine. Spix Publishing; 2006.
3. Samour J. Avian medicine. Mosby Elsevier; 2008.
4. Clark P, Boardman W, Raidal S. Atlas of clinical avian hematology. Wiley-Blackwell Publishing; 2009.
5. Campbell T, Ellis KC. Avian and exotic animal hematology and cytology. Blackwell Publishing; 2007.
6. Krautwald Kinghanns ME, Pees M, Reese S, et al. Diagnostic imaging of exotic pets. Hannover (Germany): Schlutersche Verlagsgesells; 2011.
7. Taccini E, Rossi G, Gili C, editors. Tecnica autoptica e diagnostica cadaverica. Poletto; 2006.
8. Todisco G. Gestione sanitaria e management in canaricoltura. Teramo (Italy): Giservice s.r.l; 2008.
9. Schiano C. congresso "International Congress of the Italian Association of Companion Animal Veterinarians". Rimini, May 19–21, 2006.
10. Birchard SJ, Sherding RG. Medicina e chirurgia degli animali da compagnia. Elsevier; 2009.
11. Catania S, Bilato D, Capitanio M, et al. Il controllo precova: come strumento per il miglioramento dei risultati riproduttivi nell'allevamento del canarino 62° Congresso Internazionale Multisala SCIVAC. Rimini May 30–June 1, 2009. p. 9.
12. Gobbo F, Bilato D, Sturaro A, et al. Pre-breeding check: a tool for improving the reproductive performance in the canary (Serinus canarius, Linnaeus, 1758). XVII Congress of WVPA (World Veterinary Poultry Association). Cancun, August 14–18, 2011.p. 165.
13. Glünder G, Hinz KH. (1979). Vorkommen und Bedeutung von Enterobakteriaceen bei Körnerfressern. Verhandlungsber. I. Tagung Krank. D. Vögel. Munchen: 89-95.
14. Conzo G. Medicina degli Uccelli da Gabbia. Edizioni Calderini-Edagricole; 2001.
15. Bilato D, Sturaro A, Corso C, et al. Metodologia di valutazione microbiologica delle deiezioni di canarino. 59° Congresso Internazionale Multisala SCIVAC. Rimini, May 30–June 1, 2008. p. 377.

16. Tomaszewski EK, Logan KS, Snowden KF, et al. Phylogenetic analysis identifies the 'megabacterium' of birds as a novel anamorphic ascomycetous yeast, Macrorhabdus ornithogaster gen. nov., sp. nov. Int J Syst Evol Microbiol 2003;53(Pt 4): 1201–5.

17. Ceglie L, Battanolli G, Belfanti I, et al. Biomolecular techniques applied to the diagnosis of Atoxoplasmosis in canary birds (Serinus canarius, Linnaeus, 1758). XVII Congress of WVPA (World Veterinary Poultry Association). Cancun, August 14–8, 2011.p. 166.

18. Bilato D, Gobbo F, Boscaro G, et al. Diagnosis and treatment of plasmodiosis in canary (Serinus canarius, Linnaeus, 1758). XVII Congress of WVPA (World Veterinary Poultry Association). Cancun, August 14–8, 2011.p. 174.

Acid-Base Status in the Avian Patient Using a Portable Point-of-Care Analyzer

Andrés Montesinos, lv*, María Ardiaca, lv

KEYWORDS

- Avian • Blood gas • Electrolytes • Emergency • Point of care

KEY POINTS

- The i-STAT point-of-care analyzer is easy to use and can be used as a blood analyzer in critical avian patients, although single values have to be interpreted carefully.
- The study of the acid-base status in companion birds is still in its infancy.
- Further research is needed to establish normal reference values in arterial blood gases and compare with venous blood gas, and then to determine if the formulas that deviate from small animal medicine are or are not applicable.
- Normal reference values for African Grey Parrot are shown in the text.

INTRODUCTION

Metabolic derangements and respiratory distress are common presenting problems in emergency medicine.[1] In patients whose clinical condition dictates urgent care, emergency intervention should be initiated as soon as possible. Sometimes several diagnostic tests must be postponed until the patient is stabilized, and its hydration, ventilation, and oxygenation status assessed. The patient's electrolyte levels and acid-base status (pH) provide quick results with a minimal sample volume and minimal stress to the patient.

Recent technologic advances have allowed the production and marketing of point-of-care blood gas analyzers to private practitioners. These new machines are able to run a complete analysis with small amounts of blood or plasma samples (0, 1 mL), which makes them especially useful in avian medicine. As a result, evaluation of blood gases is no longer an activity confined to academic institutions and has become a daily part of many practicing veterinarians' activities.

What Do the Numbers Tell Us?

Depending on the blood analyzers in use, more or fewer numbers will form the results. It is important to understand the various components of each of these numbers. Only

Centro Veterinario Los Sauces, Santa Engracia 63, 28010 Madrid, Spain
* Corresponding author.
E-mail address: cvsauces@cvsauces.com

Vet Clin Exot Anim 16 (2013) 47–69
http://dx.doi.org/10.1016/j.cvex.2012.10.001
vetexotic.theclinics.com

a few results are truly measured by the analyzer. The rest are calculated from various formulas or nomograms that are programmed into the analyzer. Some of the calculated values are derived using values that are appropriate and accurate for human samples but not for veterinary patients (especially avian patients). These variables may differ from analyzer to analyzer. **Table 1** is a list of the common variables found on a blood gas analysis.

Point-of-care blood gas analyzers directly measure the pH, Po_2, and Pco_2. These measured values are then used to derive the percentage of hemoglobin (Hb) saturated with oxygen (SO_2), bicarbonate (HCO_3) concentration, total CO_2 (TCO_2) concentration, and base excess of the extracellular fluid (BE). The SO_2 is usually determined by the Po_2, from the oxygen dissociation curve. The HCO_3 concentration, TCO_2 concentration, and BE are also derived from formulas and nomograms. The BE, HCO_3 concentration, and TCO_2 concentration all serve as measures of the metabolic component of the patient's acid-base status, whereas Pco_2 evaluates ventilation and represents the respiratory component of the acid-base status. Oxygenation, as calculated from the Pao_2, is also part of the assessment of respiratory function (see **Table 1**).

Why Perform a Blood Gas Analysis?

Blood gas analysis is performed to obtain information about the acid-base status of a patient and about gas exchange in the lungs. If information about the acid-base status is desired, a venous sample is most informative. Venous blood contains cellular waste products and provides a more accurate reflection of acid-base state at the cellular level. If evaluation of respiratory gas exchange is the goal, then an arterial sample is desired. Arterial blood has been through the lungs (unless there is a shunt present) but has not been exposed to any cellular uptake or waste, which allows a view of how effectively the lungs have been able to load oxygen into the blood and remove carbon dioxide.[2]

Also, most blood gas analyzers include some metabolites and main ions in the results, helping to the practitioner in the decision about what fluids need to be used.

Notes on Physiology

In birds, as in mammals, mainly two organs are responsible for maintaining normal acid-base physiology or compensating for acid-base disturbances. The lungs are responsible for regulating the CO_2 concentration of blood (more CO_2 in blood, more acidic pH). Respiratory acid-base alterations that disarrange (increase or decrease) carbon dioxide concentrations are generally a result of neurologic, respiratory musculoskeletal or extrarespiratory system dysfunction.

Table 1		
Variables that commonly form the results of a blood gas analysis		
Variable	**Definition**	**Measured or Calculated**
pH	The pH of the sample	Measured
Pco_2	The partial pressure of carbon dioxide in the sample	Measured
Po_2	The partial pressure of oxygen in the sample	Measured
SO_2	The percent of Hb saturated with oxygen	Measured or calculated
HCO_3	The concentration of bicarbonate in the sample	Calculated
BE	The base excess	Calculated
SBE	The standard base excess	Calculated

The kidney contains numerous regulatory mechanisms controlling the amount of acid or base excreted in urine. The gastrointestinal tract may be the source of increased loss of acid base through vomiting or diarrhea. Cellular metabolism, ingestion of toxins with acidic or alkaline characteristics, and liver dysfunction that alters normal metabolism could result in increases or decreases of acid or bases in the body. All these alterations in physiologic function are nonrespiratory (or metabolic) acid-base disturbances.

In general, the respiratory system attempts to compensate for derangements in the nonrespiratory system and vice versa. Because of the volatile nature of the CO_2 and that it can be exhaled from the body very quickly, the respiratory system is able to compensate rapidly for nonrespiratory disturbances. Generally, the kidney is the organ responsible for altering acid or base excretion for the body. It takes longer to compensate for respiratory disturbances but, if given enough time, renal function can be efficient at this task. If a single acid-base disturbance is present, the unaffected system begins compensating in an attempt to mitigate any severe alteration in the blood pH that could impair cellular enzymatic function. In severely ill patients, however, alterations may be present in multiple systems and compensation may be inadequate or absent, resulting in complex or mixed acid-base disturbances.

Avian Patients: Renal Contribution to Acid-Base Regulation

Most birds maintain an alkaline arterial pH of approximately 7.5, despite a constant metabolic production of acid. Most of this acid, resulting in the hydration of CO_2, is excreted as respiratory CO_2. However, nonvolatile acids (eg, H_2SO_4 and H_3PO_4) are also a threat to acid-base homeostasis and the kidneys must excrete the protons equivalent to these metabolic end products. Thus, avian urine is typically acidic, with a pH in the range of 5.5 to 7.5. The renal defense of arterial alkaline pH is presumed to consist of two components: conservation of the base (bicarbonate) and excretion of acid (H^+, largely buffered).[3]

Avian renal conservation of bicarbonate is thought to be accomplished by mechanisms similar to those existing in the mammalian kidney. That is, secreted H^+ combines in the tubule lumen with filtered HCO_3- to form CO_2 that diffuses back into the tubule cells. Overall, birds are indeed as efficient at conserving bicarbonate as are the mammals. It is likely that bicarbonate reabsorption in the avian kidney occurs in the distal nephron.

The lack of acidification of proximal tubule fluid, even in acidotic birds, suggests that H^+ secretion may also take place in distal nephron segments. Three compounds (ammonia, phosphate, and urate) serve as the primary urinary buffers in birds.

STEP-BY-STEP APPROACH TO ARTERIAL AND VENOUS BLOOD GAS ANALYSIS
Step 1: Sampling

Appropriate sampling methods should be used when analyzing blood gases to ensure that no preanalytical errors are introduced. There are numerous manufactured blood-gas specific syringes on the market. These syringes include lyophilized lithium heparin as an anticoagulant and sometimes an arterial self-filling mechanism. Some brands of these syringes cannot be used to aspirate venous blood. The dry lithium heparin is used to minimize errors in ionized calcium (iCa) that can result from the use of sodium heparin (less important if the analyzer is not running iCa).

For the practitioner, a recent study showed the following heparinization technique to be the most accurate[4]:

1. Fill a 3 mL syringe to the 3 mL mark using liquid heparin and a 22G needle
2. Depress the plunger to expel all of the heparin to the syringe

3. Aspirate 3 mL of air back into the syringe and rapidly expel the contents of the syringe
4. Repeat the air aspiration and expulsion two additional times
5. Fill the syringe with 1 mL of arterial of venous blood.

The study was developed for canine blood samples. In the case of avian samples, 1 mL can be excessively high, especially in small birds. Alternative technique is needed in smaller patients. See the article by Ardiaca and colleagues elsewhere in this issue for further exploration of this topic.

Step 2: Determine Whether the Sample is Arterial or Venous

When studying the respiratory component of a blood gas analysis, it is important to know if the sample obtained is really an arterial blood sample. The main indicators are the SO_2 and the Po_2. In small animal medicine, the following is accepted:

SO_2 >88% = arterial
PO_2 >60 mm Hg = arterial
SO_2 <88% = mixed, venous
PO_2 <60 mm Hg = mixed, venous.

Causes of arterial blood with SO_2 less than 88% could be pulmonary or Hb derangements.[5]

Step 3: Determine the Acid-Base Status of the Patient

Step 3.1 Determine whether the sample is acidotic, alkalotic, or normal (pH)

The blood pH represents the overall balance of all the acid (acidotic) and base (alkalotic) processes in the body. It is determined by the ratio between the metabolic (HCO_3^-) and respiratory (Pco_2) components of the acid-base balance.[6] In general (canine, feline, and human medicine), acidemia is defined as a blood pH below 7.35 and alkalemia as a blood pH above 7.45 (7.4 is neutral). Based on the Henderson-Hasselbalch equation, the pH can be defined by the ratio of the HCO_3^- concentration ($[HCO_3^-]$) to the dissolved CO_2 ($[\alpha Pco_2]$) concentration in the extracellular fluid.

$$pH = \frac{[HCO_3^-]\ (metabolic)}{[\alpha Pco_2]\ (respiratory)}$$

In this equation, α is the solubility coefficient for CO_2, and it equals 0.03. A good rule is that pH generally changes in the same direction as the primary disorder.[7]

Step 3.2 Determine whether the Pco2 is normal or abnormal

The Pco_2 provides information regarding ventilation, or the respiratory component of the acid-base balance. Hypoventilation is characterized by increases in the Pco_2 (>45 mm Hg) because CO_2 is retained in the blood. CO_2 is a volatile acid, so retention of CO_2 leads to respiratory acidosis. In most instances, respiratory acidosis is caused by some aspects of ventilation failure. Common causes of hypoventilation include those affecting neurologic control of the respiration (eg, anesthesia, sedation), breathing mechanics (eg, diaphragmatic hernia in mammals), or proper flow of air through the airways (eg, upper or lower airway obstruction) or the alveoli.[8]

Hyperventilation is characterized by the decreases in Pco_2 as the CO_2 is blown off from the lungs, which leads to respiratory alkalosis (Pco_2 <35 mm Hg). Causes of hyperventilation include hypoxemia, pulmonary disease, pain, anxiety, and excessive manual or mechanical ventilation. Hyperventilation may also develop as a compensation for metabolic acidosis.[9]

Step 3.3 Determine whether the HCO₃⁻ is normal or abnormal

The metabolic contribution to the acid-base balance can be assessed with the HCO_3^- and the BE. Typical reference ranges for HCO_3^- are 19 to 23 mEq/L in dogs and 17 to 21 mEq/L in cats. Value less than these ranges indicate metabolic acidosis, whereas values greater than the ranges indicates metabolic alkalosis.[10,11]

Metabolic acidosis can be caused by increases in the generation of hydrogen ions (H^+) from endogenous (eg, lactate, ketones) or exogenous (eg, salicylates) and by the inability of the kidneys to eliminate H^+ from dietary protein (renal failure). These increases in H^+ are buffered by decreases in the HCO_3. In addition, metabolic acidosis can be caused by a direct loss of bicarbonate through the gastrointestinal tract (diarrhea) or kidneys (renal tubular acidosis) or, less commonly, by the abusive use of intravenous fluids that contain no bicarbonate precursors.[10] Metabolic alkaloses can occur from a loss of H^+ (vomiting of stomach contents) or from gain of HCO_3^- (eg, sodium bicarbonate administration, hyperchloremic alkaloses caused by the use of loop diuretics).

The BE concept As mentioned previously, the HCO_3- concentration is calculated from the pH and P_{CO_2}; therefore, it is not independent of respiratory activity. In an attempt to isolate the metabolic component from respiratory influences, the concept of BE was developed by European physiologists. It is defined as the amount of strong acid or alkali required to titrate 1 L of blood to pH 7.40 at 37°C while the partial pressure of CO_2 is held constant at 40 mm Hg. In essence, the blood sample no longer has any respiratory acid-base disturbance, and the amount of acid or base required to titrate to a pH of 7.4 is representative of the summation of all nonrespiratory acid-base disturbances. The concept of standard base excess was developed because the buffering capacity of a blood sample outside of the patient is not representative of what might take place in vivo. The concept of standard base excess evaluates the acid or base that would require titration of the extracellular fluid space back to a pH of 7.4. Some analyzers may report these calculated values. These values are also often used in calculating the amount of buffer (usually bicarbonate) to administer to a patient with severe acidosis.[2] **Table 2** summarizes the four primary acid-base disturbances.

Step 3.4 Determine whether compensating is occurring

Typically, pH changes arising from one component (eg, metabolic) are opposed by changes in another component (eg, respiratory) to maintain the proper ratio of metabolic to respiratory contribution to overall pH.[6] For example, with metabolic acidosis, the HCO_3- concentration decreases, thereby lowering the HCO_3^- to P_{CO_2} ratio and resulting in alkalemia. In most instances, the body compensates by decreasing the P_{CO_2} or hyperventilating in an attempt to maintain the ratio. In other words, the respiratory component compensates for the metabolic acidosis in an attempt to raise the pH to neutral. Physiologic compensation rarely completely resolves the primary acid-base problem and never leads to overcompensation. Therefore, the pH typically

Table 2
The four primary acid-base disorders and their compensatory changes

Conditions	Primary Disorder	Compensation
Low pH and low HCO₃⁻ (low BE)	Metabolic acidosis	Decreased P_{CO_2}
High pH and High HCO₃⁻ (high BE)	Metabolic alkalosis	Increased P_{CO_2}
Low pH and High P_{CO_2}	Respiratory acidosis	Increased HCO₃⁻ (BE)
High pH and low P_{CO_2}	Respiratory alkalosis	Decreased HCO₃⁻ (BE)

deviates from neutral, even after adequate compensation, although it can be within the reference ranges in patients with mild acid-base disorders.[12]

Metabolic acidosis is the most common acid-base disturbance in canine and feline medicine. If metabolic acidosis is the primary disturbance, it will be represented by a lower pH, a negative BE or lower HCO_3^- concentration, and a compensatory decrease in the P_{CO_2} in an attempt to blow off the excess acid load. The adequacy of the compensatory response can be quantified with the use of formulas that predict the expected response to the primary disturbance (**Table 3**). These responses have not been objectively evaluated in cats or in avian patients but, in most cases, cats' responses are assumed to be similar to those of dogs.[2] Acute responses last less than 2 days, whereas chronic responses may take 2 to 5 days to reach maximal effect.

By quantifying the degree of compensatory changes and comparing with the expected (calculated) values, clinicians can assess whether the patient's values are within or outside a defined margin of error. If they are within the margin, the patient has a primary disturbance and is compensating adequately. If they are outside it, the patient likely has multiple primary acid-base disorders (a mixed acid-base disorder).[2] For example, inappropriate respiratory compensation (P_{CO_2}) for metabolic acidosis ($\downarrow HCO_3^-$) is diagnosed by comparing the measured P_{CO_2} with the expected changes in P_{CO_2} predicted for each mEq/L decreased in HCO_3^-. When the measured P_{CO_2} is lower than expected, primary respiratory alkalosis is complicating the metabolic acidosis. An example of a patient with such a mixed disturbance would be a hyperventilating parrot with kidney disease. Pain, restraint, fear, and excitement can cause hyperventilation in the excess of the calculated compensation for metabolic acidosis, which, in this patient, is a result of the hyperuricemic acidosis associated with renal disease.

Step 4: Assess the Animal's Oxygenation

Step 4.1 Is the animal breathing room air?

Hypoxemia refers to a reduction of P_{aO_2} values to below 80 mm Hg. The presence of hypoxemia can be life-threatening, and a P_{aO_2} value below 60 mm Hg warrants immediate therapeutic intervention.[13] Theoretically, in human and small animal medicine,

---

Table 3
Summary of compensatory responses in dogs with metabolic and respiratory acid-base disorders

Primary Disorder	Expected Compensation
Metabolic acidosis $\downarrow HCO_3^-$ ($\downarrow$ BE)	$\downarrow$ P_{CO_2} of 0,7 mm Hg per 1.0 mEq/L decrease in [HCO_3^-] (± 3)
Metabolic alkalosis $\uparrow HCO_3^-$ ($\uparrow$ BE)	$\uparrow$ P_{CO_2} of 0,7 mm Hg per 1.0 mEq/L increase in [HCO_3^-] (± 3)
Acute respiratory acidosis $\uparrow P_{CO_2}$	$\uparrow$ [HCO_3^-] of 0.15 mEq/L per 1.0 mm Hg increase in P_{CO_2} (± 2)
Chronic respiratory acidosis $\uparrow P_{CO_2}$	$\uparrow$ [HCO_3^-] of 0.35 mEq/L per 1.0 mm Hg increase in P_{CO_2} (± 2)
Acute respiratory alkalosis $\downarrow P_{CO_2}$	$\downarrow$ [HCO_3^-] of 0.25 mEq/L per 1.0 mm Hg decrease in P_{CO_2} (± 2)
Chronic respiratory alkalosis $\downarrow P_{CO_2}$	$\downarrow$ [HCO_3^-] of 0.55 mEq/L per 1.0 mm Hg decrease in P_{CO_2} (± 2)

Data from Autran de Morais HS, Dibartola SP. Ventilatory and metabolic compensation in dogs with acid-base disturbances. J Vet Emerg Crit Care 1991;1(2):39–49.

anytime a low Pao_2 value below 60 mm Hg is obtained from a patient breathing room air, the alveolar equation should be used to determine the alveolar-arterial (A-a) gradient:

A-a gradient = A-a.
$A = [(P_B - 47)]0.21 - P_{co2}/0.8$
$a = Po_2$.

In these equations, P_B is atmospheric pressure (760 mm Hg at sea level), and 47 is the water vapor pressure in mm Hg (which is subtracted because only dry alveolar gas pressures are measured). The figure 0.21 represents the oxygen fraction inspirited, 21% of the air composition. The factor 0.8 represents the ratio of oxygen uptake to CO_2 exhaled.

The following equation is a simplified version of the alveolar gas equation that can be used for patients breathing room air ($Fio_2 = 21\%$) at sea level ($P_B = 760$ mm Hg).

$A = 150 - (1.2 \times Paco_2)$

Clinically, a normal A-a gradient (0–20 mm Hg) excludes pulmonary disease and suggests that arterial hypoxemia (Pao_2 <80 mm Hg) is due to hypoventilation or decreased inspired oxygen. Patients with a gradient more than 25 mm Hg should be considered to have a degree of ventilation: perfusion ratio mismatch from pulmonary parenchymal disease, although cardiovascular disease can also affect this value.[14]

Step 4.2 Is the animal on supplemental oxygen?
When the animal is on supplemental oxygen, the A-a gradient is Pao_2/Fio_2. Normal values in dog medicine are above 200 (>200 mm Hg).[14]

Step 5. Determine the Anion Gap (Electrolytes Availability)

Anion Gap = $(Na^+ + K^+) - (HCO_3^- + Cl^-)$

The anion gap (AGap) is an adjunct to blood gas evaluation that helps differentiate causes of metabolic acidosis. It is calculated as the difference between the measured plasma concentration of the major positively charged ions (cations) and the major negatively charged ions (anions).[5] In reality, the body always attempts to maintain the electroneutrality, so the concentration of serum cations equals that of anions. The AGap exists because standard electrolytes panels do not measure all the anions present in serum. Therefore, in general, the AGap represents the unmeasured anions (proteins and organic and inorganic acids). Metabolic acidosis, a very common acid-base disturbance in critically ill small animal patients, causes a reduction in HCO_3^- concentration. When there is an increase in unmeasured anions or in the Cl^- concentration, the HCO_3^- decreases to maintain electrochemical balance. Thus, the AGap can be used to categorize metabolic acidosis as increased or hyperchloremic (normal AGap acidosis). Typical reference ranges are 12 to 24 mEq/L in dogs and 13 to 27 mEq/L in cats. **Table 4** shows the approximate concentrations of cations and anions in healthy dogs and cats.

Increased AGap acidosis arises when excess acid containing unmeasured anions accumulates in the blood. Examples include lactic acidosis, ethylene glycol (antifreeze) poisoning, and salicylic poisoning. These excess anions titrates the HCO_3^- downward, thus preserving electrochemical balance.[15,16]

Metabolic acidosis characterized by a normal AGap arises when chloride, which is routinely measured, is added to the blood (eg, dilutional acidosis with aggressive

Table 4
Approximate concentrations of cations and anions in healthy dogs and cats

	Na + K + Ca + Mg + Trace Elements	=	Cl + HCO₃ + Proteins + Organic Acids + Inorganic Acids
Dog	145 + 4 + 5 + 2 + 1	=	110 + 21 + 19 + 5 + 4
	Total cations = 157	=	Total anions = 157
Cat	155 + 4 + 5 + 2 + 1	=	128 + 21 + 14 + 8 + 4
	Total cations = 167	=	Total anions = 167

sodium chloride fluid administration) or when HCO_3^- loss from the body (diarrhea) is replaced with chloride to maintain electrochemical balance.[15]

Step 6. Using Venous Blood Gases to Assess the Acid-Base Status

In veterinary medicine, is not always easy to get arterial blood, especially in very small animals. Some researchers have developed equations that can calculate arterial values from measured venous blood values.

Arterial pH $= 0.039 + (0.961 \times$ venous pH$)$
Arterial $Pco_2 = 7.735 + (0.572 \times$ venous $Pco_2)$
Arterial $HCO_3^- = 0.538 + (0.845 \times$ venous $HCO_3^-)$

WHAT IS KNOWN IN AVIAN MEDICINE

In birds, only limited data are available for blood gas values. Research has been conducted on measurement of blood gases in a variety of avian species (in particular ducks and chickens[17]) with regard to anesthetic conditions,[18] exercise,[19] or change in pressure and altitude.[20] All the studies have been developed in experimental conditions and are far from the common clinical scenario of the avian practitioner. Indeed, avian physiology textbooks include normal blood gases obtained using benchtop analyzers and again in experimental conditions.

Table 5 summarized the values of arterial blood gases and pH in nonanesthetized birds breathing air that were published in a reference text on avian physiology.[21]

Hochleithner[22] describes the normal range of venous pH and Pco_2 in adults and juvenile budgerigars (Melopsittacus undulatus) and briefly report the existence of acidosis in birds with renal disease.

Schoemaker and Kitslaar[23] provided reference values of venous blood gases in 60 racings pigeons (Columba livia domestica) using a benchtop analyzer (RapidLab 248 Blood Gas analyzer; Bayer Health Care, Mijdrecht, The Netherlands) along with their core body temperature. Results from blood gas analysis can be altered by several factors, including the higher core-body temperature found in birds.[24] Blood gas analyzers have a conversion formula within its software to correct for core-body temperature differences. However, this correction formula was established for mammalian (human) individuals. It is not known whether this formula can be accurately used in avian species. Handling and storage of the obtained samples are also important aspects in obtaining valid and reliable results for blood gases.[25] In addition to reference values, Schoemaker and Kitslaar[23] transferred blood samples from 10 pigeons to a tonometer (IL Tonometer model 237; Instrumentation laboratories, Milan, Italy) to determine whether temperature correction formula could be used for avian species. By using the tonometer, they were able to determine that the calculated

Table 5
Arterial blood gases and pH in nonanesthetized birds breathing air

Bird Species	P_{O_2} (Torr)	P_{CO_2} (Torr)	pH
Female Black Bantam chicken	—	29.9	7.48
Female White Leghorn chicken	82	33	7.52
Male White Rock chicken	—	29.2	7.53
Mallard duck	81	30.8	7.56
Muscovy duck	82	38	7.49
Muscovy duck	96.1	36.9	7.46
Pekin duck	93.5	28	7.46
Pekin duck	100	33.8	7.48
Emu	99.7	33.8	7.45
Bar-headed goose	92.5	31.6	7.47
Domestic goose	97	32	7.52
Herring gull	—	27.2	7.56
Red-tailed hawk	108	27.0	7.49
Burrowing owl	97.6	32.6	7.46
White pelican	—	28.5	7.50
Adelie penguin	83.8	36.9	7.51
Chinstrap penguin	89.1	37.1	7.52
Gentoo penguin	77.1	40.9	7.49
Pigeon	77.1	40.9	7.503
Roadrunner	—	24.5	7.58
Abdim's stork	—	27.9	7.56
Mute swan	91.3	27.1	7.50
Turkey vulture	—	27.5	7.51

Data from Powell FL. Respiration. In: Caussey Whittow G, editor. Sturkie's avian physiology. 5th edition. San Diego (CA): Academic Press, Inc; 2000. p. 233–64.

values were an acceptable representation of the actual values. **Table 6** summarized the values in budgerigars obtained by Hochleithner[22] and the values in pigeons at 37°C and 42.1°C (mean core-body temperature found in pigeons) from the study of Schoemaker and Kitslaar.[23]

Table 6
Values of blood gases and pH obtained in budgerigars and in pigeons at different temperatures

Results	Budgerigars[22]	Pigeons at 37°C[23]	Pigeons at 42.1°C[23]
pH (1/H)	7.334–7.489	7.48–7.60	7.41–7.51
P_{CO_2} mm Hg	30.6–43.2	24.5–30.8	30.4–3.,0
P_{O_2} mm Hg	85–99	58.2–71,2	83.4–100.3
HCO_3 mmol/L	21–26	20–25	21–26

Data from Hochleithner M. Biochemistries. In: Ritchie BW, Harrison GH, Harrison LH, editors. Avian medicine: principles and application. Lake Worth (FL): Wingers Publishing, Inc; 1994. p. 223–7; and Schoemaker NJ, Kitslaar WJ. Venous blood gases in healthy racing pigeons. Proceedings of Association of Avian Veterinarians. 2007. p. 261–3.

Zandvliet and colleagues[26] also measured blood gases in Amazon parrots with and without respiratory distress using the same methodology as Zandvliet and colleagues[26] (**Table 7**). Venous blood gases, which were measured in three patients, revealed hypoxia in two birds. All three showed significant hypercapnia when compared with values collected in eight healthy individuals. This research indicates that collection of venous blood gases can be of additional diagnostic value in birds with respiratory disease, particularly in parrots with lung fibrosis.

Heatley and colleagues[27] also describe the use of electrolytes and blood gases to assess the health status in rehabilitated Red-tailed hawks (**Table 8**). The researchers of this study used the point-of-care analyzer Heska i-STAT (Heska Corp, Denver, CO, USA) and showed reference values for venous blood gases in healthy Red-tailed hawks (n = 40), comparing some of the results with the numbers obtained using the bench top analyzer Hitachi 911 (Roche Diagnostics, Indianapolis, IN, USA). Based on their data, Na^+ and K^+ values were significantly different based on the method of assay. Also, i-STAT determination of hematocrit (Ht) values was consistently low when compared with standard laboratory values.

In a pilot study conducted at the Sacramento Zoo with 16 Thick-billed parrots (*Rhynchopsitta pachyrhyncha*) and 9 Caribbean flamingos (*Phoenicopterus ruber*), Howard and Wack[28] studied blood gases and iCa using the CG8[+] cartridge of the i-STAT analyzer. In the flamingos, the iCa ranged from 1.3 to 1.4 mmol/L, with a concurrent pH of 7.168 to 7.465 (**Table 9**). In the Thick-billed parrots, iCa ranged from 1.03 to 1.4 mmol/L, with a concurrent pH of 7.201 to 7.446. The investigators noted that the range of iCa in avian serum may be affected by the tendency of the i-STAT to underestimate iCa greater than 1.3 mmol/L. In equine, canine, and feline blood samples, the i-STAT underestimated iCa when iCa is greater than 1.3 mmol/L.[29] Although the researchers of this pilot study used the CG8+ cartridge, no reference is made about the use of the temperature correction formula included in the software of the i-STAT analyzer.

McKinney[30] sampled 70 healthy falcons to establish normal parameters (**Table 10**). He used venous blood and the falcons were anesthetized using isoflurane administered via face mask in an Ayres T-piece circuit. All i-STAT tests were performed using heparinized blood within 5 minutes of sampling and EC8[+] cartridges.

Investigations into the acid-base status of birds of prey have suggested that acidosis is a common finding and the use of lactated ringer solution (as source of HCO_3^-) is recommended.[31] However McKinney[30] suggests that, although acidosis is seen, alkalosis (ie, a pH over 7.55) is a more common problem in trained falcons,

Table 7 Venous blood gas levels and acid-base values in Amazon parrots affected with chronic pulmonary interstitial fibrosis (Amazon 1–3) and normal Amazon parrots (n = 8)				
	Sick Amazon Parrot 1	Sick Amazon Parrot 2	Sick Amazon Parrot 3	Reference Values (n = 8)
pH	7.24	7.16	7.30	7.35 ± 0.08
P_{O_2} (mm Hg)	38.62	33.69	52.77	49.46 ± 7.62
P_{CO_2} (mm Hg)	48.77	80.08	50.16	37.92 ± 4.23
HCO_3 (mmol/L)	19.70	26.80	23.05	20.05 ± 4.62

Data from Zandvliet MM, Dorrestein GM, van der Hage M. Chronic pulmonary interstitial fibrosis in Amazon parrots. Avian Pathol 2001;30:517–24.

Table 8
Electrolytes and venous blood gases of the healthy Red-tailed hawks (n = 40)

Parameter	Units	Determination Method	Determination Method
—	—	Hitachi 911	i-STAT
Na^+	mEq/L	161.5 (4.0)	151.7 (2.1)
K^+	mEq/L	1.68 (0.749)	3.06 (0.47)
Cl^-	mEq/L	122 (2.8)	119.2 (39)
AGap	mEq/L	22.17 (7.5)	17.63 (4.8)
HCO_3^-	mEq/L	19.06 (5.7)	18.1 (4.25)
Glucose	mg/dl	379.3 (429)	369.5 (44)
Ht	%	42.8 (4)[a]	36.8 (3.2)
pH	—	—	7.43 (0.07)
Pco_2	mm Hg	—	26.78 (4.6)
BE	mmol/L	—	−6.36 (5.22)
Hb	g/dl	—	12.65 (0.98)
TCO_2	mmol/L	—	18.65 (4.25)

All values given as mean (standard deviation).
[a] Determined by microHt centrifugation.
Data from Heatley JJ, Demirjian SE, Wright JC, et al. Electrolytes of the critically ill raptor. Proceedings of Association of Avian Veterinarians; 2005. p. 23–4.

which are undergoing strenuous exercise in hot climates. In this study, improved clinical success was achieved with the use of 5% dextrose saline and 5% dextrose infusions instead of lactated ringers solution, but the investigator never discussed the osmolarity of the solutions used on the fluid therapy. Finally, this study describes some i-STAT values in some birds with aspergillosis, bumblefoot, and other diseases

Table 9
i-STAT–derived venous blood results of Caribbean flamingos at the Sacramento Zoo using the CG8+ cartridge

Parameter	Units	Mean	Minimum	Maximum	n
Na^+	mEq/L	143	136	149	9
K^+	mEq/L	4.1	3.3	5.1	9
Hb	g/dl	13	10	15	9
TCO_2	mEq/L	17	9	22	8
Po_2	mm Hg	39	30	50	9
Ht	g/dl	38	30	43	9
pH	(1/H)	7.34	7.17	7.47	8
Pco_2	mm Hg	30	23	39	8
HCO_3^+	mmol/L	16	8	21	8
BE	mmol/L	−9	−20	−3	8
Ca ion	mmol/L	1.35	1.3	1.4	9
SO_2	%	70	58	87	8

Data from Howard LL, Wack RF. Preliminary use and literature review of the i-STAT (a portable clinical analyzer) in birds. Proceedings of the American Association of Zoo Veterinarians. 2002. p. 96–100.

Table 10
i-STAT EC8+ mean, with standard deviation and the range of parameters for falcons (n = 70)

Parameter	Units	Mean	SD	Minimum	Maximum
Glucose	mg/dl	338.61	25.87	283	406
SUN	mg/dl	3.44	1.1	<3	8
Na	mEq/L	150.33	2.3	146	157
K	mEq/L	2.9	0.69	2	4.1
Cl	mEq/L	119.86	2.22	15	125
TCO$_2$	mEq/L	26.41	2.24	21	30
AGap	mmol/L	6.76	2.7	1	14
Ht	%	46.57	4.48	40	57
Hb	g/dl	15.79	1.51	14	19
pH	log10 (1/H)	7.47	0.04	7.4	7.6
Pco$_2$	mm Hg	34.96	4.2	27	49.9
HCO$_3$	mmol/L	25.34	2.19	26	29
BE	mmol/L	1.77	2.41	−3	6

Data from McKinney P. Clinical applications of the i-STAT blood analyzer in avian practice. Proceeding of the European Association of Avian Veterinarians. 2003. p. 341–6.

(**Tables 11** and **12**). Some of the sick birds had normal blood gas levels. The more curious finding of this research is the values of Ht of the falcons, which are higher than the values reported by Heatley and colleagues[27] in Red-tailed hawks and by Howard and Wack[28] in the Caribbean flamingos. Also, the values of Pco$_2$ in this study are slightly higher that the results on Red-tailed hawks and flamingos; however, it is important to keep in mind that those falcons were sampled under isoflurane anesthesia.

Also in falcons, Arca-Ruibal and colleagues[32] described blood gases and electrolytes in normal falcons (59 animals, 28 sakers, 16 peregrines, and 15 gyrfalcon hybrids). The investigators used a standard analyzer instead of the i-STAT analyzer and the falcons were sampled under ketamine-medetomidine anesthesia from the vena ulnaris. Statistical significant difference between the three species was only

Table 11
Acid-base status of critically ill falcons

Disease	pH (Range 7.37–7.55)	Pco$_2$ (Range 27–49.9 mm Hg)	HCO$_3^-$ (Range 26–29 mmol/L)
Training Stress	7.92	10.3	21
	7.88	8.2	16
	7.82	13.7	22
Pododermatitis	7.72	18.7	24
Septicemia	7.78	12.5	19
Aspergillosis, Advanced	7.54	21.2	18
	7.34	48.3	26
Aspergillosis	7.47	36.4	27
Myopathy (Creatine Kinase >4115 IU/L)	7.6	22.1	22

Data from McKinney P. Clinical applications of the i-STAT blood analyzer in avian practice. Proceedings of the European Association of Avian Veterinarians. 2003. p. 341–46.

Table 12
Blood gas values in venous blood of captive hunting falcons in the United Arab Emirates

Parameter	N	Mean	Median	SD	Minimum	Maximum	Percent 2.5%–97.5%	95% CI
pH	59	7.491	7.488	0.047	7.375	7.621	7.385–7.602	7.478–7.503
P_{CO_2} mm Hg	55	27	27.1	4.5	18.2	43.6	18.4–40.3	25.8–28.2
P_{O_2} mm Hg	54	100.9	86	48	30.8	214.6	33.2–2 12.6	—
SO_2%	59	92.7	96.7	10	57.1	99.8	59.5–99.8	—
Ht %	59	45	45	6	30	60	33–58	44–47
Na^+ mmol/L	58	151	151.1	3.1	142.8	162.6	143.5–160.8	—
K^+ mmol/L	59	3.78	3.70	0.91	1.94	9.33	2.15–7.43	—
BE mmol/L	55	−3	−3.3	2	−6.8	1.4	−6.6 to 1.2	−3.5 to −2.4
SBE mmol/L	55	−0.5	−0.6	1.7	−3.8	3.2	−3.7 to 3.1	−1 to 0
HCO_3^- mmol/L	55	20.6	20.1	2	16	25.7	16.4–25.2	20–21.1
TCO_2 mmol/L	55	21.4	20.9	2.1	16.5	27.1	16.9–26.4	20.9–22
Hb Saker g/dl	28	15.7	15.9	1	13.8	17.6	13.8–17.6	15.3–16.1
Hb Pereg g/dl	16	16.9	16.8	1.4	14.8	19.9	14.8–19.9	16.2–17.7
Hb Hybr g/dl	15	16.1	15.7	1.9	11.9	19.8	11.9–19.8	15–17.1
Cl Saker mmol/L	28	118.3	117.8	3.7	104.6	125.9	104.6–125.9	116.9–119.8
Cl Pereg mmol/L	15	121	121.2	2.1	117.7	124.7	117.7–124.7	119.9–122.2
Cl Hybr mmol/L	15	121.3	121.5	5.7	112.7	130.1	112.7–130.1	118.1–124.4
iCa Saker mmol/L	25	1.28	1.3	0.11	0.83	1.4	0.83–1.4	1.24–1.33
iCa Pereg mmol/L	11	1.26	1.26	0.06	1.18	1.36	1.18–1.36	1.22–1.29
iCa Hybr mmol/L	7	1.16	1.20	0.14	0.85	1.28	0.85–1.28	—

Abbreviations: Hybr, gyrfalcon hybrids; Pereg, peregrine falcons; Saker, saker falcons.

found for Hb, Cl$^-$, and iCa. In this study, the high variations in the Po_2, with maximum values of 214.6 mm Hg suggests that some sample could be taken inadvertently from arterial blood instead of venous blood. Vessels, arteries, and veins run very closely over the elbow joint and it is not uncommon to get blood from the artery trying to sample the vein and vice versa.[18]

Harms and Harms[33] conducted a study measuring blood gas pressures, pH, and bicarbonate and lactate concentrations in three species of birds to assess the immediate impact of mist net capture and handling for banding and venipuncture (**Table 13**). They sampled (venous blood) mourning doves (*Zenaida macroura*), Boat-tailed grackles (*Quiscalus major*), and house sparrows (*Passer domesticus*). Mourning doves and house sparrows exhibited mild alkalemia, relative to Boat-tailed grackles. House sparrows exhibited relative respiratory acidosis. All the birds captured by mist net and handled for banding and venipuncture experienced some degree of lactic alkalemia. The metabolic, respiratory, and acid-base alterations observed in this study were minor in most cases, which indicate the general safety of these important field ornithology techniques. The study was developed using the i-STAT analyzer and the CG4$^+$ cartridges.

Paula and colleagues[34] published a study done on 35 Blue-Fronted Amazon parrots using arterial blood from the superficial ulnar artery and the EG7+ cartridge of the i-STAT system as analyzer. This research was done using nonanesthetized parrots form a rescue center. The animals have been maintained captive because they did not present good physical conditions to be released. Results are summarized in **Table 14**. Mean findings of this study slightly differs from the reference values showed by Zandvliet and colleagues,[26] but different methods are used in each study. Paula and colleagues[34] found very low levels of iCa in Amazon parrots and they conclude that these low levels could be attributable to excess of heparin or to the effect of the respiratory alkalemia found in those animals.

THE I-STAT ANALYZER

The i-STAT is a compact portable clinical analyzer system that comprises a hand-held device and disposable, self-contained cartridges.[35] The hand analyzer weighs 540 g and runs on two 9-volt batteries. More than 10 different cartridge configurations offer a choice of different biochemical panels. The cartridges contain a series of thin film

Table 13
Median (minimum-maximum) venous pH, blood gas partial pressures, and bicarbonate and lactate concentrations at analyzer temperature (37°C) for birds after capture by mist net and banding

Species	N	pH	Pco_2 (mm Hg)	Po_2 (mm Hg)	HCO$_3^-$ (mmol/L)	Lactate (mmol/L)
Mourning dove	24	7.453 (7.285–7.5589)	28.6 (21–45.9)	49 (22–63)	21.2 (14.4–30.1)	7.72 (3.94–14.14)
Boat-tailed grackle	17	7.513 (7.423–7.575)	29.2 (23.1–36.69)	47 (39–56)	23.7 (15.8–30.99)	5.74 (3.09–8.75)
House sparrow	18	7.454 (7.304–7.519)	37.6 (831.8–49.69)	40 (27–49)	25.8 (16.9–30.1)	4.77 (2.66–12.03)

Data from Harms CA, Harms RV. Venous blood gas and lactate values of mourning doves (*Zenaida macroura*), boat-tailed grackles (*Quiscalus major*), and house sparrows (*Passer domesticus*) after capture by mist net, banding, and venipuncture. J Zoo Wild Med 2012;43(1):77–84.

| Table 14 |||||||
| Values of acid-base status and electrolytes of nonanesthetized Amazon parrots (*Amazona aestiva*) using EG7 + cartridges of the i-STAT PCA |||||||
Parameter	Units	Mean	SD	Minimum	Maximum
iCa	mmol/L	0.8	0.28	0.34	1.4
K	mEq/L	3.5	0.53	2.8	4.9
Na	mEq/L	147.4	2.2	141	150
pH	log10 (1/H)	7.452	0.048	7.343	7.552
P_{CO_2}	mm Hg	22.1	4	14.6	29.8
P_{O_2}	mm Hg	98.1	7.6	85	113
Ht	%	38.7	6.2	24	50
Hb	g/dl	13.2	2.1	8.2	17
HCO_3	mmol/L	14.8	2.8	9.5	21
SO_2	%	96.2	1.1	94	98
BE	mmol/L	−7.9	3.1	−15	−1
Respiration rate	Breaths/min	82	33	32	150
Temperature	°C	41.8	0.6	40.2	43

Data from Paula VV, Fantoni DT, Otsuki DA, et al. Blood and electrolyte values for Amazon parrots (*Amazona aestiva*). Pesq.Vet Bras 2008;28(2):108–12.

electrodes, or biosensors, that connect with the blood sample and send signals to the hand-held analyzer. The i-STAT requires 0.06 to 0.2 mL of sample, and produces results within 2 minutes. Ideally, whole blood stored in lithium heparin should be used. Whole blood without added anticoagulant will also produce accurate results if used in a timely manner. Blood stored in a sodium heparin tube is not recommended because of anticoagulant effects on sodium analysis. The blood sample is contained within the cartridge and does not come into contact with the analyzer anytime.[35]

Measurements of Ht, iCa, glucose, and potassium have been shown to be divergent to the point of more or less clinical significance when i-STAT results are compared with a standard laboratory analyzer.[29] Also, Steinmetz and colleagues[36] evaluated the use of i-STAT in chickens, comparing the obtained results with a validated standard analyzer. They found some divergent results in the case of the calculated BE value.

The i-STAT measures Ht by conductivity. Ht measured using the i-STAT in canine, feline, and equine patients was consistently lower than values obtained by the micro-hematocrit (microHt) method or by an automated cell counter.[29] When Ht was measured using the i-STAT analyzer in Red-tailed hawks[27] and Caribbean flamingos,[28] the results were also lower than when using standard methods. However, no differences were found in chickens[36] and falcons.[30]

Glucose is measured by the i-STAT amperometrically via the product of the glucose oxidase reaction.[33] In equine, canine, and feline samples, the i-STAT was accurate at physiologic mammalian glucose range, 60 to 120 mg/dL. At low concentrations (<50 mg/dL), the i-STAT overestimated the glucose concentration. At high concentrations (>120 mg/dL), the i-STAT underestimated glucose concentrations.[29] Underestimation of glucose at high concentrations could be problematic in avian patients because their normal glucose range is higher (180–350 mg/dL) than in mammals.[22] This was not a problem in the two studies done on falcons.[27,30] Also, glucose concentrations were not validated in the comparison between i-STAT and the standard analyzer using domestic chickens.[36]

As previously mentioned, a deep study comparing i-STAT and a benchtop analyzer was done by Steinmetz and colleagues.[36] The investigators used a total of 75 EC7+ cartridges, measuring pH, P_{CO_2}, P_{O_2}, Na^+, K^+, iCa, and packed cell volume (PCV), as well as calculating HCO_3^-, TCO_2, SO_2, BE, and Hb. The reliability and performance of the i-STAT measuring or calculating all these parameters were judged to be very acceptable, confirming earlier studies in other species.[37,38] Only K^+ and BE were out of the limits of acceptability and with significant bias between the two analyzers. The failure of K+ might be explained by the differences in sample type (whole blood vs serum) and/or by the relatively high artifactual change in plasma potassium values as has been shown in various avian species were potassium levels decreased from 30% to 60% within a 2-hour period.[22,39] The bias of BE was high and the investigators, not finding an explanation, have called for further research.

POINT-OF-CARE BLOOD GASES AND ELECTROLYTES IN AFRICAN GREY PARROTS (*PSITTACUS ERITHACUS ERITHACUS*)

As previously discussed, reference values of blood gases in psittacines are scarce in the scientific literature. In the authors' laboratory, blood samples were collected from clinically normal African Grey Parrots (AGPs) to obtain reference values in healthy parrots.

Materials and Methods

System description
The i-STAT system is composed of two main parts: the point-of-care analyzer (PCA) and the disposable cartridges with microfabricated sensors. For clinical analysis, the blood specimen is introduced into the cartridge using a syringe; the cartridge is then inserted in the PCA, and operator and patient identification are entered into the system. A calibration is automatically performed just before the sample analysis. Results are displayed on the screen and stored in the analyzer's memory. In addition, results can be sent by infrared port to a printer.

Two types of cartridges were used, the EC8+ and the CG8+. The first one has been designed for metabolic blood gas studies and the second one is designed to assess the respiratory status of the patient, including different software to correct the temperature variations. The EC8+ does not include temperature correction.

Animals
Forty-six AGPs were sampled using the EC8+ cartridge and 47 were used for the CG8+ study. All the animals were in good health status and sampling was part of an ordinary yearly health check and the AGPs' clinical records in our practice showed no relevant disease. The parrots were between 1 to 12 years old, and no distinction was made between males or females.

Sampling
To avoid the effects of handling on the core body temperature and ventilation, the sampling method follow this protocol:

1. A heparinized syringe of 1 mL was prepared using lithium heparin, following an adaptation of the technique described by Hopper and colleagues.[4]
2. The i-STAT cartridge (EC8+ or CG8+) was removed from cold storage at least 5 minutes before intended use.
3. Each parrot was taken out from his cage or carrier box using a towel.

4. Cloacal temperature was measured using a thermometer probe during 10 seconds with the bird under manual restraint. This step was omitted if the EC8+ cartridge was used.
5. 0.5 mL of venous blood was taken from the right jugular vein.
6. The whole blood sample (0.1 mL) was tested without delay on the i-STAT PCA.

The remaining blood sample was used to determine other parameters such as PCV (microHt method), Hb (Hemocue method), or other biochemical parameters.

Statistical analysis

The data was tested by a D'Ágostino-Pearson test for normal distribution. Reference values were determined by the robust method. For smaller samples sizes (fewer than 120), the robust method with a calculation of a 95% of reference range with a 90% confidence interval of the reference limits is recommended and shows good performance. MedCalc version 12.30 (MedCalc Software, Borekstraat 32, 9330 Mariakerke, Belgium) was used for the statistical analysis.

Results

The results are summarized in **Tables 15** and **16**. Data related to Ht and Hb are removed from the tables to avoid misleading conclusion. Results for Ht and PCV by i-STAT analyzer in AGPs showed considerable disparity with the real values (determined by reference methods) and were considered not useful for clinician application.

Discussion

Ht and Hb

The i-STAT measures Ht via conductivity. Erythrocytes act as insulators and decrease conductivity; therefore, measured conductivity is inversely related to Ht. Also total serum protein can affect conductance and measurement of Ht. In humans, the i-STAT measurement of Ht can be affected when Ht is less than 40% and protein is over 8 g/dL or under 6 g/dL.[40] Avian samples have total serum protein commonly lower than 6 g/dL.[22] One potential reason behind the difference in i-STAT Ht values and those of microHt tubes or automated cell counters could be related to the anticoagulant used. Tripotassium ethylenediaminetetraacetic acid (K_3EDTA) causes human red blood cells to shrink owing to an osmotic pressure gradient, artificially reducing the Ht below its true in vivo value.[40] Because K_3EDTA is the anticoagulant of choice in human laboratories, automated cells counters are calibrated to match microHt determinations based on samples anticoagulated with K_3EDTA. The i-STAT is also calibrated to match the measurements of microHt tubes containing human whole blood with K_3EDTA, making it less reflective of the in vivo Ht. In this study, Ht and Hb were measured concurrently using standard methodology (microHt method for Ht determination and Hemocue method [Hemocue, HemoCue® AB, Kuvettgatan 1, SE-262 71, Ängelholm, Sweden] for Hb concentration). The regression analysis using the Passing-Bablok method showed that Ht measured by i-STAT did not match Ht measured by microHt method. Same discrepancies were obtained for Hb concentration. For further discussion see the article by Ardiaca and colleagues elsewhere in this issue.

iCa

Calcium plays an important physiologic role in avian species and disorders of calcium metabolism in AGPs are well known.[41] Reference intervals for iCa in AGPs has been determined in a range of 0.96 to 1.22 mmol/L. Values obtained in this study are very similar to those published by Stanford[41] and the use of the i-STAT system to assess iCa in AGPs could be a good tool for the practitioner in an aviary clinic scenario.

Table 15
Results from venous samples from healthy AGPs (n = 46) analyzed with EC8+ cartridges for i-STAT analyzer

Parameter	95% Reference Range	Reference Point	Total Range (Lowest and Highest Value Registered)	Arithmetic Mean[a]	SD	Method
pH	7.204–7.511	7.353	7.205–7.486	7.353	0.075	Parametric
Pco₂ (mm Hg)	18.7–43.9	31	18.2–43.9	31	6.1	Parametric
HCO₃⁻ (mmol/l)[b]	8.3–25.5	17.4	11.9–35	17.4	4.2	Parametric
TCO₂ (mmol/l)[b]	11–25	18	12–25	18	3.4	Parametric
BEecf (mmol/l)[b]	−17 to 0	—	(−15) to (+1)	NA	NA	Nonparametric percentile method
Na (mmol/l)	136–156	—	135–156	NA	NA	Nonparametric percentile method
K (mmol/l)	2.2–4.7	3.5	2.3–5.1	3.5	0.6	Parametric
Cl (mmol/l)	106–124	115	103–124	115	4.5	Parametric
AGap (mmol/l)	5.4–27.8	—	5–28	NA	NA	Nonparametric percentile method
Hct (%)	NA	—	NA	NA	NA	
Hgb (g/dl)	NA		NA	NA	NA	
SUN (mg/dl)	<3	<3	<3	<3	0	
Glu (mg/dl)	196–312	254	205–305	254	28	Parametric

Abbreviation: NA, not available.
[a] Arithmetic mean and standard deviation are displayed only for results following a normal distribution.
[b] Calculated results.

Table 16
Results from venous samples from healthy AGPs (n = 47) analyzed with CG8$^+$ cartridges for i-STAT analyzer

Parameter	95% Reference Range	Reference Point	Total Range (Lowest and Highest Value Registered)	Arithmetic Mean^a	SD	Method
pH$_{37°C}$	7.166–7.493	7.322	7.138–7.493	7.322	0.077	Parametric
Pco$_2$ (mm Hg)$_{37°C}$	16.4–41.7	29.3	19.9–40.6	29.3	6.1	Parametric
Po$_2$ (mm Hg)$_{37°C}$	30.1–46.2	37.9	28–48	37.9	3.8	Parametric
HCO$_3$$^-$ (mmol/l)^b	9.5–19.6	15	9.7–22.3	15	2.4	Parametric
TCO$_2$ (mmol/l)^b	9.9–21.2	16.01	10–24	16.01	2.7	Parametric
BEecf (mmol/l)^b	(−18.2) to (−5.7)	—	(−17) – (−3)	NA	NA	Nonparametric percentile method
Na (mmol/l)	141–159	—	134–157	NA	NA	Nonparametric percentile method
K (mmol/l)	2.5–4.7	3.6	2.9–4.6	3.6	0.5	Parametric
iCa (mmol/l)	0.94–1.33	1.14	0.94–1.39	1.14	0.1	Parametric
SO$_2$ (%)	47.9–88.8	68.4	44–97	68.4	10.10	Parametric
Hct (%)	NA	—	NA	NA	NA	—
Hgb (g/dl)	NA	—	NA	NA	NA	—
SUN (mg/dl)	<3	—	<3	<3	0	—
Glucose (mg/dl)	197–292	246.9	196–302	246.9	24.5	Parametric
Temperature (°C)	41–42.7	41.6	41 to −42.7	41.6	0.4	Parametric
pH$_{Temperature}$^{c}	7.097–7.426	7.256	7.081–7.414	7.256	0.077	Parametric
Pco$_2$ (mm Hg)$_{Temp}$^{c}	20.1–50.6	35.7	23.8–49.7	35.7	7.5	Parametric
pO$_2$ (mm Hg)$_{Temp}$^{c}	41.3–65	52.5	39–67	52.5	5.6	Parametric

Abbreviation: NA, not available.
^{a} Arithmetic mean and SD are displayed only for results following a normal distribution.
^{b} Calculated results.
^{c} Calculated pH, Pco$_2$, and Po$_2$ after application of the correction formula within the i-STAT software.

Immediate analysis of iCa with a PCA has the potential to eliminate variables associated with sample storage and gives the clinician enough time and security margin for therapeutic help.

pH

Surprisingly, the mean pH values determined in this study for AGPs were lower than in other birds,[21,23,27,30,32,33] yet close to the values obtained for budgerigars,[22] flamingos,[28] and Amazon parrots.[26,34] Temperature-corrected values of ph are still lower. These correction formulas have been validated for use in pigeons using a tonometer and considering a core body temperature of 42.1°C.[23] Correction formulas follow an exponential curve and, at higher temperatures, there is less correlation between pH values. The range of temperature for AGPs was determined between 41 and 42.7°C. The authors assume that correction formulas are also useful in AGPs. In AGPs, values of Pco_2 and HCO_3- are lower than in dogs and cats, and the AGap is lightly higher than in these mammalian species. In psittacine birds, the osmolar gap has the same theoretical use as in mammals to diagnosing several toxicoses, but the occurrence of these types of toxicoses in pet birds (eg, ethylene glycol, methanol, and paraldehyde) is rare and largely unreported, except in *Anseriformes* and *Galliformes*.[42] Considering the higher values of Na+ and Cl-, and the lower values of HCO_3- and albumin, in parrots any other unmeasured anion, possibly the uric acid, must contribute to the high value of the AGap found in this study.

BE, being a calculated value, is also lower in AGPs compared with dogs and cats (±4 mEq/L) and also compared with raptors values (range from −6 to 1 mEq/L).[27,30,32] Again, AGPs' BE results are closer to Caribbean flamingo and Amazon parrot BE results. BE is also often used in calculating the amount of buffer (usually in the form of sodium bicarbonate) to administer to a patient with severe acidosis. Two formulas based on BE concentration have been developed to assess bicarbonate fluid therapy.[2,12] There are no studies supporting the possible application of this formula in avian medicine.

Metabolites

Blood urea nitrogen (BUN) was under the limits of detection of the i-STAT system in all the samples. SUN has a limited diagnostic value in avian medicine but can be used to assess dehydration.[22] Values greater than 3 mg/dL are expected in healthy, well-hydrated AGPs. The authors use blood gas routinely as part of the emergency analysis panel in sick parrots and, curiously, we have never found values greater than 3 mg/dL in AGPs, including very dehydrated birds. On the other hand, some values greater than 7 to 10 mg/dL have been obtained in macaws and Amazon parrots, especially in severely dehydrated chicks.

Glucose

A glucose value parameter was not included in the validation study of the i-STAT system compared with a standard analyzer and, as previously discussed, no big differences were found when i-STAT was used to measured glucose in two species of raptors. In the authors' study, glucose levels measured by the i-STAT were slightly, but consistently, lower than those measured by benchtop analyzer were. Reference values of glucose in AGPs range from 256 to 360 mg/dL.[43] However, other references could include the range showed by the i-STAT system.[22]

Electrolytes

Electrolyte status, specifically Na+, K+ and iCa, play an important role in water homeostasis and cardiac pathophysiology.[41,44] Also, knowledge of the AGap deviation helps the practitioner choose the more adequate fluid therapy.[2] Whereas calcium disorders in captive AGPs are well known, only limited reports of sodium and potassium exists.[44–46] Most reports refer to aquatic birds or show electrolytes abnormalities in experimental conditions. In the experience of the authors, expected electrolytes abnormalities occur in captive birds in the same way they occur in mammals. That is, parrots with urinary obstruction due to egg binding or cloacal stones develop hyperkalemia, or parrots with crop stasis develop hyponatremia with concurrent hypochloremia.

Oxygenation

In the second part of this study, the CG8[+] cartridge was chosen because the potential application to assess oxygenation. The ability to obtain reliable measurements with currently available methods, such as pulse oximetry and capnometry, for the assessment of oxygenation and ventilation can be limited by abnormal physiologic states commonly seen in emergency patients. In emergency situations (eg, shock or bleeding), an abnormal ventilation-perfusion relationship affects end-tidal CO_2 measurements and the absence of an adequate pulse signal can result in the failure of pulse oximetry to measure arterial Hb saturation. Therefore, gas analysis would be desirable for assessing oxygenation and ventilation in avian critical care. The main problem in avian medicine is that it is not known whether the formulas used in human and dog medicine have application in the field. Determination of the A-a gradient or the use of Pao_2 or Fio_2 could have different significances in avian patients. Further research is needed to determine the possible application and reference values for these parameters.

SUMMARY

From a practical point of view, the i-STAT PCA is easy to use and can be used as a blood analyzer in critical avian patients, although single values (Ht, Hb, K, glucose, and BE) must be interpreted carefully. The study of the acid-base status in companion birds is still in its infancy. Further research is needed to establish normal reference values in arterial blood gases, compare them with venous blood gas, and to determine if the formulas that deviate from small animal medicine are or are not applicable.

REFERENCES

1. Irizarry R, Reiss A. Arterial and venous blood gases: indications, interpretations, and clinical applications. Compendium Continuing Education for Veterinarians 2009;31:E1–8.
2. Bateman SH. Making sense of blood gas results. Vet Clin North Am Small Anim Pract 2008;38(3):542–57.
3. Goldstein DL, Skadhauge E. Renal and extrarenal regulation of body fluid composition. In: Caussey Whittow G, editor. Sturkie's avian physiology. 5th edition. San Diego (CA): Academic press, Inc; 2000. p. 265–97.
4. Hopper K, Rezende M, Haskins S. Assessment of the effect of dilution of blood samples with sodium heparin on blood gas, electrolyte, and lactate measurements in dogs. Am J Vet Res 2005;66(4):656–60.
5. Bailey JE, Pablo LS. Practical approach to acid-base disorders. Vet Clin North Am Small Anim Pract 1998;28(3):645–62.
6. Haskins SC. An overview of acid-base physiology. J Am Vet Med Assoc 1977; 170(4):423–8.
7. Roberson SA. Simple acid-base disorders. Vet Clin North Am Small Anim Pract 1969;19(2):289–306.

8. Johnson RA. Respiratory acidosis: a quick reference. Vet Clin North Am Small Anim Pract 2008;38(3):431–4.

9. Johnson RA. Respiratory alkalosis: a quick reference. Vet Clin North Am Small Anim Pract 2008;38(3):427–30.

10. De Morais HA. Metabolic acidosis: a quick reference. Vet Clin North Am Small Anim Pract 2008;38(3):439–42.

11. Foy D, de Morais HA. Metabolic alkalosis: a quick reference. Vet Clin North Am Small Anim Pract 2008;38(3):435–8.

12. Autran de Morais HS, Dibartola SP. Ventilatory and metabolic compensation in dogs with acid-base disturbances. J Vet Emerg Crit Care 1991;1(2):39–49.

13. Day TK. Blood gas analysis. Vet Clin North Am Small Anim Pract 2002;32(5): 1031–48.

14. Camps-Palau MA, Marks SL, Cornick JL. Small animal oxygen therapy. Compend Contin Educ Pract Vet 1999;21(7):587–98.

15. Irizarry R, Reiss A. Beyond blood gases. Making use of additional oxygenation parameters and plasma electrolytes in the emergency room. Compend Contin Educ Vet 2009;31:E1–5.

16. Wingfield WE, Van Pelt DR, Hackett TB. Usefulness of venous blood gases in estimating acid-base status of the seriously ill dog. J Vet Emerg Crit Care 1994;4:23–7.

17. Richardi JC, Nightingale TE. Comparison of brachial venous and mixed blood gas tensions and pH values in the chicken. Poult Sci 1982;60:1558–60.

18. Endling TM, Degernes LA, Flammer K, et al. Capnographic monitoring of anesthetized African grey parrots receiving intermittent positive pressure ventilation. J Am Vet Med Assoc 2001;219:1714–8.

19. Brackenbury JH. Blood gases and respiratory pattern in exercising fowl: comparison in normoxic and hypoxic conditions. J Exp Biol 1986;126:423–41.

20. Shams H, Scheid P. Effects of hypobaria and parabronchial gas exchange in normoxic and hypoxic ducks. Respir Physiol 1993;91:155–63.

21. Powell FL. Respiration. In: Caussey Whittow G, editor. Sturkie's avian physiology. 5th edition. San Diego (CA): Academic press, Inc; 2000. p. 233–64.

22. Hochleithner M. Biochemistries. In: Ritchie BW, Harrison GH, Harrison LH, editors. Avian medicine: principles and application. Lake Worth (FL): Wingers Publishing, Inc; 1994. p. 223–7.

23. Schoemaker NJ, Kitslaar WJ. Venous blood gases in healthy racing pigeons. Proceedings of Association of Avian Veterinarians. 2007. p. 261–3.

24. Kawashiro T, Scheid P. Arterial blood gases in undisturbed resting birds: measurements in the chicken and duck. Respir Physiol 1975;23:237–342.

25. Scheid P, Kawashiro T. Metabolic changes in avian blood and their effects on determination of blood gases and pH. Respir Physiol 1975;23:291–300.

26. Zandvliet MM, Dorrestein GM, van der Hage M. Chronic pulmonary interstitial fibrosis in Amazon parrots. Avian Pathol 2001;30:517–24.

27. Heatley JJ, Demirjian SE, Wright JC, et al. Electrolytes of the critically ill raptor. Proceedings of Association of Avian Veterinarians. 2005. p. 23–4.

28. Howard LL, Wack RF. Preliminary use and literature review of the i-STAT (a portable clinical analyzer) in birds. Proceedings of the American Association of Zoo Veterinarians. 2002. p. 96–100.

29. Grosenbauch DJ, Gadawski J, Muir W. Evaluation of a portable analyzer in a veterinary hospital setting. J Am Vet Med Assoc 1998;213:691–4.

30. McKinney P. Clinical applications of the i-STAT blood analyzer in avian practice. Proceedings of the European Association of Avian Veterinarians. 2003. p. 341–6.

31. Redig PT. Fluid therapy and acid-base balance in the critically ill avian patient. In: Redid PT, editor. Medical management of birds of prey. A collection of notes on selected topics. St Paul, Minnesota: Minnesota Univ Press; 1993. p. 39–54.
32. Arca-Ruibal B, Aguilar-Sanchez V, Silvanose C, et al. Blood gas values in venous blood of captive hunting falcons in the United Arab Emirates. Proceedings of the European Association of Avian Veterinarians. 2007. p. 459–61.
33. Harms CA, Harms RV. Venous blood gas and lactate values of mourning doves (*Zenaida macroura*), boat-tailed grackles (*Quiscalus major*), and house sparrows (*Passer domesticus*) after capture by mist net, banding, and venipuncture. J Zoo Wildl Med 2012;43(1):77–84.
34. Paula VV, Fantoni DT, Otsuki DA, et al. Blood and electrolyte values for Amazon parrots (*Amazona aestiva*). Pesq Vet Bras 2008;28(2):108–12.
35. Erikson K, Wilding P. Evaluation of a novel point-of-care system, the i-STAT portable clinical analyzer. Clin Chem 1993;39:283–7.
36. Steinmetz HW, Vogt R, Kästner S, et al. Evaluation of the i-STAT portable clinical analyzer in chickens (*Gallus gallus*). J Vet Diagn Invest 2007;19:382–8.
37. Silverman SC, Birks EK. Evaluation of the i-STAT hand-held chemical analyzer during treadmill and endurance exercise. Equine Vet J Suppl 2002;34:551–4.
38. Verwaerde P, Malet C, Lagente M, et al. The accuracy of the i-STAT portable analyzer for measuring blood gases and pH in whole-blood samples from dogs. Res Vet Sci 2002;73:71–5.
39. Harr KE, Raskin RE, Heard DJ. Temporal effects of 3 commonly used anticoagulants on hematological and biochemical variables in blood samples from macaws and Burmese pythons. Vet Clin Pathol 2005;34:383–8.
40. The i-STAT technical bulletin 2012. Hematocrit determination in the i-STAT system and comparison to other methods. 2012:433–8.
41. Stanford M. Calcium metabolism. In: Harrison GH, Lightfoot TL, editors. Clinical avian medicine. Palm Beach (FL): Spix Publishing; 2006. p. 141–51.
42. Beaufrere H, Acierno M, Mitchell M, et al. Plasma osmolality reference values in African grey parrots (*Psittacus erithacus erithacus*), Hispanolian Amazon parrots (*Amazona ventralis*) and Red-fronted macaws (*Ara rubrogenys*). J Avian Med Surg 2011;25(2):95–6.
43. Fudge AM. Laboratory references ranges for selected avian species. In: Fudge AM, editor. Laboratory medicine: avian and exotic pets. Philadelphia: WB Saunders Company; 2001. p. 376–88.
44. Genao A, Seth K, Schmidt U, et al. Dilated cardiomyopathy in turkeys: an animal model for the study of human heart failure. Lab Anim Sci 1996;46:399–404.
45. Tuttle AD, Andreadis TG, Frasca S Jr, et al. Easter equine encephalitis in a flock of African penguins maintained at an aquarium. J Am Vet Med Assoc 2005;226(12):2059–62.
46. Chitty J. Hyponatremia in a flock of Humboldt penguins. Proceedings of the European Association of Avian Veterinarians. 2007. p. 72–7.

Overview of Psittacine Blood Analysis and Comparative Retrospective Study of Clinical Diagnosis, Hematology and Blood Chemistry in Selected Psittacine Species

Raffaella Capitelli, Dr Med Vet[a],*, Lorenzo Crosta, Dr Med Vet, PhD[b]

KEYWORDS

- Psittacines • Hematology • Biochemistry • Psittacines diseases
- Abnormal and normal blood values

KEY POINTS

- Avian blood cells are fragile and samples should be processed as soon as possible after collection.
- It is important how the samples are taken, transported, and processed; therefore it is essential that suitable structures are available before taking samples.
- Mistakes when collecting, processing, and shipping the sample can cause many artifacts and can make a normal panel abnormal, or mask out the abnormalities caused by various pathologies.
- Avian hematology and clinical chemistry are important in the diagnosis of many diseases in psittacine species, but a proper interpretation of the results of a sample from a particular species can only be achieved if its reference values are available and were obtained using the same methods.

PART I
Introduction

Avian patients are not showing clear symptoms, therefore hematology and biochemistry are important aids in the diagnostic process of birds, including the species belonging to the order Psittaciformes. Our need to widen diagnostic investigations is made more difficult by the many differences among the various psittacine species and the physiologic differences with the mammals.

[a] CSV-Labvet, via Kennedy 10, 23873 Missaglia, Lecco, Italy; [b] Clinica Veterinaria Valcurone, via Kennedy 10, 23873 Missaglia, Lecco, Italy
* Corresponding author.
E-mail address: capitelli@libero.it

Vet Clin Exot Anim 16 (2013) 71–120
http://dx.doi.org/10.1016/j.cvex.2012.10.002
1094-9194/13/$ – see front matter © 2013 Elsevier Inc. All rights reserved.
vetexotic.theclinics.com

Avian laboratory medicine is relatively new to veterinary medicine. Before 1980, avian hematology was primarily used as a research tool in the poultry industry.[1] The first description of avian hematology was by Lucas and Jamroz in 1961.[2] Their atlas is the basis of avian hematology and it describes the various hemic cells in poultry.[2] In 1980, the Association of Avian Veterinarians reported a gradual increase in the numbers of pet birds (primarily psittacines) being presented to their clinical practices.[1]

Blood Analysis

Avian blood cells are fragile and samples should be processed as soon as possible after collection. It is important how the samples are taken, transported, and pro-cessed, therefore it is essential that suitable structures are available before taking samples.[3] Mistakes when collecting, processing, and shipping the sample can cause many artifacts and can make a normal panel abnormal or mask out abnormalities caused by various pathologies.[4–6]

It is important to know whether the referring laboratory, either an in-house or external laboratory

- is equipped to process avian blood samples, using specific and validated tech-niques for the different avian species, working with smaller blood collection size;
- has knowledge of the normal reference values for many species, including pet birds, and provides a chemistry panel suitable for each avian species/group;
- is prepared to give information about the correct methods for blood collection, sampling, and shipping and good professional advice for the interpretation of the results.[6]

Blood Sampling

Animals differ in sex, age, environment, and possible stress factors, and sampling conditions are also different making it difficult to interpret the data.[4] Blood sampling should be done with minimal stress. The practitioner should have the skill to obtain a blood sample without anesthesia.[4,5] A blood volume representing 1% or less of the body weight can usually be withdrawn from healthy birds without risk. The sample size taken from severely ill birds, however, must be reduced. For routine hematologic evaluations in birds, a sample size of 0.2 mL is usually adequate. A variety of collection methods has been used to obtain blood from birds, and the choice of method depends on the size of the bird, peculiarities of the species, preference of the collector, volume of blood needed, and the physical condition of the patient.[1,3–5,7] Some examples are show in **Table 1**.

Routinely it would be safe to collect a blood volume that ranges between 0.5% and 0.7% of the patient's body weight. The method of restraint to a safely collection of

Table 1		
Maximum blood sample volume for selected Psittaciformes		
Species	Body Weight (g)	Maximum Volume of Blood Sample (1% Body Weight) (mL)
Amazon	250–600	4.5–2.5
Cockatoo	250–800	5.0
Cockatiel	40–80	0.4
African gray parrot	450	4
Macaw	200–1800	2.5–5

blood sample is dependent on the size of the bird, its capacity to inflict an injury, its familiarity with humans, and the skills of the practitioner. Most birds require physical restraint and it can be useful to use a towel or cloth to wrap them in order to prevent self-inflicted injuries such as wing fractures. The three available sites for blood collection from psittacines birds, in order of preference, are the right jugular vein, the cutaneous ulnar (brachial) or wing vein, and the medial metatarsal vein. For tame birds, it is possible to collect a blood sample from the jugular vein with a minimal amount of restraint.

The right jugular vein is the most commonly used for blood collection in psittacine birds. The right jugular vein is large and easy to locate and access in the featherless area of the neck (apterium), providing a quick and easy method for collection of adequate amounts of blood with minimum restraint even in small psittacines. The disadvantage is that the jugular vein is mobile and must be well stabilized.[7–10]

An alternative site for blood collection in medium-large psittacine birds is the cutaneous ulnar (brachial) vein. Most parrots and cockatoos have short tarsometatarsi, which makes access to the medial metatarsal vein difficult (**Table 2**).[7]

Because psittacine birds are small to medium in size and the total blood collected cannot exceed a milliliter, not even a drop of the blood collected can be wasted. To optimize the results, and using Psittaciformes as an example, the blood collected should be used as follows:

- 2 drops of whole blood to make 2 blood smears at the time of collection using nonanticoagulated blood and possibly using precleaned, bevel-edged microscope slides
- 2 drops of whole blood to soak absorbent paper diskettes for Chlamydia Immunocomb
- 2 to 3 drops of whole blood into a tube with a preserving solution suitable for polymerase chain reaction analysis (PCR) (depending on the laboratory techniques available)
- 2 to 3 drops of whole blood to fill a microhematocrit capillary tube for measuring packed cell volume (PCV) and total plasma protein
- The surplus into a lithium heparin container or other tests as needed

The best device to collect blood from a bird is a syringe with a 22- to 25-gauge hypodermic needle. Thinner needles may cause hemolysis and it is advisable to avoid a heparinized syringe.[1,3–5,7,8,10,15] In smaller psittacine species, insulin syringes are frequently used, better with detachable needles. Ejecting blood through a 25-gauge or smaller needle may cause moderate to marked hemolysis, and this can invalidate most biochemical analyses.[16,17]

Samples are collected in microhematocrit capillary tubes, EDTA tubes, lithium heparin tubes, and serum separator tubes. EDTA tubes are not used for hematology

Table 2		
Reported sites for the collection of blood from selected species of psittacines		
African gray parrot	Brachial	Hawkey et al,[11] 1982
Amazon parrot	Cutaneous ulnar, jugular	Tell & Citino,[12] 1992
Budgerigar	Right jugular	Scope et al,[13] 2005
Red lory	Right jugular	Scope et al,[14] 2000

The terminology to describe the vein is as used in the original publication.
Data from Clark P, Boardman W, Raidal SR. Atlas of clinical avian hematology. Oxford (United Kingdom): Wiley-Blackwell; 2009.

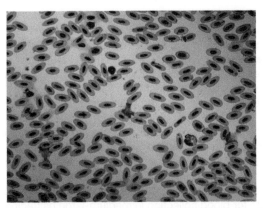

Fig. 1. Normal avian erythrocytes and some nondifferentiable leukocytes due to adverse effects on the morphology and staining by lithium heparin in a blood film of a healthy *Psittacus erithacus* (Hemacolor, 400×).

because they can cause adverse effects in some avian species, although many authors advise them for hematology in psittacines because they allow for proper staining of cells and leukocytes tend not to clump.[1,4,5,8,15,18,19] Heparin is useful for chemistry and is widely used in avian hematology.[4,5,9,20] Many authors state that heparin has adverse effects on the morphology and staining of avian hemic cells (**Fig. 1**) and that, after 12 hours, it can cause leukocytes and thrombocytes to clump so interfering with manual and automated cell counts.[1,8,15,18] Blood samples collected without anticoagulant require immediate processing because whole blood ships poorly and cellular degeneration takes places quickly.[1] Unseparated, clotted, or hemolyzed samples frequently cause unreliable values. Lumeij[21] noted that serum potassium levels decrease in samples that are left unseparated for more than 2 hours. Fudge says that samples shipped unseparated for 12 hours or longer results in increased values of lactate dehydrogenase (LDH), potassium, and total proteins, decreased values of glucose, and variable changes to calcium and phosphorus levels.[4] Lumeij[22] suggests that lithium heparin is the best method for biochemistry although in pigeons, serum bile acid levels are higher. Lipemia is a normal finding in ovulating birds and can severely alter most photometric analyses. Lipemia is also present in certain pathologies, such as some liver diseases. Fasting is not usually necessary before blood sampling in a bird. In excitable or roughly handled pet birds, or for intramuscular injections, creatine phosphokinase (CPK) levels can increase.

Unfortunately, bacterial contamination of avian samples received by laboratories can easily occur, causing cloudiness in serum or plasma, which can affect photometric assays of various analytes such as marked decrease in CPK and glucose levels.[4,5]

A blood film should be made immediately after collection. An air-dried thin smear provides superior morphology compared with samples stored in EDTA or heparin. The use of precleaned, bevel-edged microscope slides minimizes cell damage. The wedge smear or slide and long coverglass techniques normally used by general practitioners can produce damaged cells (smudged cells). The presence of numerous smudged cells, which are probably granulocytes, causes inaccurate hematologic results.[4,5] Blood films can be prepared by using a slide and coverslip or by using 2 coverslips.[4,15,23] Conventional Romanosvsky stain (Wright and Giemsa stains) usually gives good results for avian blood smears. Quick stains can also produce good quality blood films.[1,9,20]

Hematology

The blood of avian psittacines contains nucleated erythrocytes, nucleated thrombocytes, heterophils, eosinophils, basophils, lymphocytes, and monocytes. The main difference between avian blood and mammalian blood is that the avian blood contains nucleated erythrocytes and nucleated thrombocytes, which can interfere with automated blood counting procedures.[9] Moreover, avian white blood cell morphology differs from that of mammals because the predominant avian granulocyte is the heterophil versus the neutrophil in mammalian species. The other leukocytes are morphologically similar to their mammalian counterparts. There also are some physiologic factors that can influence the hematologic results such as age, gender, anesthesia, nutrition, environmental conditions, physiologic status, and genetic factors (species).

Measurement techniques for avian hematology

The laboratory evaluation of psittacine blood involves the same routine procedures used for mammalian hematology with some modifications.[1]

PCV or hematocrit PCV or hematocrit expresses the proportion of the volume of the corpuscular part in whole blood.[7] The standard method for determination of the hematocrit (PCV) uses a microhematocrit tube that is centrifuged at 12,000×g for 5 minute or at 3000×g for 30 minutes.[1] Normal values for PCV range from 35% to 55% in most psittacine species. A decreased PCV suggests anemia, whereas an increased PCV indicates dehydration if total proteins are increased or erythrocytosis if total proteins are normal or low.

Hemoglobin Hemoglobin concentration is determined using spectrophotometric analysis of cyanmethemoglobin at 540 nm, after centrifugation to remove the free nuclei from lysed erythrocytes to avoid overestimation. Recent reports have used a colorimetric method assessed at both 570 and 880 nm to compensate for turbidity of the sample.[7,24,25]

The normal hemoglobin concentration is 11 to 18 g/dL in most psittacine species. The hemoglobin of mature birds contains myoinositol pentophosphate and not 2,3-diphosglycerate, as in mammals. In avian erythrocytes, the phosphate compounds differ from those of mammals and therefore avian tissues can extract oxygen more readily from hemoglobin than mammalian tissues.[1]

Hemic cell counts

A major limiting factor in avian hematology is the lack of a validated automated method for the measuring hemic cell counts, and in particular for analyzing leukocytes. Thus, manual counting methods have been well described and are the most common techniques used in all birds. These methods are often time consuming, not accurate, and suitable only for laboratories that handle many avian samples. Impedentiometric electronic cell counters are the gold standard in mammalian hematology but they cannot be used in birds.[20] Since 1990, studies performed in avian hematology (particularly on ostriches and chickens), using laser and impedance technologies (Cell-Dyn 3500), have given encouraging and reproducible results for erythrocyte and leukocyte counts.[26–30] The Cell-Dyn 3500 hematology system (Abbot laboratories, Abbot Park, IL, USA) has veterinary software with a special application for avian species.

The most common techniques used in birds for erythrocyte and leukocyte counts are manual by hemacytometer. The total red blood count (TRBC) is done using Natt-Herrick solution or the erythrocyte Unopette system. For total white blood cell counts (TWBC), direct methods with Natt-Herrick solution and indirect methods with the eosinophil Unopette system are used. In the direct method, blood is diluted with Natt-Herrick solution. The advantage of this method is that using the same charged hemocytometer, total erythrocyte and thrombocyte counts can also be obtained.[20] The disadvantage is that differentiating thrombocytes from small lymphocytes is often difficult, thus count errors are common. However, staining the blood for 60 minutes in Natt-Herrick solution improves the ability to differentiate between different cells.[31]

The Unopette eosinophil system uses a 1% phloxine B solution, a standard Neubauer hemocytometer, and a rectangular coverglass. It is based on the principle that phloxine B stains the eosinophils and heterophils red. With this system, only granulocytes (eosinophils and eosin-stained heterophils), which appear as round, refractile, and red-orange cells, can be counted in both chambers of the hemocytometer. A differential cell count on a stained blood film is performed by obtaining the percentage of eosinophils and heterophils. The TWBC count is calculated using the following formula[1,8,30]:

TWBC (cells/μL)

$$= \frac{\text{total eosin} - \text{stained cells counted in 18 squares} \times 1760 \ (\text{or } 1.1 \times 16 \times 100)}{\% \text{ heterophils} + \% \text{ eosinophils (from differential count)}}$$

Alternatively, when it is not possible to obtain a sufficient volume of blood to perform a quantitative count of TWBC or when the count cannot be performed within a few hours, some investigators have suggested estimating the WBC count from a blood smear. This technique does not require special equipment and is available to most practitioners. The estimated WBC count can be obtained from a stained blood smear, and requires only a drop of blood. This method is based on the ratio of RBCs to WBCs, and the total estimated WBC count is determined by counting all leukocytes in 10 microscope fields (40$\times$) of a monolayer blood smear and multiplying the mean number by 2000.[4,5,9,20] A comparison of the leukocyte concentrations, obtained by a quantitative hemacytometer method, have found significant differences between these 2 methods, with greater values recorded for the hemacytometer counts.[32] On the other hand both the direct and indirect method can be inaccurate due to many reasons: manual dilution, the use of a hemacytometer, the difficulty in identifying the hemic cells (leukocytes vs erythrocytes and thrombocytes), and the possibility of an incorrect differential count, which can change the final result of the Unopette eosinophil count.[9]

A reliable thrombocyte count is difficult to determine because they tend to clump. For this reason, their concentration is often indicated as normal, increased, or decreased depending on estimates from peripheral blood films. In a blood film of a healthy psittacine, it is normal to see 1 to 5 thrombocytes in a monolayer $\times$1000 (oil immersion) field unless thrombocytes clump excessively.[1,10]

Erythrocyte morphology

Evaluation of avian erythrocyte morphology is based on observation of the cells in monolayer $\times$1000 fields.[1,33] Avian erythrocytes should be evaluated for their size, shape, color, nucleus, and cellular inclusions.[1,34,35] Mature psittacine erythrocytes are elliptical with an elliptical, centrally positioned nucleus, and vary in size depending on the species.

The hemoglobin within the cytoplasm stains a light orange-pink color. During maturation, the erythrocyte assumes its characteristic oval shape and hemoglobinization occurs. Nuclear chromatin is evenly clumped and becomes increasingly condensed

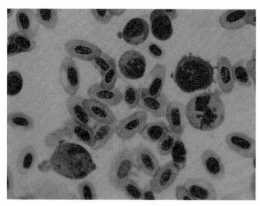

Fig. 2. Presence of increased polychromasia, anisocytosis, immature erythrocytes at different stages of erythrocyte maturation and 1 mitotic figure in the blood smear from an anemic *Ara ararauna* with 12% of PCV as part of a regenerative response (Hemacolor, 1000×).

with cellular aging; small numbers of polychromatophils (less than 5%) may be present. They are characterized by a slightly larger and more rounded appearance. The nucleus is less condensed and the cytoplasm is bluish.[1,8–10]

Avian erythrocytes have a short lifespan compared with mammalian erythrocytes. Erythropoiesis is controlled by circulating levels of erythropoietin, which is produced in the kidney in response to blood oxygen and cortical, estrogen, and androgen hormone levels.[9]

The degree of erythrocyte polychromasia and reticulocytosis, the presence of binucleate immature erythrocytes, and an increase of immature erythrocytes in the peripheral blood are evidence of active erythropoiesis (**Figs. 2** and **3**). However, these cells indicate abnormal erythropoiesis in nonanemic birds and may suggest the stimulation of the hematopoietic tissue following an anoxic insult or toxicity.[1] The presence of a large number of hypochromatic erythrocytes indicates an erythrocyte disorder, such as iron deficiency or iron sequestration caused by infectious diseases.

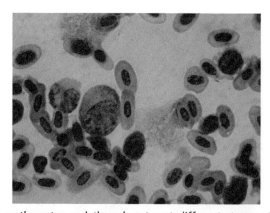

Fig. 3. Immature erythrocytes and thrombocytes at different stages of erythrocyte and thrombocyte maturation, in the blood smear from the same birds as in **Fig. 2**. The cytoplasm of immature erythrocytes (large cells) contains spots of pink material due to the development of hemoglobin (Hemacolor, 1000×).

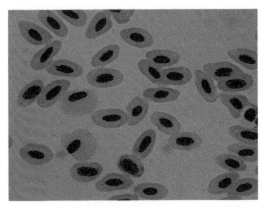

Fig. 4. The blood film reveals abnormal erythrocyte shape with increased membrane fragility (ballooning). The presence of atypical erythrocytes should not be confused with artifacts of slide preparation (Hemacolor, 1000×).

A slight anisocytosis is considered normal for psittacine birds, but marked anisocytosis is usually observed in birds with regenerative anemia associated with polychromasia. Similarly, a slight poikilocytosis (variation of the shape) (**Fig. 4**) is normal in the peripheral blood of birds, whereas marked poikilocytosis may indicate erythrocytic dysgenesis.

Anuclear erythrocytes (erythroplastids) or cytoplasmic fragments are occasionally observed in the peripheral blood of healthy birds. Mitotic activity associated with erythrocytes in blood films suggests a marked regenerative response (**Fig. 5**) or erythrocytic dyscrasia.[10] Binucleate erythrocytes rarely occur in blood smears of normal birds; however, the presence of large numbers of binucleated erythrocytes plus other features of RBC dyscrasia is suggestive of neoplastic, viral, or genetic diseases.[10,36]

RBC indexes
The RBC indexes are calculated from the PCV, hemoglobin level, and TRBC count. Using the measured values, additional characteristics of erythrocytes can be

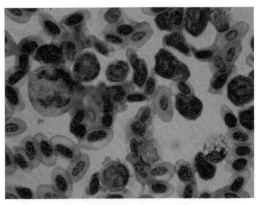

Fig. 5. Immature erythrocytes and thrombocytes at different stages of erythrocyte and thrombocyte maturation in the blood smear from the same birds as in **Fig. 2**. On the right side of the image, an activated thrombocyte may be observed (Hemacolor, 1000×).

Table 3
Morphologic classification of anemia based on the RBC indexes

	Normal MCH and MCHC	Less Than MCH and MCHC
Normal MCV	Normocytic normochromic	Normocytic hypochromic
>MCV	Macrocytic normochromic	Macrocytic hypochromic
<MCV	Microcytic hypochromic	Microcytic hypochromic

calculated. The mean corpuscular volume (MCV) and mean corpuscular hemoglobin (MCH) values in birds are larger than in mammals, due to a wider red cell size in birds, whereas the MCH concentration (MCHC) is smaller than in mammals due to the presence of an erythrocyte nucleus. The evaluation of the RBC indexes gives additional information on erythrocytes that may help in the morphologic classification of anemia (as summarized in **Table 3**).

Response and abnormalities of the erythrogram

Absolute anemia (decreased PCV and TRBC) in psittacine birds can be caused by blood loss (hemorrhagic anemia), increased destruction of erythrocytes (hemolytic anemia), and decreased or no cell production (depression/aplastic anemia).[9] The most common causes of hemorrhagic anemia are trauma and hemorrhagic lesions of internal organs, such as ulcerated neoplasms and gastric ulcerations. Less common causes of blood loss anemia in psittacines include heavy infestation with blood-sucking ectoparasites or gastrointestinal endoparasites, coagulopathies associated with toxins, septicemic and viral infections, neoplasms, coagulation factor deficiencies, or severe liver diseases. With increasing chronicity, hemorrhagic anemia can be normocytic normochromic, macrocytic hypochromic, and microcytic hypochromic. Hemolytic anemia can result from parasitemia, bacterial septicemia, heavy metal toxicosis, acute aflatoxicosis, and extensive burns. Although rare, immune-mediated anemia may result in hemolysis with red cell agglutination present in the blood film. Hemolytic anemia is mostly regenerative characterized by marked polychromasia, macrocytosis, anisocytosis, reticulocytosis, and hypochromasia.[1,8–10,19,36–39] Depression anemia indicates decreased erythropoiesis and is therefore nonregenerative, and can commonly develop in birds with chronic inflammatory diseases, mainly those caused by infectious agents (**Fig. 6**). Psittacines can develop anemia due to decreased erythropoiesis much faster than mammals do, possibly because of the relatively short half-life of avian erythrocytes.[10,24,40] Disorders frequently associated with depression anemia in psittacine birds include chlamydiosis, aspergillosis, egg yolk peritonitis, mycobacteriosis, chronic air sacculites, chronic hepatic or renal disease, hypothyroidism, hyperestrogenism, protein and iron deficiency, starvation, neoplasia, and other chronic inflammatory diseases.[10,41] Depression anemia is usually normocytic normochromic and can be associated with the presence of hypochromasia, anisocytosis, and poikilocytosis.[9]

Hypochromasia is associated with nutritional deficiencies, especially iron deficiency anemia, and can be found in birds with chronic inflammatory diseases, presumably related to iron sequestration as part of the bird's defense against infectious agents.[1]

Erythrocytosis (polycythemia) is characterized by an increase in circulating red cells and is rarely reported in psittacines.[1,42] Absolute polycythemia can be primary (polycytemia vera) or secondary, caused by hypoxia resulting in increased circulating RBCs, and often occurs in chronic respiratory, circulatory, and cardiac diseases.[9,10]

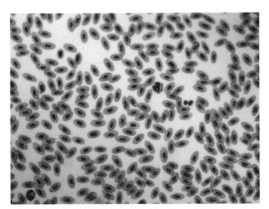

Fig. 6. The blood film reveals poor erythrocytic regenerative response in an anemic *Psittacus erithacus* affected by PBFD (Hemacolor, 400×).

Leukocyte morphology

The leukocytes in avian peripheral blood smears include granulocytes and mononuclear cells. Granulocytes are classified as heterophils, eosinophils, and basophils, and mononuclear cells as monocytes and lymphocytes.[1]

Heterophils are the predominant leukocyte in the peripheral blood of most psittacines, whereas lymphocytes are the most abundant in some species. This could be due to the variation associated with the different interpretation of the leukocyte differential count performed in several laboratories.[10] Heterophils are round cells with a bilobed or trilobed nucleus that stains poorly. Its cytoplasm is clear or colorless with numerous prominent eosinophilic granules (orange-pink, brick-red, or brown). The cytoplasmic granules are typically spindle, rod, or spiculated shaped, but may appear oval to round in some species (**Figs. 7** and **8**). Heterophil granules degranulate with many stains showing clear cytoplasmic vacuoles containing a distinct round orange granule (central body). Heterophils are the main phagocyte and are involved in bacterial killing by chemotaxis, opsonization, phagocytosis, and lysis. These

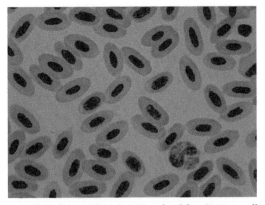

Fig. 7. A normal heterophil and erythrocytes in a healthy *Cacatua alba*. The heterophils, larger in size than erythrocytes, can vary among the species. The differences are observed predominantly on the affinity of dyeing granules and on their form (Hemacolor, 1000×).

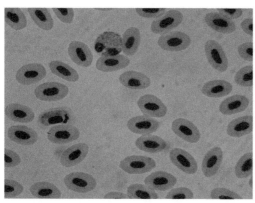

Fig. 8. A normal heterophil and erythrocytes in an asymptomatic *Psittacus erithacus*. The erythrocyte on the left side of the image shows a *Haemoproteus* gametocyte within the cytoplasm (Hemacolor, 1000×).

granulocytes increase due to inflammatory conditions. Abnormal heterophils include immature and toxic heterophils. Immature heterophils are large round cells and have increased cytoplasmic basophilia, nonsegmented nuclei, and round cytoplasmic eosinophilic (secondary) and basophilic (primary) granules. Immature heterophils possibly seen in the blood are myelocytes and metamyelocytes.[1,2,7,9,10]

Eosinophils are the least common granulocyte in psittacines. Eosinophils are medium-sized round cells with a clear or light-blue cytoplasm in contrast to the color-less cytoplasm of normal mature heterophils. They have a bilobed nucleus character-ized by clumped chromatin that stains more intensely than heterophils. Most psittacine eosinophils are the same size as heterophils but have round, strongly eosin-ophilic, cytoplasmic granules. The cytoplasmic granules of eosinophils lack the central refractile body seen in heterophils and stain more intensely than heterophil gran-ules.[1,7–9] The term eosinophil is incorrect for many psittacines species, such as the cockatoo, which has eosinophils that lack the classically eosinophilic cytoplasmic granules. The granules of eosinophils may stain differently in the various species and may be eosinophilic, aqua, light blue or gray, or dark blue, and they can be round or rod-shaped.[7] The real function of these cells is unknown.[1,7,24]

Basophils of psittacines are smaller than heterophils, round with a round to oval nonlobed nucleus and contain many round deeply metachromic granules that can frequently degranulate; they fill the cytoplasm and obscure the nucleus. Basophils seem to be involve in the initial phase of acute inflammation.[1,9]

Lymphocytes are the most common leukocyte in some psittacine species,[10] and they are similar to mammalian lymphocytes. Avian lymphocytes can be divided into 3 groups[1,2,8–10,24] according to their size (small, medium, and large lymphocytes). Most lymphocytes in peripheral blood smears are small and medium sized and are smaller than the average heterophil; large lymphocytes are rare and are larger than heterophils. The lymphocyte is typically a round cell, sometimes irregular when its margins are in contact with surrounding cells or when it shows cytoplasmic blebs or pseudopodes on the periphery. Normal small lymphocytes have a homogeneous weakly basophilic cytoplasm, without a perinuclear area (Golgi apparatus) and lack vacuoles and granules. In reactive lymphocytes, the cytoplasm tends to be strongly basophilic and can have a perinuclear area (**Figs. 9** and **10**). Medium and large lymphocytes have a moderate amount of blue-pale cytoplasm and may contain

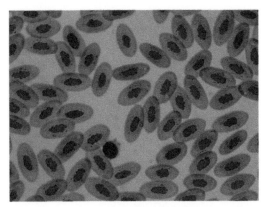

Fig. 9. Mature erythrocytes and a small mature lymphocyte with irregular cytoplasmic protrusions in pancytopenic *Psittacus erithacus* affected by chronic virus disease (PBFD) (Hemacolor 1000×).

a few distinct azurophilic granules or magenta bodies. The nucleus is centrally placed and shows an increased nucleus to cytoplasm ratio (except in large lymphocytes). Cytoplasmic appearance is important to differentiate small lymphocytes from thrombocytes or medium and large lymphocytes from monocytes. Abnormal psittacine lymphocytes are classified as reactive or blast-transformed lymphocytes. The function of lymphocytes is the same as in mammals. B lymphocytes (depending on the bursa of Fabricius) are involved in humoral immunity and T lymphocytes (depending on the thymus) are involved in cell-mediated immunity.[1,2,8,24,43]

In peripheral blood films of psittacine birds, the monocyte is typically the largest leukocyte and has an irregular to round shape, a gray–pale blue vacuolated cytoplasm with fine eosinophilic dustlike granules (a pinkish tinged cytoplasm), and an irregular and eccentric nucleus (sometimes with a flat or smoothly indented side). Monocytes are involved in cell-mediated immunity.[1,2,8,9,24,43]

Differential leukocyte count
The differential WBC count is obtained on a monolayer blood smear by microscopic observation at ×100 and oil immersion of the central third of the blood film, counting

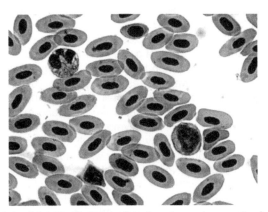

Fig. 10. A toxic heterophil, a small mature lymphocyte, and a reactive lymphocyte among mature erythrocytes in a young *Ara ararauna* with chlamydiosis (Hemacolor, 1000×).

at least 100 leukocytes and differentiating and calculating the relative (percentage) and absolute number. The avian differential WBC count is technically more difficult to interpret than the mammals one, because of some problematic cell pairs such as heterophils versus eosinophils, monocytes versus large lymphocytes, small lymphocytes versus thrombocytes, reactive lymphocytes versus rubricytes, toxic heterophils versus immature heterophils and basophils.

The distinction between eosinophils and heterophils is the first difficulty to be overcome by the hematologist. The heterophils are the major avian granulocytes, whereas eosinophils are uncommon in many psittacine species. Eosinophils do not degranulate as quickly as heterophils and their granules appear brighter and rounder than heterophils; their cytoplasm is blue and the nucleus is deeper blue, whereas, in heterophils, the cytoplasm is clear or colorless and the nucleus is less condensed.[1,8,9,18,19,24,30,43] The distinction between large lymphocytes and monocytes is based on fact that monocytes have a homogeneous blue-gray cytoplasm, usually vacuolated, and have an irregular shape and eccentric nucleus, whereas large lymphocytes have a pale blue unvacuolated cytoplasm and a centrally located nucleus.[1,8,9,18,19,24,30,43] Small lymphocytes and reactive lymphocytes may be confused with thrombocytes and rubricytes. The lymphocytes are typically round and with homogeneous pale blue cytoplasm and only rarely have magenta granules scattered throughout the cytoplasm, whereas thrombocytes are oval with a colorless, vacuolated cytoplasm and often have eosinophilic bipolar bodies (**Fig. 11**). The rubricytes are numerous when a marked regenerative response is present; the cytoplasm is basophilic, gray or eosinophilic-gray depending on the maturation stage and is darker than reactive lymphocytes (**Fig. 12**). Toxic mature heterophils have a recognizable nuclear lobulation and sometimes a swollen appearance with nuclear karyolysis in severe cases, whereas immature heterophils lack any lobulation. A high basophil count can indicate an inaccurate result, probably caused by mistakenly counting toxic heterophils as basophils. The differential count achieved on low-quality smears gives incorrect results.[1,8,9,18,19,24,30,43] The smudge cells are probably granulocytes and an increase in the relative count of lymphocytes could also depend on smudging artifacts.[4,5,30]

Response and abnormalities of the leukogram

In the interpretation of a leukogram, the variations compared with normal reference values can have physiologic causes (sex, environment, diet, and stress), pathologic

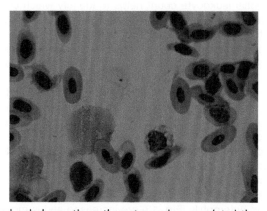

Fig. 11. Mature and polychromatic erythrocytes and a vacuolated thrombocyte in an *Ara ararauna*. The blood film also reveals some ruptured cells that can cause inaccurate hematologic results (Hemacolor, 1000×).

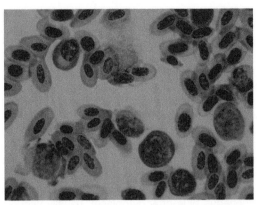

Fig. 12. Rubriblasts, prorubrocytes, basophilic rubricytes, polychromatophilic rubricytes, and polychromatic erythrocytes in a peripheral blood smear of an anemic *Ara ararauna* (Hemacolor, 1000×).

causes (leukocytosis, leucopenia, and myeloproliferative disorders) and causes unrelated to the patient such as differential and total WBC count performed by various laboratories, inadequate techniques leading to inaccurate results, and artifacts due to improper blood collection, sampling, and processing.

As already mentioned, avian leukograms can vary widely between normal psittacines of the same species. Many young normal psittacines have mature heterophilia.[9,18,19,39] Normal TWBC count reference intervals reported in psittacine birds are generally broad, therefore only significant variations from normal ranges have a diagnostic meaning. Most psittacine birds get frightened or excited when handled for blood sampling, causing a physiologic leukocytosis resulting in an increase of the concentration of heterophils and lymphocytes in the peripheral blood .This effect (mature heterophilia) decreases within 24 hours if the stressor is removed.[1,9,10]

Leukocytosis is more frequently due to increased heterophils or lymphocytes rather than monocytes, eosinophils, or basophils.[9,18,19,39] The principal causes of leukocytosis in psittacines include inflammation with infectious or noninfectious causes, exposure to toxins, hemorrhages in the body cavity, rapidly growing neoplasms, and leukemia. A differential leukocyte count helps to identify which component is most responsible. Heterophils are responsible for the first defense against microbial infection and inflammatory reactions and heterophilia is generally seen when leukocytosis is caused by inflammation.[1,9,18,19,39] Heterophilia is found as a response to systemic or local inflammation caused by infectious agents and noninfectious causes such as trauma or toxicity. The severity of heterophilia is dependent on the degree of inflammation and the cause of disease.[10,44,45] Slight to moderate leukocytosis and lymphopenia can occur with excess endogenous or exogenous glucocorticoids (stress leukogram). Early or mild bacterial infection, metabolic disease, neoplasm, trauma, and surgery can cause mature heterophilia. Marked leukocytosis and heterophilia are often seen in psittacines with infections caused by common pathogens such as *Chlamydia, Mycobacterium,* and *Aspergillus.*[1]

Heterophil morphology is more important than the absolute number to evaluate the severity of disease and to make a prognosis. A left-shift leukocytosis is mild "regenerative" if only band heterophils (**Fig. 13**) are increased and is moderate to severe if metamyelocytes and myeloblasts are also increased, whereas if the band heterophils and immature cells are larger than mature heterophils, the left shift is referred to as

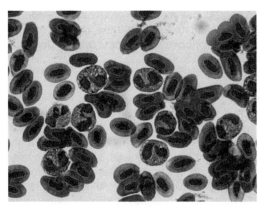

Fig. 13. Marked heterophilia in the blood film of an *Amazona aestiva* affected by acute chlamydiosis (Hemacolor, 1000×).

"degenerative", indicating a severe inflammatory response. Regenerative left shifts are correlated with severe or chronic bacterial, fungal, and chlamydial infection, and less with toxins and neoplasms, but they can occur in severe blood loss anemia associated with erythroid regeneration.[9]

Degenerative left shifts occur in septicemia, toxins, and some viral diseases. Marked increases in immature heterophils may also result from granulocytic leukemia, which is a rare condition in birds[1,10] Toxic heterophils occur with severe systemic illness such as septicemia, viremia, chlamydiosis, mycotic infections, and severe tissue necrosis. The degree of heterophil toxicity characterizes the severity of disease and a marked grade (4+) indicates a poor prognosis.[1,9,10]

Eosinophilia is rare in birds. The true functions of avian eosinophils are unknown and so eosinophilia is difficult to interpret in psittacine birds.[1,10] Basophilia is also rare and has been related to tissue necrosis occurring in chlamydiosis, respiratory diseases, autoimmune hemolytic anemia, and traumas; it could also suggest early inflammation or an immediate hypersensitivity reaction, because avian basophils produce, store, and release histamine.[1,9,18,19,39,46]

Lymphocytosis is not common when compared with heterophilia and is related to antigenic stimulation. A few reactive lymphocytes in the peripheral blood smear of healthy psittacines may be normal, but the presence of many reactive lymphocytes is suggestive of lymphocytosis with chronic antigenic stimulation associated with infectious diseases, or during convalescence from infections. Severe lymphocytosis can also occur with lymphocytic leukemia. In some cases of lymphocytic leukemia, immature atypical lymphocytes may be present in the blood film.[1,9,10,19,36,39] Anemia, mitotic figures, and marked lymphocytosis, when most small mature lymphocytes have scalloped cytoplasm, may also be present.[1,8,10,19]

Monocytosis is often associated with infectious diseases related to granulomatous inflammation with necrosis (*Mycobacterium, Chlamydia*, and fungi) and massive tissue loss. Monocytosis is often accompanied by heterophilia.[1,9]

Leukopenia can depend on pancytopenia, panleukopenia, granulocytopenia, and lymphopenia. Heteropenia is the most frequent leukopenia and is associated with severe septicemic and endotoxemic infections or with some viral diseases such as Pacheco parrot disease.[1,9,10,47] Other causes could be toxemia (drugs, plants, and chemical substances), nutritional disease anaphylaxis, radiation, and autoimmune disorders.[9] Leukopenia, heteropenia, immature heterophils, and toxic heterophils suggest a degenerative response and poor prognosis. In these cases, it is useful to monitor the decrease in leukocyte count and the variation in leukocyte morphology with serial leukograms. Lymphopenia can occur with endogenous and exogenous steroid excess and viremia.[1,8–10]

Eosinopenia is difficult to assess in psittacines because of their low normal values.

Thrombocyte morphology and abnormalities

Avian thrombocytes originate from mononuclear precursors in the bone marrow, and occasionally immature thrombocytes are present in the peripheral blood.[1,10] Mature thrombocytes are round to oval cells with a round or oval centrally placed nucleus with densely clumped chromatin. The nucleus is rounder, more dense, and bigger than the erythrocyte nucleus, and thrombocytes have a high nucleus to cytoplasm ratio. Their cytoplasm appears clear or colorless or pale gray-blue and often has a reticulated aspect. In activated or phagocytic thrombocytes, numerous vacuolations may be found depending on the degree of the reaction. Thrombocytes can frequently have some distinct small eosinophilic granules located in the polar area of the cell. Thrombocyte cells are usually aggregated in clumps of 2, 3, or more and show degranulation of polar bodies, cellular degeneration, and nuclear pyknosis.[1,2,9,19,24,43]

Avian thrombocytes have an important function in blood clotting and in phagocytosis, participating in the removal of foreign materials from the blood.[10,48] They can become reactive in chronic conditions.[43] Thrombocytosis is frequently present in a marked regenerative response after anemia. Thrombocytopenia is a result of a depressed bone marrow production either due to excessive peripheral consumption or destruction, and it is seen in psittacines with severe septicemia and/or diffuse intravascular coagulation.[9,10]

Clinical Chemistry

Clinical chemistry is important in the diagnosis of many diseases in psittacine species, but a proper interpretation of the results of a sample from a particular species can only be achieved if its reference values are available and were obtained using the same methods.[49] Plasma is preferred for routine blood biochemical evaluations, and lithium heparin is the preferred anticoagulant.[4,5]

Avian plasma samples are frequently yellow due to the presence of carotenoid pigments and not bilirubin.[16,50] Pink or red plasma is generally caused by hemolysis.[50] Common causes of hemolysis are forcing whole blood through a small needle (25–26 gauge), mixing too vigorously or improperly storing the sample (freezing, exposing to high temperatures or maintaining at room temperature for a long time).[5,16] Furthermore, lipemia can interfere with many biochemical analysis. It is not routinely possible to obtain fasting samples from birds because of the particular nature of their digestive physiology and anatomy, and because it is not advisable to subject a sick bird to fasting.[4,5,51]

Veterinary laboratories, clinical pathologists, and practitioners must develop the techniques and services needed for avian biochemical analysis and interpretation. Biochemical reference ranges for common species of psittacines have been obtained by specialized laboratories and published.[11–14,49,52–56] A computerized database can be downloaded (www.isis.org). The physiologic and anatomic conditions in birds are different from mammals and require the use of different tests. Correct knowledge of avian physiology is important for the proper interpretation of routine chemistry values.[16]

Nitrogenous waste products

The role of the avian kidney is to eliminate nitrogenous waste products and regulate homeostasis with water and electrolytic exchanges. Birds are uricotelic animals and are able to eliminate or accumulate large amounts of uric acid with little water. The avian kidney has two different types of nephrons: the mammalian-type nephron and the "reptilian" nephron. The reptilian nephron (uricotelic) lacks the Henle's loop and receives blood from the renal portal system. The mammalian-type nephron instead contains the Henle's loop and is involved in the osmotic gradient process. A single avian nephron has a lower glomerular filtration rate (GFR) than a mammalian nephron but birds have a higher number of nephrons resulting in an overall similar GFR. Avian kidneys bypass blood from reptilian to mammalian-type nephrons if the GFR is reduced, improving the ability to concentrate urine. The ability to concentrate urine is inverse with size, so that smaller birds have a greater ability to concentrate urine.[16,57–59]

Uric acid

Uric acid is the major nitrogenous waste product and is an oxidized form of hypoxanthine.[16] It is synthesized predominantly in the liver from purine metabolism and, in a lesser amount in the renal tubules. In normal conditions, most of the uric acid (80%–90%) is secreted actively in the proximal convoluted tubules, whereas a small part (10%) is filtered by the glomerulus.[59] Uric acid secretion is active through the renal tubules and is not affected by dehydration until it is severe that is when the flow of urine is insufficient to get the condensed uric acid into the convolute tubules. The blood levels of uric acid can be influenced by species, age, and diet. In young birds, the levels are lower than in adults. The concentration of uric acid can increase only with serious kidney damage (<30% functionality) or severe dehydration. In general, a concentration of uric acid in the blood greater than 15 mg/dL indicates renal impairment from a variety of causes such as nephrotoxic aminoglycoside antibiotics or lead toxicity, urinary tract obstruction, nephritis, nephrocalcinosis, and nephropathy associated with hypovitaminosis A. It can also increase after a hyperproteic meal intake or with severe tissue necrosis or starvation (increased nitrogenous catabolism). Uric acid levels in the blood are the sum of production and secretion and can be normal even if the kidney function is compromised when the bird is not eating or has a liver disease at the same time. Furthermore, in polyuric and polydipsic nephropathic birds, the filtration of urine can increase compensating the decreased secretory capacity.[16,51,59]

Evaluation of uric acid levels is useful for monitoring treatment or progress of disease when used with serial blood tests. When the plasma uric acid concentration exceeds the solubility of sodium urate, uric acid (in the form of urate crystals) precipitate in the tissues (especially in the synovial joint and on the visceral surface) and cause gout. In these cases, blood uric acid levels are greatly increased (eg, fivefold greater than normal) and result from severe renal dysfunction.[51]

Creatinine and urea

Both urea and creatinine levels in birds are low compared with those of mammals and may be less than the minimum assay level for standard laboratory techniques. Normally, creatinine plasma concentrations in African gray parrots and macaws are higher than in Amazons and cockatoos. Increased levels are rare and occur in severe kidney disease. Routine estimations of this constituent have poor diagnostic value in avian medicine.[49,60]

Urea and uric acid, together, can be useful to evaluate the urea to uric acid ratio to differentiate between dehydration, postprandial effects, and renal pathologies. This ratio, as well as being an indicator of the state of dehydration, may also be useful as an indicator of urinary fluid flow, being markedly increased in cases of renal failure with reduced urinary flow.[16,49]

Enzymes in liver and muscle tissue

Experimental studies on *Melopsittacus ondulatus* and *Psittacus erithacus* involving the sensitivity and specificity of the enzymes in liver and muscle have been performed. The specificity and sensitivity of these enzymes may vary with the species and the type of disease because the organ distribution of these enzymes is different among the species. Generally, the normal activity of a specific enzyme is a reflection of the amount of tissue that contains it and increased enzyme values give a measure of the damage of an organ and not of a decrease in its function.[61]

Aspartate aminotransferase High aspartate aminotransferase (AST) activity has been found in a multitude of tissues but mainly in liver and muscle tissues, and its distribution among tissues can vary with the species. Plasma AST activity is sensitive but not specific for hepatocellular damage and muscle injury, and is frequently evaluated with CPK (a muscle-specific enzyme) to differentiate between liver and muscle damage.[16,61] Increases in plasma AST activity in birds are moderate when greater than 350 IU/L (depending on different species and reference laboratory values) and can result from hepatic or muscle damage. Increased plasma AST activity is marked when greater than 800 IU/L. Increases of this magnitude may occur in severe hepatic damage in the presence of biliverdinuria or biliverdinemia.[16,51,61] In psittacines, increases in AST activity occur with all liver diseases, including Pacheco disease, chlamydiosis, exposure to toxic chemicals, the use of some drugs (eg, doxycycline injection and antifungal drugs such as ketoconazole, fluconazole, and itraconazole).[60]

Lactate dehydrogenase Lactate dehydrogenase (LDH) isoenzymes are found in most avian tissues and they are not specific for hepatocellular disease. Plasma LDH activity is often markedly increased in association with hepatocellular disease or muscle damage, but compared with plasma AST and alanine aminotransferase (ALT) activity, it increases and declines more rapidly. Hemolysis causes a high increase in plasma LDH activity because avian red cells have a high LDH activity.[16,51,61]

CPK Increased plasma CPK activity is found only in muscle tissue and is a muscle-specific enzyme to detect muscle cell damage in birds. The normal plasma CPK activity in most psittacine species is between 100 and 500 IU/L.[51] Plasma CPK activity is higher if any muscle cell damage is present, even with marked exertion or in birds struggling during blood collection or suffering from seizure disorders. Muscle tissue damage can happen with trauma, intramuscular injection of irritating fluids, or systemic infections that affect the skeletal or cardiac muscles. It can be useful for comparison with AST activity to differentiate muscle injury from hepatocellular injury, which can be a cause of increased AST activity. When AST, CPK, and LDH are increased, skeletal muscle injury should be considered. When the plasma CPK activity is increased due to intramuscular injection, forced exercise, handling, and traumatic injuries, AST and LDH activity can be lower. Under these conditions, if a bird has a pre-existing hepatocellular injury, it could have an increase in both AST and the CPK activity leading to misinterpretation. Plasma AST has a longer half-life than CPK, and after a single muscle injury, as with an intramuscular injection of an irritating drug, CPK activity may return to normal before the AST activity. In these cases, an erroneous diagnosis of hepatobiliary disease may be made.[16,61]

Amylase Amylase is not a specific enzyme. Information and studies on birds are poor and pancreatic diseases are rare. Amylase activity is greatly increased in pancreatic disease but also in other pathologies. Zinc toxicosis can cause pancreatitis and the higher the toxic levels, the more it is associated with the increases in plasma amylase levels.[53,62]

Electrolytes

Potassium Potassium concentrations can increase or decrease, if blood samples not separated immediately and the degree of artifactual changes depends on the species.[53] In macaws the potassium levels in blood samples increase by approximately 30% within 4 hours.[16] Decreased values have been associated with chronic diarrhea, starvation, and alkalosis. True hyperkalemia is possible in renal disease, acidosis, and severe tissue necrosis.[16,51]

Sodium Sodium is the primary osmotically active electrolyte in avian plasma and urine.[51,63] Dietary sodium is absorbed in the intestinal tract, carried to the kidneys and excreted by glomerular filtration. According to the bird's need for sodium, it may be reabsorbed into the plasma or secreted by the renal tubules, and then excreted.[51] Hyponatremia (<130 mEq/L) can be associated with an excessive loss of sodium, such as in renal disease and diarrhea, or with excessive hydration, such as polydipsia or iatrogenic low-sodium intravenous fluids. Hypernatremia (>160 mEq/L) is seen rarely with excessive dietary salt intake, dehydration due to decreased water intake, or increased water loss such as in diarrhea, renal failure, or rarely, diabetes insipidus.[51]

Calcium The values of total calcium can be much higher than the normal physiologic values tolerated by mammals. Marked increases in plasma total calcium levels are seen in oviparous females in the reproductive phase, due to estrogen stimulation for the production of calcium-binding proteins such as vitellogenin and albumin.[16,63] The calcium metabolism is controlled by parathyroid hormone (PTH), calcitonin, and vitamin D_3 (ie, 1,25-dihydrocholecalciferol, calciferol). Estrogens, corticosteroids, total thyroxine (T_4), and glucagon also influence calcium metabolism.

PTH maintains normal calcium plasma levels affecting bone, kidney, and intestinal mucosa; it mobilizes the calcium from bones, increases calcium absorption by the intestinal mucosa and calcium reabsorbtion by the renal tubules, aiding in the maintenance of the normal plasma concentration of ionized calcium. Calcitonin has the opposite action to PTH, to prevent excessive calcium reabsorbtion from bones.[51,63] The normal plasma calcium levels in nonlaying females is around 8 to 11 mg/dL and one-third or one-half of this calcium is bound to albumin. Consequently, the total plasma calcium concentration is influenced by plasma albumin levels and can decrease with hypoalbuminemia and increase with hyperalbuminemia.[51] A significant relationship was only observed between albumin and calcium concentrations in African gray parrots and correction formulas have been developed (adjusted Ca (mmol/L) = Ca (mmol/L) − 0.015 albumin (g/L) + 0.4).[52] The ionized calcium (active fraction) is not affected by changes in the albumin plasma level and could differentiate pathologic from physiologic increases in total calcium concentration. Some avian veterinarians use ionized calcium considering the normal range values to be between 1.0 and 1.3 mmol/L (P. Gibbons, personal communication)[16] or between 0.96 and 1.22 mml/L in African gray parrots.[64] Blood samples for ionized calcium assay should be tested as soon as possible because pH changes can affect this parameter.[65] Hypocalcemia (<8.0 mg/dL) in most psittacine species may be caused by dietary calcium and vitamin D_3 deficiency, excessive dietary phosphorus, alkalosis, and hypoalbuminemia.[51] Marked hypocalcemia may be caused by malnutrition or reproductive abnormalities such as chronic egg laying.[16] African gray parrots often are affected by a hypocalcemic syndrome rarely seen in other psittacines[64,65] with a plasma calcium concentration of less than 6.0 mg/dL that results in seizure disorders.[51,63]

Hypercalcemia (>11 mg/dL) in most psittacine species has been correlated with hypervitaminosis D_3, osteolytic bone lesions secondary to neoplasm, and hyperalbuminemia.[51]

Phosphorus Plasma phosphorus is primarily maintained by renal excretion. Young birds have a normal plasma phosphorus level higher than adults. Hypophosphatemia is present with hypovitaminosis D_3, malabsorption, or starvation, and even long-term corticosteroid therapies. Hyperphosphatemia can occur with severe renal diseases and hypervitaminosis D_3. Artifactual hyperphosphatemia may be caused by hemolysis and unseparated whole blood can produce a leakage of intracellular phosphorus.[51]

Metabolites

Biliverdin and bilirubin The major bile pigment in birds is biliverdin and not bilirubin (due to a lack of biliverdin reductase); it is a green pigment and biliverdinuria is responsible for the green discoloration of the urates often seen in avian liver disease.[16,51,66] Biliverdin is not currently measured in clinical laboratories, only in research laboratories.[16,67] The presence of green serum or plasma occurs in severe hepatobiliary diseases and is associated with a poor prognosis.[51,66]

Bile acids The determination of bile acids is a sensitive test for liver function in some species of birds. Bile acids are synthesized in the liver from cholesterol and excreted in the bile; more than 90% of these acids are reabsorbed by the jejunum and ileum into the portal circulation, and carried from the blood by the hepatocytes.[16,66] This process is referred to as the enterohepatic circulation.[51,66] Unlike mammals, a single sample after fasting for 12 hours overnight is preferred to eliminate random postprandial increases in bile acids, but in debilitated birds and smaller species fasting is not recommended.[16,66] Fasting plasma bile acid concentrations do not differ with or without a gallbladder.[22,66] The bile acid concentration can vary depending on the analytical method used (radioimmumoassay test or enzymatic colorimetric method).[16,51,66] The enzymatic method for determination of bile acids is preferable but has been only validated in a few species and lipemia and hemolysis can interfere with this spectophotometric method.[16,66] The reference range for bile acids has been obtained using the enzymatic method.[49] The reference range for African gray parrots, cockatoos and macaws is 18 to 71 μmol/L. In healthy Amazon parrots, normal fasting bile acid levels are slightly higher than in other psittacines, between 19 and 144 μmol/L.[49,51] In other references, the normal plasma values of bile acids in Amazons and African gray parrots differ slightly from these.[66] The increases in fasting plasma bile acid concentrations are suggestive of abnormal hepatic uptake, bile acid storage, excretion, or hepatic perfusion.[51] In one report, some psittacine species were tested to evaluate bile acid levels, AST and CPK activity, and electrophoresis. The results showed that enzymatic activities correlate poorly with high levels of bile acids, whereas bile acids have the highest association with the positive results of hepatic biopsies.[68] This suggests that liver disease can be present without increases in enzyme activity but it is probably present with high plasma levels of bile acids. Bile acids levels cannot differentiate the kind of liver disease but they can be useful to detect the presence of a hepatic disease and to assess the need for a liver biopsy or to monitor birds undergoing therapy for liver disease.[66]

Cholesterol Plasma cholesterol is eliminated in the form of bile acids and its concentration increases in extrahepatic biliary obstruction, hepatic fibrosis, and bile duct hyperplasia. Hypercholesterolemia can also be caused by hypothyroidism, high-fat diets, and lipemia. Hypocholesterolemia may be associated with end-stage liver failure, maldigestion or malabsorption, and starvation.[51]

Glucose Glucose metabolism in birds is controlled by insulin and glucagon as in mammals. Healthy psittacines have blood glucose concentrations greater than

150 to 200 mg/dL. In mammals, insulin has a primary role in glucose homeostasis; in birds this role belongs to glucagon with some differences among the species.[16,51,63]

Diabetes mellitus in psittacines is attributed to increased glucagon secretion but there are some reports describing a decreased blood insulin concentration and a significant response to insulin therapy. Therefore, either hyperglucagonemia or hypoinsulinemia can be involved in diabetes in psittacines.[51] Hypoglycemia (<150–200 mg/dL) occurs with prolonged starvation, severe liver disease (eg, Pacheco disease), septicemia, enterotoxemia, endocrine disorders such as hypothyroidism, and maldigestion or malasbsorption. The artifactual decrease in glucose levels caused by nonseparation of plasma or serum from blood as in mammals, is not significant in birds, because avian erythrocytes use fatty acids rather than glucose for energy. A mild to moderate hyperglycemia (>500–600 mg/dL) may be induced by high levels of endogenous or exogenous glucocorticoids as in exertion, excitement, extreme temperature, stress, or glucocorticoid administration.[16,51,64] Marked hyperglycemia in psittacines (>700 mg/dL and in budgerigars also >900 mg/dL) raises the suspicion of diabetes mellitus.[51,63]

Total proteins The normal total protein levels in birds are substantially lower than those of mammals[16,51,63] and generally range from 2.5 to 4.5 g/dL.[51] The plasma proteins consist of albumin, transport proteins, proteins of coagulation, fibrinogen, enzymes, hormones, and immunoglobulins.[63] An essential function of plasma protein levels is preservation of the normal colloidal osmotic pressure, which maintains the normal blood volume and pH.[51]

Some differences exist among psittacine species when different protein standards and different methods are used in the various laboratories.[52] The refractometer method (easiest and common technique to test total proteins) in psittacines can produce inaccurate results caused by interference from high concentrations of other refractive substances such as blood glucose (higher in Psittacines) or lipemia and hemolysis that can alter the accuracy of the refractometric method.[16,51,63,69,70] The Biuret method (BCG) is more accurate and gives reliable results when the total protein levels are between 1 and 10 g/dL, but it has not been validated in birds.[16,51] The comparison between results obtained using the BCG method and gel electrophoresis has shown many differences, probably caused by the use of human albumin standards and controls, whose binding affinity with the dye is different from avian albumin. The difference between the total protein levels in psittacines is probably caused by the use of bovine or human standards lacking species-specific protein standards.[16,49,53] The total protein concentration obtained with a BCG method combined with gel electrophoresis represents an absolute accurate concentration of the plasma protein[51] and can be used to determine albumin concentration and globulin distribution.[16] Electrophoresis is useful for staging acute and chronic inflammatory conditions and for monitoring therapeutic response in birds.[16,63,68] The primary plasma protein fractions include prealbumin, albumin, α-globulins (α_1 and α_2), β-globulins, and γ-globulins. The prealbumin fraction may be found in some psittacines. Albumin migration differs among the species. These different migration patterns are related to variable conformation and surface charge distribution of albumin molecules; this may also explain the differential binding of BCG, and inaccurate results using human standards.[16,71] These difference were also present in globulin fractions with a lower normal concentration of γ-globulins and an increase primarily in the α- and β-globulin fractions (rather than the γ-globulin fraction) in acute inflammatory disease.[72]

A recent study has compared electrophoresis results using 3 different commercial electrophoresis systems in African gray parrots, and has found many differences in protein fraction migration.[73] Normal concentrations for albumin, α-globulin, β-globulin, and γ-globulin obtained with protein electrophoresis in psittacine birds ranged from 1.5 to 3.0 g/dL, 0.1 to 0.5 g/dL, 0.2 to 0.6 g/dL, and 0.2 to 0.7 g/dL, respectively. The normal albumin to globulin (A/G) ratio for most psittacine birds is between 1.5 and 3.5.[51] Reference intervals for each species of bird should be established in each laboratory and because the results for protein fractions from psittacine species are variable in terms of migrations pattern, they should be interpreted with caution.[73–75] Hypoalbuminemia has been found in birds with maldigestion, malabsorption, protein-losing enteropathy or nephropathy, and liver disease.[16,51,75] Hypoproteinemia in birds is frequently associated with hypoalbuminemia (decreased A/G ratio) and occurs with marked external hemorrhage, renal disease with chronic proteinuria, or protein-losing enteropathies.[16,51,63] A physiologic decrease in A/G ratio is recurrent in egg-laying females with estrogen-induced hyperproteinemia to complete egg formation because most of the yolk and chalazae proteins are globulins and cause a marked increase in globulin fractions.[16,51,53,63,75] The acute phase proteins (α- and β-globulin fractions) are typically increased during inflammation. Chronic inflammatory disorders such as active hepatitis may increase the α- and β-globulin fractions.[51,75] Immunoglobulins (IgM and IgG) may migrate in the latter fractions. The γ-globulin peak contains IgA, IgM, IgG, and IgE immunoglobulins. In many chronic infections (eg, *Chlamydia*, *Aspergillus*, and *Mycobacterium* spp.), polygammopathy can be seen indicating active chronic inflammatory diseases. Immunodeficiency may be present when γ-globulin fractions are lowered.[51] Hyperproteinemia can be found in dehydration (normal A/G ratio), in acute or chronic inflammation (decreased A/G ratio), or in a preovulatory condition. In chronic disturbances, γ-globulins are the most increased fraction. Hyperproteinemia associated with hyperalbuminemia and hypoglobulinemia with an increased A/G ratio is suggestive of dehydration, chronic stress, or other immunosuppressive conditions (virus such as psittacine beak and feather disease [PBFD]).[16,51,75]

Several organ-specific and species profiles used in our clinic and laboratory to evaluate the patient in a more complete way are given in **Tables 4** and **5**.

PART II

This part of the article considers whether there are significant changes in hematologic and biochemical parameters and if these abnormalities have similarities with those reported in literature. Possible analytical errors, diagnostic omissions, and potential risks of overestimated or underestimated diagnoses in some clinical cases presented to our practice are also considered.

Materials and Methods

A list of all tests evaluated are summarized in **Table 6**. Blood samples were collected over 5 years from 150 different psittacines of 29 different species and grouped into 7 genera as summarized in **Tables 7** and **8**. The study is limited to those birds for which we had a complete set of results for analysis that could lead to a proper diagnosis. Most birds were adult (128 of 150 birds ranged between 1 and 25 years); a small number of birds was young (8 birds were between 3 months and 12 months of age), or were aging (14 birds were aged between 25 and 50 years). Gender was not determined in all patients. Usually in our practice a venous blood sample is collected from the right jugular or subcutaneous ulnar (wing) vein and the selected site depends on bird species, age, and size; the veterinarian's/technician's experience is also an issue. Some samples were collected from anesthetized birds (isoflurane), others from unanesthetized

Table 4
Examples of biochemical profiles of organs

Complete	Renal	Liver	Pancreas	Feather Picker
Uric acid	Uric acid	Uric acid	Glucose	Uric acid
LDH	LDH	LDH	Lipase	LDH
CPK	CPK	CPK	Amylase	CPK
AST	AST	ALT	Cholesterol	AST
Glucose	Glucose	AST	Triglycerides	Glucose
Creatinine	Creatinine	Glucose	Zinc	Creatinine
Electrophoresis	Electrophoresis	Bile acid	Complete CBC	Plasma proteins
Calcium	Calcium	Electrophoresis		Calcium
Ionized calcium	Sodium	Complete CBC		Phosphorus
Sodium	Phosphorus			Fecal examination
Phosphorus	Potassium			Gram stain
Potassium	Complete CBC			Total thyroxine
Bile acids				Complete CBC
Amylase				Zinc
Complete blood count				

Abbreviations: ALT, alanine aminotransferase; AST, aspartate aminotransferase; CBC, complete blood count.

patients, using 1- or 2-mL syringes and 23- to 25-gauge detachable needles. The samples (from 0.8 to 2.0 mL of whole blood) were mixed immediately with lithium heparin in pediatric collection tubes. Two monolayer blood smears were made with non-heparinized fresh blood immediately after collection. Most of the blood tests were run

Table 5
Some biochemical profiles for selected species

Amazon	Macaw	Cockatiel	Cockatoo	African Gray	Budgerigar
Uric acid	Uric acid	Uric acid	Uric acid	Uric acid	Bile acids
Calcium	Calcium	AST	AST	Glucose	Fecal stain
AST	Phosphorus	Glucose	Plasma proteins	AST	CBC
Glucose	Chloride	Plasma proteins	Microbiology	Ionized calcium	
Cholesterol	LDH	Microbiology	CBC	Sodium	
Plasma proteins	AST	*Chlamydophila psittaci* AC		Potassium	
Microbiology	CPK	CBC		Plasma proteins	
Chlamydophila psittaci AC	Glucose	Fecal stain		Microbiology	
CBC	Plasma proteins			CBC	
	Cholesterol				
	CBC				

Abbreviations: ALT, alanine aminotransferase; CBC, complete blood count.

Table 6 Total number of tests performed	
Test	**Number**
Hematocrit	134
Total protein	125
Hemoglobin	115
TRBC	115
TWBC	150
Lymphocytes (%)	150
Monocytes (%)	150
Heterophils (%)	150
Eosinophils (%)	150
Basophils (%)	150
Anisocytosis/poikilocytosis	150
Polychromasia	150
Band heterophils	150
Toxic heterophils	20
Zinc	31
Calcium	68
Ionized calcium	37
Phosphorus	51
Sodium	51
Potassium	55
Bile acids	74
Glucose	128
Uric acid	130
Amylase	41
Creatinine	41
CPK	107
Cholesterol	39
LDH	103
AST	129
Prealbumin	75
Albumin	75
α_1-Globulin	74
α_2-Globulin	74
β-Globulin	74
γ-Globulin	74
A/G ratio	75
Total data number	3465

within 4 to 12 hours after collection, with the exception of samples collected from birds located in other premises. Our laboratory stains blood smears with Giemsa stain; once the stained smears are dried, they are fixed and mounted with a coverslide glass. For each sample, a microhematocrit tube is filled with blood with lithium heparin and centrifuged at 12,000 × g for 5 minutes to determine the PCV. The erythrocyte total count, the hemoglobin, and granulocyte total count were performed using an automated analyzer

Table 7
Total number of selected psittacine species

Species	Number
Amazona aestiva	13
Amazona amazonica	2
Amazona auropalliata	1
Amazona autumnalis	1
Amazona brasiliensis	2
Amazona farinosa	1
Amazona festiva	1
Amazona finschii	1
Amazona ochrocephala	10
Amazona o. panamensis	6
Amazona vinacea	2
Amazona xantholora	2
Hybrid Amazon	2
Ara ararauna	18
Ara chloroptera	10
Ara macao	4
Ara militaris	2
Diopsittaca nobilis	4
Ara severa	5
Cacatua alba	8
Cacatua ducorpsii	2
Cacatua galerita	5
Cacatua sanguinea	1
Cacatua s. citrinocristata	2
Eclectus roratus	1
Aratinga solstitialis	1
Aratinga (Nandayus) nenday	1
Nymphicus hollandicus	3
Psittacus erithacus	39
Total	150

(Cell-Dyn 3500 hematology system; Abbot Laboratories, Abbott Park, IL, USA) updated with specific veterinary software. The hemoglobin concentration needs to be corrected. The Cell-Dyn analyzer uses the correction factors from the Vet 2.3 software, which are adapted for some genus/groups or species of psittacines (*Ara* spp, *Amazona* spp, *Cacatua* spp, *Psittacus erithacus, Melopsittacus undulatus*) using adequate correction factors previously developed. For the granulocyte total count, only the optical leukocyte count (WOC) is used, or (in the presence of interference by erythrocytes and thrombo-cytes nuclei) the absolute count of neutrophils that corresponds to heterophils. The esti-mated TWBC count is routinely performed for all samples to evaluate the number of lymphocytes to compare it with the automated TWBC count and to double check any abnormal results. The estimated TWBC count and WBC differential count are always performed by the same operator. The biochemical results were obtained (see **Table 6**) using standard spectrophotometric methods, according to the standard

| Table 8 | |
| Number of specimens for each group of selected psittacines | |
Group	Number
Amazons	44
Macaws	43
Eclectus	1
Conures	2
Cockatoos	18
Cockatiels	3
African gray parrots	39
Total number of birds sampled	150

protocol provided with the system. Colorimetric methods were used to evaluate calcium, phosphorus, glucose, cholesterol, creatinine, and uric acid concentrations. Total bile acids were also measured using an enzymatic colorimetric method; total proteins were assessed with the BCG method using a human standard. All enzymes were measured with a kinetic optimized Scandinavian Committee on enzymes (SCE) method. Sodium, potassium, and ionized calcium have all been tested with ion selective electrode (ISE). Albumin, prealbumin, and globulin fractions were obtained by plasma protein electrophoresis using a manual method (cellulose acetate membranes, barbiturate buffer, for 30 minutes at 180 V and stained with Coomassie Blue). The biochemical analysis were run using the Roche Cobas Mira Classic chemistry analyzer (Roche Diagnostics) and AVL 9180 electrolyte analyzer (Roche Diagnostics). The data collected over a 5-year period were compared with the published reference values for psittacines, as summarized in **Tables 9–11**. These results were correlated with the suspected diagnosis proposed by the different practitioners and the list of the diagnosed diseases as summarized in **Box 1**. The diseases are grouped to facilitate the understanding of the data.

Results

Table 12 summarizes the correlation between the species/group and the diagnosis. **Table 13** summarizes the rating for each parameter evaluated (total number and percentage of the hematologic and biochemical normal, decreased, and increased values, in comparison with the reference range).

Tables 14–16 present a score for each hematologic or blood chemistry parameter (mild, moderate, marked, decreased, or increased). Data referring to conditions with less than 3 specimens are excluded from the tables. The 2 cases of neurologic disorders, regarding the same bird (African gray parrot), revealed mild heterophilia and, in the first control, marked total hypocalcemia and decreased ionized calcium, mild hyperphosphatemia, marked hypokalemia, moderate hypoglycemia, and an increase in all muscle enzymes. In the 2 cases of osteomalacia, we observed a marked total hypocalcemia and marked decreased ionized calcium with light hyperphosphatemia and moderate increase in amylase, CPK, and LDH activity. In the 2 cases of trauma, 1 only had moderate heteropenia; the other showed marked hyperkalemia. In the only neoplasm observed, the bird showed moderate hyperproteinemia, leukocytosis with lymphocytosis and monocytosis, moderate hyperphosphatemia and high amylase activity, mild increase of CPK activity, a marked decrease in A/G ratio with mild albumin decrease and severe increase in α_2-globulin and β-globulin fractions.

Discussion

This study refers only to psittacines living in Italy. According to our data, Amazons as a group, seem to be more susceptible to bacterial infections and are the second group for sensitivity to psittacosis. On the other hand, Amazons are less prone to be infected by viruses compared with macaws. Macaws are apparently more susceptible to infectious disease; specifically, they seem more prone to chlamydiosis and viral infections, followed by bacterial, mycotic infections, and air sac infections (aerosacculitis). African gray parrots are more susceptible to aerosacculitis and fungal infections and are the second group for sensitivity to bacterial infections; conversely they seem to be less sensitive to viruses and chlamydiosis as reported in the literature.[65] Cockatoos are less susceptible to bacterial and viral infections; they also seem to be more resistant to psittacosis compared with other large parrots.[65]

As suggested in the literature,[65] organ-related diseases are more typically diagnosed in Amazons; liver diseases are the most represented followed by renal disease. In macaws, there are some cases of enteritis, cloacal diseases, and reproductive disorders but liver diseases are rare. African gray parrots are the second group of parrots most susceptible to organ-related diseases and particularly to heart disease, neurologic disorders, and osteomalacia. The latter two may be related to the typical hypocalcemic syndrome of African gray parrots.[51,52,63–65] The other psittacine species show no evidence of these diseases. The last group is represented by some typical psittacine issues and miscellaneous diseases. The most susceptible group is the African gray parrots, which have the most dietary disorders followed by some cases of feather and beak disorders, behavioral disorders, trauma, and gizzard foreign bodies according to Rosskopf and Woerpel.[65] Cockatoos are more susceptible to feather and beak disorders and macaws seem to be more susceptible to behavioral disease and zinc toxicosis. Even though there is only 1 Eclectus in our study, and thus it is not useful from a statistical point of view, it is interesting that the bird was referred for zinc toxicosis. It is reported in the literature that Eclectus parrots and cockatoos have higher normal levels of zinc in plasma or serum than other psittacines. The authors suggest taking into consideration the species of parrots when evaluating zinc toxicosis.[76] The rest of the organ-related pathologies are rare or absent in the other psittacine species. The group of diseases referred to as check are not considered in this evaluation because they do not have any specific diagnostic value.

Considering the data summarized in **Table 13**, all the abnormal values obtained may have an explanation compatible with what has been described earlier; that the hemoglobin level is higher than the PCV and RBC count might depend on an artifactual increase due to lysis of erythrocytes and thrombocytes. Leukocytosis, which is commonly observed in psittacines, is normally seen with heterophilia.[9,18,19,39] Leukopenia is rarely observed in birds, and is normally caused by a low number of heterophils (heteropenia). Monocytosis is less common than heterophilia, but is more common than lymphocytosis.[1,9] As frequently reported, sick parrots are brought to the veterinarian at an advanced, chronic stage of the disease; this could explain the frequency of birds presenting with monocytosis. Eosinophilia and eosinopenia are rarely observed in birds, as highlighted in **Table 13**. Also basophils are rare or absent.[1,9] Banded and toxic heterophils are observed less frequently and this happen because it is not easy to recognize them and because they are not often present unless in severe inflammatory diseases.[1,9,10] Electrolytes (Na, K, phosphorus) show a higher percentage of abnormal values but they are also the parameters most affected by artifactual interference.[4,5,16,21,53] Glucose and uric acid have lesser percentages of abnormal values and are decreased most of the time; that can

Table 9
Reference values for hematology and clinical chemistry parameters in selected psittacine species

	Units	Psittacus erithacus (African Gray Parrot)	Amazona Group (Amazon Parrots)	Ara Group (Macaws)	Nymphicus hollandicus (Cockatiel)	Cacatua Group (Cockatoos)	Cacatua galerita (Sulfur-Crested Cockatoo)	Cacatua sanguinea (Little Corella)	Cacatua sulphurea (Yellow-Crested Cockatoo)	Eclectus roratus (Eclectus Parrot)	Nandayus nenday (Nanday Conure)	Aratinga solstitialis (Sun Conure)
Hematocrit	%	43–51[a]	44–56[a]	45–55[a]	45–57[a]	40–54[b]	41–49[a]	—	—	35–47[c]	39–49[c,d]	39–49[c,d]
Red blood cells	×10^6/μL	3.0–3.6[a]	2.6–3.5[a]	2.5–4.5[a]	2.5–4.7[a]	2.5–2.95[b]	2.4–3.0[a]	—	—	2.4–3.9[c]	2.5–4.0[c,d]	2.5–4.0[c,d]
White blood cells	×10^3/μL	6.0–12[b]	5.0–17[b]	6.0–13.5[a]	5.0–10[a]	5.0–13[b]	12–16[b]	7.0–13[b]	9.0–16[b]	9.0–15[b]	5.0–11[b]	6.0–11[b]
Hemoglobin	g/dL	14.2–17.0[a]	13.8–17.9[a]	14.8–18.9[a]	—	12.0–14.8[b]	13.8–17.1[a]	—	—	11.5–16.0[c]	12.0–16.0[c,d]	12.0–16.0[c,d]
Lymphocytes	%	19–50[b]	20–67[b]	20–50[a]	25–55[a]	20–50[b]	22–56[b]	22–51[b]	21–56[b]	23–57[b]	24–47[b]	20–49[b]
Monocytes	%	0–2[b]	0–2[b]	0–3[a]	0–2[a]	0–2[b]	0–2[b]	0–1[b]	0–2[b]	0–1[b]	0–1[b]	0–1[b]
Heterophils	%	45–73[b]	31–71[b]	45–70[a]	40–70[a]	45–72[b]	44–75[b]	45–72[b]	44–79[b]	46–70[b]	48–71[b]	44–72[b]
Eosinophils	%	0–1[b]	0–0[b]	0–2[a]	0–2[a]	0–2[b]	0–1[b]	0–2[b]	0–2[b]	0–1[b]	0–1[b]	0–1[b]
Basophils	%	0–1[b]	0–2[b]	0–5[a]	0–6[a]	0–1[b]	0–1[b]	0–1[b]	0–1[b]	0–1[b]	0–2[b]	0–2[b]
MCV	fL	137–155[a]	156–194[b]	90–185[c]	—	154–170[b]	145–187[a]	—	—	95–220[c]	90–190[c,d]	90–190[c,d]
MCH	pg	41.9–52.8[a]	44.7–58.6[a]	27–53[c]	—	45.0–55.5[b]	53.8–60.6[a]	—	—	27.0–55.0[c]	28.0–55.0[c,d]	28.0–55.0[c,d]
MCHC	g/dL	28.9–34.0[a]	28.9–35.8[a]	23.0–32.0[c]	—	24.1–32.9[b]	33.3–37.6[a]	—	—	22.0–33.0[c]	23.0–31.0[c,d]	23.0–31.0[c,d]
Thrombocytes	K/μL	11–42[a]	10–67[a]	—	11–34[a]	11–34[a]	7–24[a]	—	—	—	—	—
Amylase	U/L	415–626[b]	184–478[b]	239–564[b]	113–870[b]	228–876[b]	—	273–536[b]	136–750[b]	150–645[c]	—	—
AST	U/L	110–340[b]	150–344[b]	65–168[b]	128–396[b]	140–360[b]	120–208[b]	140–350[b]	134–276[b]	144–339[b]	147–378[b]	138–355[b]

Bile acids	μmol/L	12-96[b]	33-154[b]	7-100[b]	44-108[b]	34-112[b]	24-98[b]	15-96[b]	24-95[b]	30-110[b]	—	12-92[b]
Calcium	mg/dL	8-14[b]	8-13.9[b]	8.4-11.9[b]	8.2-10.9[b]	8.2-11.5[b]	8-12[b]	8-11.4[b]	8.1-10.3[b]	7-13.0[c]	8-11[b]	8-11.2[b]
Cholesterol	mg/dL	100-250[b]	148-228[b]	96-264[b]	—	96-212[b]	146-248[b]	—	113-206[b]	100-261[b]	117-228[b]	112-255[b]
CPK	U/L	140-411[b]	117-425[b]	88-361[b]	160-420[b]	147-418[b]	164-396[b]	144-439[b]	157-408[b]	132-410[b]	135-400[b]	153-372[b]
Creatinine	mg/dL	0.1-0.4[c]	0.1-0.4[c]	0.1-0.5[c]	0.1-0.4[c]	0.1-0.4[c]	—	—	—	0.1-0.4[c]	—	—
Ionized calcium	meq/L	0.96-1.22[e]	—	—	—	—	—	—	—	—	—	—
Glucose	mg/dL	256-360[b]	246-378[b]	210-360[b]	228-440[b]	206-418[b]	200-345[b]	220-412[b]	138-304[b]	216-396[b]	231-393[b]	167-380[b]
LDH	U/L	154-378[b]	160-368[b]	70-220[b]	122-378[b]	208-414[b]	118-374[b]	198-452[b]	178-398[b]	198-386[b]	204-396[b]	155-346[b]
Phosphorus	mg/dL	3.2-5.4[c]	3.1-5.5[c]	2.0-12.0[c]	3.2-4.8[c]	2.5-5.5[c]	—	—	2.9-6.5[c]	—	—	—
Potassium	meq/L	2.9-4.6[c]	3.0-4.5[c]	2.0-5.0[c]	2.4-4.6[c]	2.5-4.5[c]	—	—	3.5-4.3[c]	—	—	—
Sodium	meq/L	157-165[c]	125-155[c]	140-165[c]	130-153[c]	130-155[c]	—	—	130-145[c]	—	—	—
Total protein	g/dL	2.7-4.4[b]	2.6-4.5[b]	2.4-4.4[b]	2.1-4.8[b]	2.6-4.8[b]	2.4-4.8[b]	2.4-4.3[b]	2.8-4.6[b]	3.2-4.3[b]	1.9-3.7[b]	2.4-4.5[b]
Uric acid	mg/dL	2.2-11[b]	2.2-10[b]	1.8-12[b]	3.4-11[b]	3.8-11[b]	2.2-11[b]	3.5-11[b]	2.1-11[b]	2.0-11[b]	2.3-11[b]	2.2-12[b]

[a] Data for adults of both sexes, as obtained from Hawkey CM, Samour JH. The value of clinical hematology in exotic birds. In: Jacobson ER, Kollias GV, Jr, editors. Exotic animals: contemporary issues in small animal practice. London: Churchill Livingstone; 1988.

[b] Data for adults of both sexes, as obtained from The Californian Avian Laboratory, Citrus Heights, CA 95621. Reference range 1998 from Fudge AM. Laboratory reference ranges for selected avian, mammalian, and reptilian species. In: Fudge AM, editor. Laboratory medicine: avian and exotic pets. Philadelphia: WB Saunders; 2000. p. 376-400.

[c] Data for adults of both sexes, as obtained from The Avian and wildlife Laboratory, University of Miami School Medicine, Miami, FL 33136.

[d] The data are referred to the Conure group.

[e] Data for adults of both sexes, as obtained from Stanford M. The significance of serum ionized calcium and 25-hydroxy-cholecalciferol (vitamin D3) assays in African grey parrots. Exotic DVM 2003;5(3):1-6.

Table 10
Reference values for hematology and clinical chemistry in selected macaws and Amazon species

	Units	Amazona aestiva (Blue-Fronted Amazon)	Amazona amazonica (Orange-Winged Amazon)	Amazona auropalliata (Yellow-Naped Amazon)	Amazona autumnalis (Red-Lored Amazon)	Amazona farinose (Mealy Amazon)	Amazona ochrocephala (Yellow-Crowned Amazon)	Ara ararauna (Blue and Gold Macaw)	Ara chloroptera (Green-Winged Macaw)	Ara macao (Scarlet Macaw)	Ara militaris (Military Macaw)	Ara severa (Severe Macaw)	Diopsittaca nobilis (Red Shouldered Macaw)
Hematocrit	%	44–56[a,b]	44–56[a,b]	44–56[a,b]	44–56[a,b]	44–56[a,b]	44–56[a,b]	41–51[a]	41–56[a]	46–52[a]	44–50[a]	45–53[a]	41–51[a,b]
Red cells	$\times 10^6/\mu L$	2.6–3.5[a,b]	2.6–3.5[a,b]	2.6–3.5[a,b]	2.6–3.5[a,b]	2.6–3.5[a,b]	2.6–3.5[a,b]	2.7–3.5[a]	2.8–3.3[a]	2.7–3.2[a]	2.7–3.1[a]	3.1–3.6[a]	2.7–3.5[a,b]
White cells	$\times 10^3/\mu L$	6.0–13[c]	7.0–16[c]	6.0–17[c]	6.0–16[c]	9.0–16[c]	8.0–15[c]	8.0–16[c]	11.0–16.0[c]	10.0–14.0[c]	12.0–20.0[c]	9.0–14.0[c]	8.0–22.0[c]
Hemoglobin	g/dL	13.8–17.9[a,b]	13.8–17.9[a,b]	13.8–17.9[a,b]	13.8–17.9[a,b]	13.8–17.9[a,b]	13.8–17.9[a,b]	14.8–18.9[a]	14.7–18.8[a]	15.8–18.4[a]	14.8–19.6[a]	16.0–17.1[a]	14.8–18.9[a,b]
Lymphocytes	%	22–65[c]	20–64[c]	20–67[c]	22–66[c]	23–65[c]	18–63[c]	18–53[c]	22–60[c]	23–50[c]	25–40[c]	25–47[c]	32–66[c]
Monocytes	%	0–1[c]	0–1[c]	0–1[c]	0–1[c]	0–1[c]	0–1[c]	0–2[c]	0–2[c]	0–2[c]	0–2[c]	0–2[c]	0–1[c]
Heterophils	%	33–72[c]	31–73[c]	31–73[c]	33–73[c]	38–76[c]	37–69[c]	49–71[c]	49–73[c]	48–73[c]	58–85[c]	45–80[c]	34–63[c]
Eosinophils	%	0–1[c]	0–0[c]	0–0[c]	0–0[c]	0–0[c]	0–1[c]	0–1[c]	0–2[c]	0–1[c]	0–1[c]	0–1[c]	0–1[c]
Basophils	%	0–1[c]	0–2[c]	0–2[c]	0–2[c]	0–1[c]	0–1[c]	0–1[c]	0–1[c]	0–1[c]	0–1[c]	0–2[c]	0–1[c]
MCV	fL	156–194[a,b]	156–194[a,b]	156–194[a,b]	156–194[a,b]	156–194[a,b]	156–194[a,b]	132–157[a]	141–174[a]	143–175[a]	154–160[a]	145–156[a]	132–157[a,b]
MCH	pg	44.7–58.6[a,b]	44.7–58.6[a,b]	44.7–58.6[a,b]	44.7–58.6[a,b]	44.7–58.6[a,b]	44.7–58.6[a,b]	49.4–56.4[a]	50.5–57.7[a]	51.1–64.2[a]	40.6–59.6[a]	47.9–55.2[a]	49.4–56.4[a,b]
MCHC	g/dL	28.9–35.8[a,b]	28.9–35.8[a,b]	28.9–35.8[a,b]	28.9–35.8[a,b]	28.9–35.8[a,b]	28.9–35.8[a,b]	34.7–39.8[a]	29.1–38.3[a]	32.6–38.5[a]	34.7–37[a]	32.1–35.6[a]	34.7–39.8[a,b]
Thrombocytes	K/μL	10–67[a,b]	10–67[a,b]	10–67[a,b]	10–67[a,b]	10–67[a,b]	10–67[a,b]	11–34[a]	8–15[a]	17–30[a]	19–30[a]	10–13[a]	11–34[a,b]
Amylase	U/L	184–478[c,b]	184–478[c,b]	187–546[c]	156–472[c]	36–574[c]	184–478[c,b]	239–516[c]	239–564[c,b]	239–564[c,b]	239–564[c,b]	239–564[c,b]	239–564[c,b]
AST	U/L	146–408[c]	114–389[c]	150–390[c]	150–408[c]	138–377[c]	150–380[c]	64–168[c]	62–168[c]	74–177[c]	76–166[c]	72–170[c]	126–215[c]

Analyte	Units												
Bile acids	μmol/L	34-140ᶜ	29-157ᶜ	36-144ᶜ	24-120ᶜ	31-145ᶜ	59-188ᶜ	27-86ᶜ	15-78ᶜ	21-100ᶜ	24-130ᶜ	25-82ᶜ	7-100ᶜˑᵇ
Calcium	mg/dL	8.2-13.8ᶜ	8-14.5ᶜ	8.4-13.2ᶜ	8-13.2ᶜ	8.6-12.9ᶜ	8.6-11.7ᶜ	8.4-11.8ᶜ	8.4-11.8ᶜ	8.4-10.9ᶜ	8.4-10.9ᶜ	8.4-10.8ᶜ	8.4-11.9ᶜˑᵇ
Cholesterol	mg/dL	100-270ᶜ	180-254ᶜ	100-256ᶜ	150-228ᶜ	111-249ᶜ	125-246ᶜ	96-249ᶜ	—	—	—	100-252ᶜ	96-264ᶜ
Creatinine kinase	U/L	130-417ᶜ	120-455ᶜ	132-402ᶜ	136-420ᶜ	208-348ᶜ	260-490ᶜ	92-380ᶜ	96-368ᶜ	98-366ᶜ	126-321ᶜ	123-356ᶜ	88-361ᶜˑᵇ
Creatinine	mg/dL	0.1-0.4ᵈˑᵇ	0.1-0.4ᵈˑᵇ	0.1-0.4ᵈˑᵇ	0.1-0.4ᵈˑᵇ	0.1-0.4ᵈˑᵇ	0.1-0.4ᵈˑᵇ	0.1-0.5ᵈˑᵇ	0.1-0.5ᵈˑᵇ	0.1-0.5ᵈˑᵇ	0.1-0.5ᵈˑᵇ	0.1-0.5ᵈˑᵇ	0.1-0.5ᵈˑᵇ
Ionized calcium	meq/L	—	—	—	—	—	—	—	—	—	—	—	—
Glucose	mg/dL	246-389ᶜ	249-482ᶜ	249-377ᶜ	250-388ᶜ	201-337ᶜ	170-316ᶜ	210-368ᶜ	210-360ᶜ	210-333ᶜ	214-340ᶜ	220-368ᶜ	231-300ᶜ
LDH	U/L	158-366ᶜ	148-451ᶜ	160-360ᶜ	150-412ᶜ	159-381ᶜ	171-265ᶜ	69-220ᶜ	72-224ᶜ	60-210ᶜ	72-216ᶜ	66-210ᶜ	70-220ᶜˑᵇ
Phosphorus	mg/dL	3.1-5.5ᵈˑᵇ	3.1-5.5ᵈˑᵇ	3.1-5.5ᵈˑᵇ	3.1-5.5ᵈˑᵇ	3.1-5.5ᵈˑᵇ	3.1-5.5ᵈˑᵇ	2.0-12.0ᵈˑᵇ	2.0-12.0ᵈˑᵇ	2.0-12.0ᵈˑᵇ	2.0-12.0ᵈˑᵇ	2.0-12.0ᵈˑᵇ	2.0-12.0ᵈˑᵇ
Potassium	meq/L	3.0-4.5ᵈˑᵇ	3.0-4.5ᵈˑᵇ	3.0-4.5ᵈˑᵇ	3.0-4.5ᵈˑᵇ	3.0-4.5ᵈˑᵇ	3.0-4.5ᵈˑᵇ	2.0-5.0ᵈˑᵇ	2.0-5.0ᵈˑᵇ	2.0-5.0ᵈˑᵇ	2.0-5.0ᵈˑᵇ	2.0-5.0ᵈˑᵇ	2.0-5.0ᵈˑᵇ
Sodium	meq/L	125-155ᵈˑᵇ	125-155ᵈˑᵇ	125-155ᵈˑᵇ	125-155ᵈˑᵇ	125-155ᵈˑᵇ	125-155ᵈˑᵇ	140-165ᵈˑᵇ	140-165ᵈˑᵇ	140-165ᵈˑᵇ	140-165ᵈˑᵇ	140-165ᵈˑᵇ	140-165ᵈˑᵇ
Total protein	g/dL	3.5-6.5ᶜ	2.7-4.9ᶜ	2.8-4.7ᶜ	2.3-4.4ᶜ	2.4-4.2ᶜ	3.2-4.6ᶜ	2.5-4.2ᶜ	2.7-4.2ᶜ	2.4-3.8ᶜ	3.0-3.9ᶜ	2.3-3.9ᶜ	2.4-4.4ᶜˑᵇ
Uric acid	mg/dL	2.3-10ᶜ	2.3-11ᶜ	2.3-11ᶜ	2.2-9.9ᶜ	2.3-12ᶜ	2.3-11ᶜ	1.9-11ᶜ	1.5-11ᶜ	2.0-11ᶜ	2.2-11ᶜ	2.2-12ᶜ	2.2-10ᶜ

[a] Data for adults of both sexes, as obtained from Hawkey CM, Samour JH. The value of clinical hematology in exotic birds. In: Jacobson ER, Kollias GV, Jr, editors. Exotic animals: contemporary issues in small animal practice. London: Churchill Livingstone; 1988.

[b] The data are referred to the *Amazona* and *Ara* groups.

[c] Data for adults of both sexes, as obtained from The Californian Avian Laboratory, Citrus Heights, CA 95621, Reference range 1998 from Fudge AM. Laboratory reference ranges for selected avian, mammalian, and reptilian species. In: Fudge AM, editor. Laboratory medicine: avian and exotic pets. Philadelphia: WB Saunders; 2000. p. 376-400.

[d] Data for adults of both sexes, as obtained from The Avian and Wildlife Laboratory, University of Miami School Medicine, Miami, FL 33136.

Table 11
Reference ranges for protein electrophoresis in some psittacines species/groups

Fraction	Reference Range (g/dL)
Amazona spp.	
Prealbumin	0.35–1.05
Albumin	1.9–3.52
Alpha-1	0.05–0.32
Alpha-2	0.07–0.32
Beta	0.12–0.72
Gamma	0.17–0.76
Ratio A/G	1.9–5.9
Ara spp.	
Prealbumin	0.05–0.7
Albumin	1.24–3.11
Alpha-1	0.04–0.25
Alpha-2	0.04–0.31
Beta	0.14–0.62
Gamma	0.1–0.62
Ratio A/G	1.6–4.3
Cacatua spp.	
Prealbumin	0.24–1.18
Albumin	1.8–3.1
Alpha-1	0.05–0.18
Alpha-2	0.04–0.36
Beta	0.22–0.82
Gamma	0.21–0.65
Ratio A/G	2.0–4.5
Nymphicus hollandicus	
Prealbumin	0.8–1.6
Albumin	0.7–1.8
Alpha-1	0.05–0.4
Alpha-2	0.05–0.44
Beta	0.21–0.58
Gamma	0.11–0.43
Ratio A/G	1.5–4.3
Psittacus erithacus	
Prealbumin	0.03–1.35
Albumin	1.57–3.23
Alpha-1	0.02–0.27
Alpha-2	0.12–0.31
Beta	0.15–0.56
Gamma	0.11–0.71
Ratio A/G	1.6–4.3
Eclectus	
Prealbumin	0.4–1.04
Albumin	2.3–2.6

(continued on next page)

Table 11 (continued)	
Fraction	Reference Range (g/dL)
Alpha-1	0.09–0.33
Alpha-2	0.11–0.27
Beta	0.17–0.43
Gamma	0.18–0.55
Ratio A/G	2.62–4.05
Conure	
Prealbumin	0.18–0.98
Albumin	1.9–2.6
Alpha-1	0.04–0.23
Alpha-2	0.08–0.26
Beta	0.07–0.47
Gamma	0.12–0.61
Ratio A/G	2.2–4.3

Values from the Avian and Wildlife Laboratory, University of Miami, School Medicine, Miami, FL 33136. Beckman Paragon system protein electrophoresis.

mean an aspecific pathologic condition if the data are considered by themself. Bile acids have a medium percentage of abnormal values and show increased values. The muscle enzymes except AST/GPT have a higher percentage (highest LDH) of abnormal values. This fact may also depend on intramuscular injection, forced exercise, handling and traumatic injuries while travelling to the practice or during restraint. The marked artifactual effects that can affect LDH plasma activity should not be forgotten. Creatinine values are nearly always within the range. This confirms that this test is rarely useful in routine profiles.[60] Considering protein electrophoresis, there is a higher percentage of abnormal decreased values of prealbumin, whereas the percentage of abnormal decreased values of albumin are much lower. This could also be an analytical error because of the different chemical and molecular features of the different protein fractions (prealbumin) of different species of psittacines and different methods.[72–74] α- and β-globulin fractions have a higher percentage of increased values that are compatible with leukocytosis and heterophilia (acute-subacute inflammatory condition), and a high percentage of decreased values of the A/G ratio. We have only seen 2 cases of increased A/G ratio in relation to a decrease in globulin fractions and an increase in albumin. The γ-globulins have a higher percentage of marked decreased values. This could be explained by the fact that the normal γ-globulin fractions are usually lower[72] or by a state of chronic stress or immunodeficiency.[16,51,75] The percentage of total proteins with increased values (24%) is not increased and the percentage of decreased values is even less (7%).

Considering the abnormal results of hematologic and biochemical tests found in different diseases, in the first group of infectious diseases (as seen in **Table 14**), during air sac infection, there are only abnormal values for the total leukocyte count with 1 case of heteropenia and 2 cases of moderate heterophilia, marked monocytosis, and lymphopenia. Toxic heterophils are always present to a marked degree and this suggests a degenerative response and poor prognosis.[1,8–10] We observed hypoglycemia (compatible with severe anorexia and/or septicemia), an increase in plasma levels of uric acid (dehydration or secondary renal disorders),[16,51,59] and 1 case of

---

Box 1
List of diseases diagnosed

Infectious diseases

Air sac infection (4)

Bacterial infection (13)

Fungal infection (3)

Chlamydiosis (22)

Viral infection (14)

Organic-related diseases

Enteritis (5)

Cloacal disease (3)

Liver disease (12)

Renal disease (3)

Heart disease (3)

Neurologic disorders (2)

Osteomalacia (2)

Reproductive disorders (3)

Miscellaneous diseases

Feather and beak disorders (8)

Behavioral disorders (8)

Dietary disorders (11)

Gizzard foreign bodies (6)

Zinc toxicosis (4)

Pediatric pathologies (4)

Trauma (2)

Neoplasia (1)

Check (17)[a]

Total (150)

[a] The check group represents the data obtained for those psittacines (for the most part from breeding centers or pet shops) with a high risk of disease but still without symptoms.

---

marked increase in all globulin fractions and marked decrease in the A/G ratio (compatible with a heavy inflammatory and antibody stimulus).[75] In the second group (bacterial infections), (where there are more cases), we observed 5 cases of marked anemia with only 2 of them showing a regenerative response and almost every time moderate to marked leukocytosis with heterophylia, monocytosis, lymphopenia and 2 cases of heteropenia.

Biochemical parameters did not provide useful information about the abnormal serum biochemistry values due to organ infection, as reported in the literature,[77] except the plasma glucose levels and electrophoretic patterns. The plasma glucose levels were severely decreased in 4 cases (similar to aerosacculitis) and there were 3 cases of hypoalbuminemia with a markedly decreased A/G ratio; in 1 of them, the

Table 12
Comparison between different psittacine species and different diseases

Infection Disease	Amazons (44)	Macaws (43)	Ecletto (1)	Conures (2)	Cockatoos (18)	Cockatiels (3)	African Grays (39)	Total
Air sac infection (4)	0	2	0	0	0	0	2	4
Bacterial infection (13)	5	2	0	0	2	1	3	13
Chlamydiosis (22)	7	14	0	0	0	0	1	22
Fungal infection (3)	0	1	0	0	0	0	2	3
Viral infection (14)	2	8	0	0	2	0	2	14
Organ-related disease								
Enteritis (5)	1	2	0	0	0	0	2	5
Cloacal disease (3)	1	1	0	0	0	0	1	3
Liver disease (12)	10	1	0	0	1	0	0	12
Renal disease (3)	2	0	0	0	0	0	1	3
Hearth disease (3)	1	0	0	0	0	0	2	3
Neurologic disorders (2)	0	0	0	0	0	0	2	2
Osteomalacia (2)	0	0	0	0	0	0	2	2
Reproductive disorders (3)	1	2	0	0	0	0	0	3
Miscellaneous diseases								
Feather and beak disorders (8)	1	1	0	0	4	0	2	8
Behavioral disorders (8)	0	3	0	0	1	2	2	8
Dietary disorders (11)	2	0	0	1	2	0	6	11
Gizzard foreign bodies (6)	1	0	0	1	2	0	2	6
Zinc toxicosis (4)	0	2	1	0	0	0	1	4
Pediatric pathologies (4)	0	2	0	0	2	0	0	4
Check (17)[a]	9	2	0	0	2	0	4	17
Total (150)	44	43	1	2	18	3	39	150

[a] The group named check represents data that were obtained in psittacines (for the most part from breeding centers or pet shops) at high risk of disease but still without symptoms.

Table 13
Total absolute number and percentage for tests with normal, decreased, and increased values

Test	Total	Decreased Value	Increased Value	n	% Decreased	% Increased	% Abnormal
Hematocrit	134	29	28	77	22	21	43
Total protein	125	9	30	86	7	24	31
Hemoglobin	115	16	57	42	14	50	64
RBC	115	27	21	67	24	18	42
WBC	150	30	67	53	20	45	65
Lymphocytes (%)	150	38	27	85	25	18	43
Monocytes (%)	150	0	67	83	0	45	45
Heterophils (%)	150	31	56	63	21	37	58
Eosinophils (%)	150	0	3	147	0	2	2
Basophils (%)	150	0	0	150	0	0	0
Anisocytosis/ poikilocytosis	150	0	13	137	0	9	9
Polychromasia	150	0	24	126	0	16	16
Band heterophils	150	0	23	127	0	15	15
Toxic heterophils	20	0	21	129	0	14	14
Zinc	31	0	21	10	0	67	67
Calcium	68	3	19	46	4	28	32
Ionized calcium	37	8	8	21	22	22	44
Phosphorus	51	10	15	26	20	29	49
Sodium	51	4	21	26	8	41	49
Potassium	55	20	15	20	36	28	64
Bile acids	74	12	26	36	16	36	52
Glucose	128	43	2	83	34	1	35
Uric acid	130	31	12	87	24	9	33
Amylase	41	6	20	15	15	49	64
Creatinine	41	3	7	31	7	17	24
CPK	107	9	50	48	8	47	55
Cholesterol	39	1	16	22	3	41	44
LDH	103	18	54	31	17	52	69
AST	129	18	32	79	14	25	39
Prealbumin	75	27	2	46	36	3	39
Albumin	75	17	3	55	23	4	27
α_1-Globulin	74	9	14	51	12	19	31
α_2-Globulin	74	9	27	38	12	36	48
β-Globulin	74	7	25	42	10	34	44
γ-Globulin	74	29	12	33	39	16	55
A/G ratio	75	30	2	43	40	3	43

globulin fractions were all increased. In another case, we observed a decrease in γ-globulin. This can be explained by the fact that in bacterial infections, the changes are most evident in the acute phases, whereas the changes tend to be moderate in the chronic phases.[72,75] Moreover, the continued stress of some chronic forms can lead to a decrease in the γ-globulin fractions. According to literature, there have been the greatest number of abnormalities in chlamydiosis cases occurring in more parameters.[78] Even in this case the complete blood cell counts have given useful indications. In 5 cases the hematocrit was higher and in 4 cases hyperproteinemia was present. This may indicate dehydration and/or inflammation. No cases of regenerative or depressive anemia have been observed although they are reported in literature.[1,10,78] More severe leukocytosis than in bacterial diseases has been observed with lymphocytosis and monocytosis. It is reported that in Amazons the classic chlamydial leukogram shows marked leukocytosis with monocytosis; lymphocytosis with reactive lymphocytes may be seen. In macaws, leukocytosis can be important and in acute case can exceeded 100,000/mm³.[78] Leukopenia with marked heteropenia was also observed. The high-grade toxic heterophils were not always present, but when present, they confirm the severity of the disease, especially in ocular and upper respiratory tract, chronic forms or in sepsis. Major changes in biochemical parameters were also seen in this disease. Uric acid and glucose plasma levels seem to be markedly decreased in half of the cases and AST and CPK plasma activity markedly increased. Increased levels of bile acids in plasma were less frequent. Seeing such a large variety of abnormalities should induce the clinician to widen the investigation to confirm or exclude chlamydiosis. Even the electrophoretic pattern is often altered with peaks in α- and β-globulins (acute phase proteins and acute inflammatory process), hyperproteinemia, and decreased A/G ratio. In some cases, the electrophoresis test helps in the interpretation of serologic antibody tests for the diagnosis of this disease, because the globulin fractions may increase before the antibody response does.[75]

In fungal diseases, (only 3 cases) we have found 2 cases of heterophilic leukocytosis with toxic heterophils and 1 case of degenerative heteropenia. These diseases affect the respiratory system and they are often nonresponsive to treatment and have a poor prognosis. The only abnormality concerning biochemical parameters was the marked decrease of ionized calcium, which could be due to alkalosis,[64] artifactual errors, or to the many causes of organ-related loss.

In cases of viral disease, we have seen some increases in PCV together with increased proteins (severe dehydration). There were more cases of leukocytosis with lymphocytosis and monocytosis or heterophilia (antibody stimulation and/or viral infection complicated by other diseases), but there were also cases of leukopenia with heteropenia and monocytosis and/or lymphopenia with monocytosis (as reported in the literature on viral diseases).[1,8–10,47] In this case, we have observed hypoglycemia and marked increases in both muscular and hepatic enzyme activities. These increases may be caused by neurologic disorders or vomiting (muscle enzymes) or concomitant liver disease (AST). Alterations in potassium, phosphorus, and sodium could be explained by the involvement of the kidneys or gastrointestinal tract. These data are not specific, but might be useful to guide nutritional support and therapy. Furthermore, we have observed 4 cases showing increased β; and γ-globulin fractions, but rare increases in α-globulin fractions, and no hypoalbuminemia and decreases in the A/G ratio. These results can be related to acute-subacute forms in the presence of an immune response. In enteritis, we found only rare outliers represented by the frequent increase in LDH activity (LDH activity is a nonspecific test because it is present in all organs) and a decrease in glucose and uric acid levels (prolonged fasting). In cloacal diseases (even though there were few cases), we observed alterations caused by chronic damage (mostly papillomatosis with chronic prolapses). Leukocytosis with moderate heterophilia and marked monocytosis were registered and severe leucopenia and heteropenia was seen only in 1 case (cloacal calculi). In the electrophoretic pattern, the authors noted a decreased A/G ratio with increased β- or α₁-globulin fractions (acute phase inflammatory proteins). Occasional increases

Table 14
Hematologic and biochemical data grouped by infectious disease

	Air Sac Infection (4)						Bacterial Infection (13)						Chlamydiosis (22)						Funfal Infection (3)						Viral Infection (14)					
	-1	-2	-3	+1	+2	+3	-1	-2	-3	+1	+2	+3	-1	-2	-3	+1	+2	+3	-1	-2	-3	+1	+2	+3	-1	-2	-3	+1	+2	+3
Hematocrit	1							4	1					2		5		1			1						4	1	
TRBC			—					4	1						2								1	3			1			
TWBC	1			2			2			3	3	3	4			6	1	6	1			2				3		5	1	1
Hemoglobin			—					1	3	1			3			9			1			1				6				
Lymphocytes	1						5		3	3	2	1	1			2	2	1	1							1	3	2		
Monocytes						3				3	2	1					4	6												3
Heterophils		1					1					6	6			3		5		1		2				3			3	2
Eosinophils						1			—						—						—						—			
Amylase			—									3				1		2						1		2				1
AST	2			2				2				4	6			4	2	2	2			1				3	2			1
Bile acid	1			1					1			6	6			1		1				—							1	1
Calcium			—					1					7		1			2				—								
Cholesterol			—				1	1					1					1				—						1		
CPK				1			1					4	2			2	2	3				2				1		1	1	6

Creatinine	—				1		1				—
Ionized calcium	—	1					2				2
Glucose	2	2	2	3	3	2		3	2	1	
LDH		1	1	4	3		—	2		1	4	2
Phosphorus		—	1		3			2	1	1	2
Potassium	1	4				1	1	2	1	1	2
Sodium	—		2	1		—		3			
Total protein	—	2		1	2	2	1	1	3	2
Uric acid	1	1	1	3	1	3	1	1	1	1	1
Zinc	1	—		2	1					
Prealbumin	1	1		1	1	1	1	1
Albumin	1	2		1	2	2	1	1
α₁-Globulin	1		2	1	—	2	2	1
α₂-Globulin	1	1	1	1	2	2	1	1
β-Globulin	1		1	1	3	4	1	2
γ-Globulin	1	2	1	3	3	1		2	2
A/G ratio	1	2	2	5	1	1	2	1	2

Score: −1, low decrease; −2, mild decrease; −3, severe decrease; +1, low increase; +2, mild increase; +3, severe increase.

Table 15
Hematologic and biochemical data grouped by organ-related disease

	Enteritis (3)						Cloacal Disease (3)						Liver Disease (12)						Heart Disease (3)						Renal Disease (3)						Reproductive Disorders (3)					
	−1	−2	−3	+1	+2	+3	−1	−2	−3	+1	+2	+3	−1	−2	−3	+1	+2	+3	−1	−2	−3	+1	+2	+3	−1	−2	−3	+1	+2	+3	−1	−2	−3	+1	+2	+3
Hematocrit	1	1							—				3	1	3			1						1			—									1
TRBC	1								1				3	1							—						1	1					1			
TWBC	—							1	2				3							1						2	1				2					
Hemoglobin		1							1					6						1						2					3					
Lymphocytes	1								2					1						1						2			1			2				
Monocytes				2					1	1					2	2								3					3							1
Heterophils		1						1	2						3											2	1		1							
Eosinophils	—								—								1		—						—						—					
Amylase	—								—						1		2		—										1				1			
AST		2						1	3						3		2		—						—									1		
Bile acid		—							1						3	3		1		1	1				—						—					
Calcium	1								1						1										—				1				—			
Cholesterol	—								—						1				—						—				1		—					
CPK	1							1	2						1	2							2						1							1

Parameter	Scores
Creatinine	— — 2 1 2 1 1
Ionized calcium	— — 2 1 1 1 1 1 1
Glucose	2 1 1 2 1 2 1 1 1 1 — —
LDH	1 3 1 2 2 2 2 1 1 1 —
Phosphorus	1 1 1 2 1 1 1 2
Potassium	— 1 1 2 1 2 1 3 3
Sodium	— 1 1 3 3 2
Total protein	1 1 3 1 1 1 1
Uric acid	2 1 1 2 3 1 1 2 1 1
Zinc	1 1 2 1
Prealbumin	— — — — —
Albumin	— 1 1 1 1
α_1-Globulin	— 1 1 —
α_2-Globulin	1 1 2 1 1 1 1
β-Globulin	— 1 2 2 1 — 2
γ-Globulin	— 1 2 1 —
A/G ratio	2 2 1 2 2 — —

Score: −1, low decreased; −2, mild decreased; −3, severe decreased; +1, low increased; +2, mild increased; +3, severe increased.

Table 16
Hematologic and biochemical data grouped by miscellaneous disease

	Feather and Beak Disorders (8)						Behavioral Disorders (8)						Dietary Disorders (8)						Gizzard Foreign Bodies (6)						Zinc Toxicosis (4)						Pediatric Pathologies (4)					
	−1	−2	−3	+1	+2	+3	−1	−2	−3	+1	+2	+3	−1	−2	−3	+1	+2	+3	−1	−2	−3	+1	+2	+3	−1	−2	−3	+1	+2	+3	−1	−2	−3	+1	+2	+3
Hematocrit	1			2			1		3	2					3	2					1	2					1	1						2		
TRBC	1			3					3	3					1	3						1					—	1					—			
TWBC	3		1	5					3	3					5	1		1				3					—	1						4		
Hemoglobin	1			4					2	3					2	2						3						1								1
Lymphocytes	2							2	3	3					3	3		3	3			1						2								1
Monocytes				3	1			2	2	3						3						2	2						2							2
Heterophils	1	1		1			1			1	1	4	2		1	5			1			3		2				1	1					1		
Eosinophils	—							—						—				1				—				—						—				
Amylase	—									1				—						—								1							2	
AST	2						4									3		1					1		—			1			—					
Bile acid	2						1									1		1			—			1				1			—					
Calcium	1								1					1							—						—									
Cholesterol				1					—							3					—						—									
CPK			3					3		3						3						3					1								1	
Creatinine	—							—						—						—																—

Ionized calcium	—		—		—		—		—		—		—		—
Glucose	1		1		1		1		2		4				
LDH	1 1		1		5 1		1		2 1		2	—	1		2
Phosphorus	—		—		—		—								1
Potassium	2		1		1		1								1
Sodium	—		—		—		—		3				—		4
Total protein	1		1		3		3		2		3		—		3
Uric acid	2 1		1		1 1		3		1				1		1
Zinc	2		1		3		3		2		1 3				
Prealbumin	1		3		1		1					1			
Albumin	1		—		1 1		—					—			
α_1-Globulin	—		1		1 1		1					—		2	
α_2-Globulin	—		1		3 2		—					2		2	
β-Globulin	1		—		1 1		1					1			1
γ-Globulin	1 1		—		2		2		1			1		1	
A/G ratio	1		4		1 1		1		1			1		1	

Score: −1, low decreased; −2, mild decreased; −3, severe decreased; +1, low increased; +2, mild increased; +3, severe increased.

in enzyme muscle activities and glucose could depend on chronic stress and/or on the muscular effort for defecation.

Liver disease may not always have an inflammatory cause and therefore may not induce hematologic changes. We observed both anemia and false polycythemia (dehydration). Moderate heterophilia (25%) and marked leukopenia and heteropenia (25%) were not constant findings, whereas we always found relative monocytosis. Marked leukopenia and heteropenia may indicate a poor prognosis and may occur in viral diseases (eg, Pacheco parrot disease).[47] The most common alteration was increased bile plasma levels (50%); this value cannot differentiate the kind of liver disease but it always means hepatic damage.[9] These increases are not necessarily accompanied by increases in AST activities.[75] They can increase in cases of multiorgan lesions, such as in chlamydiosis or in bacteremia and septicemia, but sometimes they do not increase in liver disease as shown here. We have reported 2 cases of reduction of these enzyme activities as reported in the case of hepatic mass reduction.[4] The sporadic increases of other enzymes were certainly nonspecific. Plasma levels of uric acid (as expected) were found increased, decreased, and in most cases normal; this metabolite in the blood is the sum of secretion by the liver and renal elimination. Electrophoresis can help in the diagnosis of hepatitis and in monitoring this disease. As reported in literature, not all increases in all globulin fractions have been highlighted, and the highest incidence was in the increase of α_2-globulin and β-globulin, with a consequent decrease in the A/G ratio.[75] Two cases of increase in the A/G ratio due to a decrease in the β- and γ-globulin fractions (possible virus infection or analytical error for an altered migration of the bands) should also be noted.[16,51,75]

In kidney disease, we observed an increase in those parameters traditionally linked to kidney disorders (creatinine and phosphorus), although these could be possible artifactual increases in both tests.[4,5,49,79] The decreases in electrolytes, such as K, Na and phosphorus, may depend on the marked polydipsia and polyuria. All these parameters do not allow a diagnosis of kidney disease and certainly the most useful test could be the electrophoresis.[75] In our study, we noted a single case of increased α_1-globulin fractions without other changes.

In heart disease, we only observed increases in muscle enzyme activities (CPK and LDH), always relative to monocytosis and marked reduction of plasma levels of uric acid. These data show that aspecific muscle damage is possibly related or not related to this disease.[79]

In neurologic disorders and osteomalacia (not shown in **Table 15** because of the low number of cases), the psittacine species most affected were African gray parrots and there was a marked decrease both in total calcium and ionized calcium plasma levels and a marked increase in muscle enzyme activities. This confirms what is reported in the literature, that an assessment of ionized calcium is useful for confirming hypocalcemia, which, in this case, was also responsible for neurologic disorders.[16,64]

Regarding reproductive disorders, there are no significant alterations. We have reported only 1 marked increase in plasma levels of potassium and uric acid in the absence of any marked abnormalities. It is possible that in reproductive phases or reproductive disorders, lipemic plasma arose[4,5,53] creating an analytical error.

In the third group (miscellaneous diseases as in **Box 1**), we found some typical parrot diseases such as feather and beak disorders. In these conditions, the TWBC counts showed moderate decreases or increases and the most variable component was lymphocytes followed by heterophils and monocytes. A possible explanation for lymphocytosis may be a continuous immune stimulus or an immune-mediated form, whereas lymphopenia may be caused by a chronic stressor (prolonged sexual feather picking or severe feather picking) or viruses (PBFD).[1,8–10,64] Apart from an increase in CPK activity (caused by forced exercise or excitement), we did not observe anything else.

In behavioral disorders, which can be a cause of feather picking or at least be linked to this, no significant abnormalities were registered, besides 1 case where there was leukocytosis with lymphocytosis and others presenting stress leukograms. Monocytosis was always present. There were also increases in CPK plasma enzyme activities, which can be due to excess exercise. So, being cautious and because the issue is manifold and still misunderstood, we could observe some small differences in the leukogram (lymphocytosis or lymphopenia vs stress leukogram) between feather destructive behaviors and pure behavioral disorders.

In the hematologic and biochemical values of dietary disorders, there were a high number of cases of moderated leukopenia with lymphopenia or heteropenia and only 1 case of moderated leukocytosis with lymphocytosis and heterophilia. This occurrence may not even have any diagnostic usefulness. We have also noted moderate increases in bile acids and an increase in cholesterol in 3 cases, which so often appears only in this disease. High cholesterol levels may be observed in metabolic and liver disease and are frequently related to dietary disorders.[51,60,79] We also reported increases in α_1- and α_2-globulin fractions with decreases in the A/G ratio in 35% of cases. This occurrence could correlate with the increase in cholesterol, possible liver disease, or with underlying hormonal conditions such as hypothyroidism.

In gizzard foreign bodies, we often found leukocytosis with heterophilia and monocytosis and lymphopenia. The absence of banded heterophils suggests that they are stress leukograms and monocytosis can be caused by a penetrating injury and irritation of the tissues. Other abnormal data found were decreased plasma levels of uric acid and a case of hypoglycemia, both probably connected to prolonged starving and/or absorption disorders. There were marked increases in muscle enzymes (with exclusion of AST) caused by possible perforations through the muscle layer or excessive efforts related to dysphagia and vomiting. The finding of increased of plasma levels of zinc, often feared in gizzard metallic foreign bodies, does not show differences with increased values found in other diseases. As reported by Fudge,[79] the identification of a metal foreign body in the gastrointestinal tract is not specific for zinc or heavy metal toxicosis. Evaluation of plasma levels of zinc, if not markedly increased and accompanied by typical symptoms, can be misleading and in this case must be assessed with care, also considering the different species and their feeding habits; for example, cockatiels, typical seed eaters, normally show lower levels of zinc than Amazons.[80] In the 4 cases reported as suspected zinc poisoning, abnormal hematologic and blood chemistry values were absent or nonspecific, such as moderate heterophilia as reported in the literature.[80] In these cases, the zinc value exceeded 400 µg/dL and the animals showed symptoms of zinc poisoning. Some species such as cockatoos and the Eclectus parrots already mentioned have higher plasma levels of zinc even in healthy birds.[76] In 3 cases that do not belong to this group, we found nonspecific increases in plasma levels of zinc, even though the birds did not have symptoms of zinc toxicosis; in 2 of these cases, the diagnosis was feather picking in accordance with what it is reported.[80]

With regard to pediatric diseases, all patients showed heterophilia and 1 bird had marked lymphocytosis. These data should be critically evaluated and considered pathologic when marked and in young healthy birds, there can also be a higher total white cell count with heterophilia. Lymphocytosis is usually rare in young animals but can be caused by stimulation of the immune system. The total proteins were also increased. This, however, can indicate inflammation or dehydration because normally young birds have lower values. In the 2 cases, a high PCV can suggest dehydration, whereas an increase in α_1- and α_2-globulin in the same patient could suggest a problem of acute inflammation. The 2 cases of trauma did not give any indications, but excluded the presence of severe bleeding and needed more controls. The case of neoplasm, even though unique, showed a marked increase in α_2- and β-globulin fractions and a marked decrease in the A/G ratio. In this case, the animal had a neoplasm but also a serious bacterial infection with a granulomatous process; furthermore, we believe this had been ongoing for a long time. This bird also had marked leukocytosis and lymphomonocytosis as a response to a chronic bacterial process and malignant neoplasm. The other values were not specific to add useful information for the diagnosis and prognosis. Clearly in this case, as in others, the final diagnosis was histologic for the neoplasm and microbiologic for the bacterial infection. In this article, the results of histology, serology (antibody test), microbiology for bacterial and fungal diseases, and PCR tests, are not fully described although these, along with other diagnostic tests, have often allowed a diagnosis to be confirmed that would not otherwise be made.

In the cases in the check group, the abnormal values are not specific, for example, moderated leukopenia with heteropenia (23%) and moderated leukocytosis with heterophilia and/or lymphocytosis (23%). The other abnormalities that can be highlighted are nonspecific moderate decreases in many parameters and moderate increases in plasma levels of LDH. These results could be artifactual decreases, because most of these blood samples were collected from birds located in other premises and consequentially were processed 12 hours after collection. For this reason, these data should be critically evaluated and eventually rechecked to clarify the underlying pathologies. The laboratory must remember that it is not the blood sample that is sick, but the patient, and the veterinarian needs to understand that sure and universal analytical information cannot be obtained from a single sample of blood, maybe even badly taken.

ACKNOWLEDGMENTS

We are grateful to the staff of the CSV laboratory for their assistance in testing the psittacine blood samples and particularly to Silvia Lubelli and Simona Eterno as well as the clinical pathologist Gabriele Ghisleni for improving this article. We are extremely grateful to Enrico Parravicini for his contribution in writing the text.

REFERENCES

1. Campbell TW. Hematology of birds. In: Thrall MA, editor. Veterinary hematology and clinical chemistry. Philadelphia: Lippincott Williams &Wilkins; 2004. p. 225–58.
2. Lucas AJ, Jamroz C. Atlas of avian hematology. USD A monograph 25. Washington, DC: US Department of Agriculture; 1961.
3. Howlett JC. Clinical and diagnostic procedures. In: Samour JH, editor. Avian medicine. 1st edition. London: Mosby; 2000. p. 28–50.
4. Fudge AM. Blood testing artifacts: interpretation and prevention. Semin Avian Exotic Pet Med 1994;3:2–4.
5. Fudge AM. Avian blood sampling and artifact considerations. In: Fudge AM, editor. Avian laboratory medicine. Philadelphia: WB Saunders; 2000. p. 1–8.

6. Ivey ES. A selecting a commercial diagnostic laboratory. Semin Avian Exotic Pet Med 2001;10:72–6.
7. Clark P, Boardman WS, Raidal SR. Atlas of clinical avian hematology. Oxford (United Kingdom): Wiley- Blackwell; 2009.
8. Campbell TW. Hematology of birds. In: Campbell TW, Ellis CK, editors. Avian and exotic animal hematology and cytology. 3rd edition. Ames (IA): Blackwell; 2007. p. 3–50.
9. Van der Heiden N. Evaluation and interpretation of the avian hemogram. Semin Avian Exotic Pet Med 1994;3:5–13.
10. Campbell TW. Normal hematology of psittacines. In: Feldman BF, Zinkl JG, Jain NG, editors. Schalm's veterinary hematology. 5th edition. Baltimore (MD): Lippincott Williams & Wilkins; 2000. p. 1155–60.
11. Hawkey CM, Hart MG, Knight JA, et al. Hematological findings in healthy and sick African grey parrots (*Psittacus erithacus*). Vet Rec 1982;111:580–2.
12. Tell LA, Citino SB. Hematologic and serum chemistry reference intervals for Cuban Amazon parrots *(Amazona leucocephala leucocephala)*. J Zoo Wildl Med 1992;23:62–4.
13. Scope A, Schwendenwein I, Frommlet F. Influence of outlying values and variations between sampling days on reference ranges for clinical chemistry in budgerigars (*Melopsittacus undulatus*). Vet Rec 2005;156:310–4.
14. Scope A, Schwendenwein I, Enders F, et al. Hematologic and clinical chemistry reference values in red lories (*Eos* spp.). Avian Dis 2000;44:885–90.
15. Dein FJ. Laboratory manual of avian hematology. East Northport (NY): Association of Avian Veterinarians; 1984.
16. Harr KE. Clinical chemistry of companion avian species: a review. Vet Clin Pathol 2002;31:140–51.
17. Meyer DJ, Harvey JW. Veterinary laboratory medicine: interpretation and diagnosis. 2nd edition. Philadelphia: WB Saunders; 1992.
18. Hawkey CM, Dennett TB. Color atlas of comparative veterinary hematology. London: Wolfe Medical Publications; 1989.
19. Campbell TW. Avian hematology and cytology. Ames (IA): Iowa State University Press; 1988.
20. Walberg J. White blood cell counting techniques in birds. Semin Avian Exotic Pet Med 2001;10:72–6.
21. Lumeij JT. A contribution to clinical investigative methods for birds, with special reference to the racing pigeon (*Columbia livia domestica*) [thesis]. Utrecht (Netherlands): Proefschrift; 1987.
22. Lumeij JT. Fasting and postprandial bile acid concentrations in racing pigeons *(Columbia livia domestica)* and mallards *(Anas platyrhynchus)*. J Assoc Avian Vet 1991;5:197–200.
23. Davidson I, Henry JB. Todd-Sanford clinical diagnosis by laboratory methods. 15th edition. Philadelphia: WB Saunders; 1974.
24. Campbell TW, Dein FJ. Avian hematology: the basics. Vet Clin North Am Small Anim Pract 1984;14:223–48.
25. Samour JH, Naldo JL, John SK. Normal haematological values of captive gyr falco (*Falco rusticolus*). Vet Rec 2005;157:844–7.
26. Fudge AM. Laboratory reference ranges for selected avian, mammalian, and reptilian species. In: Fudge AM, editor. Laboratory medicine: avian and exotic pets. Philadelphia: WB Saunders; 2000. p. 376–400.
27. Lilliehook I, Wall H, Tauson R, et al. Differential leukocyte counts determined in chicken blood using the Cell-Dyn 3500. Vet Clin Pathol 2004;33:133–8.

28. Green RA, Blue-Mclendon A. Ratite hematology. In: Feldman BF, Zinkl JG, Jain NG, editors. Schalm's veterinary hematology. 5th edition. Baltimore (MD): Lippincott Williams & Wilkins; 2000. p. 1201–6.
29. Fudge AM. Clinical hematology and chemistry of ratites. In: Tully TN, Shane SM, editors. Ratite management, medicine & surgery. Malabar (FL): Kreiger; 1996.
30. Fudge AM. Avian complete blood count. In: Fudge AM, editor. Avian laboratory medicine. Philadelphia: WB Saunders; 2000. p. 9–18.
31. Robertson GW, Maxwell MH. Modified staining techniques for avian blood cells. Br Poult Sci 1990;31:881–6.
32. Russo EA, McEntee L, Applegate L, et al. Comparison of two methods for determination of white blood cell counts in macaws. J Am Vet Med Assoc 1986;189:1013–6.
33. Weiss DJ. Uniform evaluation and semiquantitative reporting of hematologic data in veterinary laboratories. Vet Clin Pathol 1984;13:27–31.
34. Rebar AH, Lewis HB, De Nicola DB, et al. Red cell fragmentation in the dog: an editorial review. Vet Pathol 1981;18:415–26.
35. Bessis M. Blood smears reinterpreted. Berlin: Springer-Verlag; 1977.
36. Zinkl JG. Avian hematology. In: Jain CJ, editor. Schalm's veterinary hematology. Philadelphia: Lea & Febiger; 1986. p. 256–73.
37. Romagnano A, Barnes HJ, Perkins P, et al. Binucleate erythrocytes and erythrocytic dysplasia in a cockatiel. Proc Assoc Avian Vet 1994;10:83–6.
38. Fudge AM. Disorders of avian erythrocytes. In: Fudge AM, editor. Avian laboratory medicine. Philadelphia: WB Saunders; 2000. p. 28–34.
39. Dein FJ. Hematology. In: Harrison GJ, Harrison LR, editors. Clinical avian medicine and surgery. Philadelphia: WB Saunders; 1986. p. 174–91.
40. Sturkie PD. Blood: physical characteristics, formed elements, hemoglobin and coagulation. In: Sturkie PD, editor. Avian physiology. New York: Springer-Verlag; 1976. p. 53–75.
41. Gaskin JM. Psittacine viral diseases: a perspective. J Zoo Wildl Med 1989;20:249–64.
42. Taylor M. Polycythemia in the blue and gold macaw a case report of three cases. Proceedings of the First International Conference on zoological and avian medicine. Oahu, HI: Association of Avian Veterinarians and American Association of Zoo Veterinarians; 1987. p. 95–104.
43. Lane R. Basic techniques in pet avian clinical pathology. Vet Clin North Am Small Anim Pract 1991;21:1157–79.
44. Topp RC, Carlson HC. Studies on avian heterophils, II: histochemistry. Avian Dis 1972;16:369–73.
45. Topp RC, Carlson HC. Studies on avian heterophils, III: phagocytic properties. Avian Dis 1972;16:374–80.
46. Carlson HC, Hacking MA. Distribution of mast cells in chicken, turkey, pheasant, and quail and their differentiation from basophils. Avian Dis 1972;16:574–7.
47. Rosskopf WJ, Woerpel RW, Howard EB, et al. Chronic endocrine disorder associated with inclusion body hepatitis in a Sulfur crested Cockatoo. J Am Vet Med Assoc 1981;79:1273–6.
48. Grecchi R, Saliba AM, Mariano M. Morphological changes, surface receptors and phagocytic potential of fowl mononuclear phagocytes and thrombocytes in vivo and in vitro. J Pathol 1980;130:23–31.
49. Lumeij JT, Overduin LM. Plasma chemistry reference values in Psittaciformes. Avian Pathol 1990;19:235–44.
50. Campbell TW. Avian hematology and cytology. 2nd edition. Ames (IA): Iowa State University Press; 1995.

51. Campbell TW. Clinical biochemistry of birds. In: Thrall MA, editor. Veterinary hematology and clinical chemistry. Philadelphia: Lippincott Williams &Wilkins; 2004. p. 479–92.
52. Lumeij JT. Relation of plasma calcium to total protein and albumin in African grey *(Psittacus erithacus)* and Amazon *(Amazon spp)* parrots. Avian Pathol 1990;19: 661–7.
53. Lumeij JT. Avian clinical biochemistry. In: Kaneko JJ, Harvey JW, Brass ML, editors. Clinical biochemistry of domestic animals. San Diego (CA): Academic Press; 1997. p. 857–84.
54. Rosskopf WJ, Woerpel RW, editors. Diseases of cage and aviary birds. 3rd edition. Baltimore (MD): Williams & Wilkins; 1996. p. 1057–63.
55. Ritchie BW, Harrison GJ, Harrison LR, editors. Avian medicine: principles and application. Lake Worth (FL): Wingers Publishing; 1994. p. 1004–20.
56. Clubb SL, Schubot RM, Wolf S. Hematologic and serum biochemical reference intervals in juvenile macaws (*Ara* sp.). J Assoc Avian Vet 1991;5(1):16–26.
57. Braun EJ. Comparative aspects of the urinary concentrating process. Ren Physiol 1985;8:249–60.
58. Goldstein DL, Braun EJ. Structure and concentrating ability in the avian kidney. Am J Physiol 1989;256:501–9.
59. Phalen DN. Avian renal disorders. In: Fudge AM, editor. Avian laboratory medicine. Philadelphia: WB Saunders; 2000. p. 61–8.
60. Krautwald-Junghanns M. Aids to diagnosis. In: Cole BH, editor. Essential of avian medicine and surgery. 3rd edition. Oxford (United Kingdom): Blackwell; 2007. p. 56–102.
61. Lumeij JT. Avian clinical enzymology. Semin Avian Exotic Pet Med 1994;3:14–24.
62. Fudge AM. Avian liver and gastrointestinal testing. In: Fudge AM, editor. Avian laboratory medicine. Philadelphia: WB Saunders; 2000. p. 47–55.
63. Jenkins JR. Avian metabolic chemistries. Semin Avian Exotic Pet Med 1994;3: 23–52.
64. Stanford M. The significance of serum ionized calcium and 25-hydroxy-cholecalciferol (vitamin D_3) assays in African grey parrots. Exotic DVM 2003;5(3):1–6.
65. Rosskopf WJ, Woerpel RW. Pet avian conditions and syndromes. In: Rosskopf WJ, Woerpel RW, editors. Diseases of cage and aviary birds. 3rd edition. Baltimore (MD): Williams & Wilkins; 1996. p. 260–82.
66. Hoefer H. Bile acid testing in psittacine birds. Semin Avian Exotic Pet Med 1994; 3:33–7.
67. Itoh S, Imai T, Kondo M. Relationships between serum (ZZ)-bilirubin, its subtractions and biliverdin concentrations in infants at one-month check ups. Ann Clin Biochem 2001;38:323–8.
68. Cray C. Changes in clinical enzyme activity and bile acid levels in psittacine birds with altered liver function and disease. J Avian Med Surg 2008;22:17–24.
69. Lumeij JT, Maclean B. Total protein determination in pigeon plasma and serum: comparison of refractometric methods with the Biuret method. J Avian Med Surg 1996;10:150–2.
70. Lumeij JT, De Bruijne JJ. Evaluation of refractometric method for the determination of total protein in avian plasma or serum. Avian Pathol 1985;14:441–4.
71. Spano JS, Whitesides JF, Pedersoli WM, et al. Comparative albumin determinations in ducks, chickens, and turkeys by electrophoretic and dye-binding methods. Am J Vet Res 1988;49:325–6.
72. Cray C, Rodriguez M, Zaias J. Protein electrophoresis of psittacine plasma. Vet Clin Pathol 2007;36:64–72.

73. Cray C, Decker LS. Differences in protein fraction of avian plasma among three commercial electrophoresis system. J Avian Med Surg 2011;22:102–10.

74. Rosenthal KL, Johnston MS, Shofer FS, et al. Assessment of the reliability of plasma electrophoresis in birds. Am J Vet Res 2005;66:375–8.

75. Cray C, Tatum L. Applications of protein electrophoresis in avian diagnostics. J Avian Med Surg 1998;12:4–10.

76. Puschner B, Leger JS, Galey FD. Normal and toxic concentration in serum/plasma and liver of psittacines with respect to genus differences. J Vet Diagn Invest 1999;11:522–52.

77. Reavill D. Bacterial disease. In: Rosskopf WJ, Woerpel RW, editors. Diseases of cage and aviary birds. 3rd edition. Baltimore (MD): Williams & Wilkins; 1996. p. 596–612.

78. Fudge A. Avian chlamydiosis. In: Rosskopf WJ, Woerpel RW, editors. Diseases of cage and aviary birds. 3rd edition. Baltimore (MD): Williams & Wilkins; 1996. p. 573–85.

79. Rosskopf WJ, Woerpel RW. Using clinical pathology results in avian clinical medicine with case reports. In: Rosskopf WJ, Woerpel RW, editors. Diseases of cage and aviary birds. 3rd edition. Baltimore (MD): Williams & Wilkins; 1996. p. 836–51.

80. Fudge AM. Selected controversial topics in avian diagnostic testing. Semin Avian Exotic Pet Med 2001;10:96–101.

Diagnosis of Liver Disease in Domestic Ferrets (Mustela Putorius)

Minh Huynh, DVM*, Flora Laloi, DVM

KEYWORDS

- Ferret • Liver • Gallbladder • Hepatopathy • Hepatitis • Lipidosis
- Hepatic neoplasia • Biliary obstruction

KEY POINTS

- Liver disease in ferrets is often subclinical and underdiagnosed.
- Clinical pathology and diagnostic imaging are needed to guide clinicians but definite diagnosis is based on histopathologic lesions.
- Inflammatory digestive conditions can lead to ascending tract infection and hepatobiliary inflammation.
- Ferrets have a specific sensitivity to hepatic lipidosis.
- Incidence of hepatic neoplasia is high in ferrets.

INTRODUCTION

Liver diseases have been extensively described in small animal species and are believed common in pet ferrets (*Mustela putorius furo*). The disease remains often subclinical, which may lead to difficulties in diagnosing those conditions accurately. Blood examination and serum chemistry evaluation are useful tools in screening hepatic pathology and monitoring response to treatment. Diagnostic imaging allows visualization of liver abnormalities, especially gallbladder and bile duct disease. Ultimately, histopathology is often required for definitive diagnosis and staging of the lesions. Various diseases have been reported: inflammatory, infectious and toxic hepatitis, and hepatic lipidosis. Less commonly, neoplasia or other pathology may be seen. After a summary of anatomy and physiology of the ferret liver, hepatic diseases known in ferret species are reviewed with their subsequent diagnostic procedures.

Exotic Department, Centre Hospitalier Vétérinaire Fregis, 43 Avenue Aristide Briand, Arcueil 94110, France
* Corresponding author.
E-mail address: nacologie@gmail.com

Vet Clin Exot Anim 16 (2013) 121–144
http://dx.doi.org/10.1016/j.cvex.2012.10.003
1094-9194/13/$ – see front matter © 2013 Elsevier Inc. All rights reserved.

ANATOMY AND PHYSIOLOGY
Anatomy

The liver is the largest visceral organ in all vertebrates. The ferret has a large liver compared with other companion mammals, representing 4.3% of the body weight, compared with 3.4% for a dog.[1,2] Normal weight ranges from 35 g to 59 g.[1] Anatomy and physiology of biliary tract in ferrets are similar to those of others mammals.[2] There are 6 lobes recognized in ferrets: left and right medial, left and right lateral, and quadrate and caudate lobes.

The gallbladder is located in a fossa formed by the quadrate lobe on the left and the right medial lobe. As in the other mammals, it is pear-shaped, is approximately 1 cm × 2 cm, and holds a volume of 0.5 mL to 1 mL.[2] Hepatocytes secrete bile that is drained by capillaries between cells. Bile capillaries join to form interlobular ducts, then bile duct. The cystic duct joins the right, central, and left ducts to form the common bile duct. The pancreatic duct usually joins the common bile duct, entering the lumen of the duodenum at the duodenal papilla approximately 2.8 cm caudal to the cranial duodenal flexure. Occasionally, an accessory papilla is present.[2] Accessory gallbladder has been reported in 2 ferrets without any concurrent clinical signs.[3]

Physiology

The liver is a key organ involved in many metabolic processes, including digestion, regulation, and mobilization of carbohydrate, lipid, and protein. Other important roles include detoxification, vitamin storage, and immunoregulation. The liver has a central anatomic topography, receiving a dual blood supply from the hepatic arteries and the portal vein, draining most of the abdominal organs. For those reasons, any systemic disease (infection or neoplasia) has potential detrimental effects on hepatic function.

Bile, which is secreted by the liver, helps digestion of fats in food and is the route of excretion of bilirubin (the product of degradation of red blood cells). It also has some bactericidal activity and helps buffer stomach acid.

SIGNALMENT
History Findings

Because of its unspecific signs, diagnosis of liver disease in ferrets can be challenging. When liver disease is suspected, the clinician has to go through a thorough questionnaire to find history of toxin or medication exposure, diet imbalance, or past episode of viral infection in the household. A high-fat diet can induce lipid hepatic accumulation in ferrets because of their specific liver metabolism.[4] Any sign of inflammatory bowel disease, especially *Coronavirus* infection, must be recorded.[5] Ferrets affected by liver disease are usually middle-aged to old ferrets.[5]

Clinical Signs

Hepatic disease in ferrets is often subclinical.[5] If present, clinical signs are usually discrete and unspecific, such as lethargy, anorexia, fever, gastrointestinal disorders, and weight loss.[5] Icterus can be a strong sign of liver disease; however, ferrets are rarely icteric because of rapid renal excretion of bilirubin.[6,7] Additionally, yellow sebaceous secretions can mask subtle icterus.[5] In reports of severe bile duct obstruction, liver cirrhosis, or copper toxicosis, icterus has been observed.[5,8–10] The nose, ear, and oral cavity are suggested as sites for searching for icterus (**Fig. 1**).[5] In cases of extrahepatic bile duct obstruction (EHBO) and ruptured gallbladder, acute abdominal pain can be detected on palpation.[9,11]

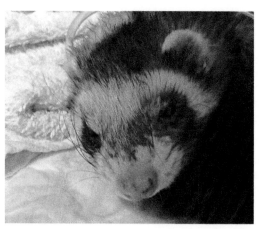

Fig. 1. Icteric ferret with jaundice observed on the nose and both ears.

In cases of severe liver dysfunction, it is expected that ferrets experience the same clinical signs as dogs, such as hepatic encephalopathy, ascites, and bleeding disorder, but such disorders have not been reported to the authors' knowledge. Several reasons may explain this fact. Because cats rarely have ascites due to chronic liver disease, similar findings can be suggested in ferrets.[12] Ascites and hemoperitoneum in ferrets have only been reported with hepatic tumors.[13,14] Polyuria-polydipsia is also a clinical sign of liver disease in cats and dogs but has not been reported in ferrets.

CLINICAL PATHOLOGY
Biochemistry

Biochemistry testing can reveal hepatocellular change, reflecting damage in the parenchyma or the biliary tract, or used to diagnose hepatic dysfunction, such as abnormal bile elimination and coagulation disorder. Normal ranges are referenced in **Table 1**.[15–17]

Table 1 Reference range for liver biochemistry values in ferrets	
Reference Range	**Values**
ALT (IU/L)	110 (49–242.8)[15]
AST (IU/L)	74 (40.1–142.7)[15]
Bilirubin (mg/dL)	1.1 (0–3.3)[15]
GGT (IU/L)	4 (0.2–14)[15]
Cholesterol (mg/dl)	165 (64–296)[16]
Protein, total (g/dL)	6.8 (5.5–7.8)[15]
Albumin (g/dL)	3.6 (2.8–4.4)[15]
Bile acids (μmol/L)	5.7 (0–28.9)[15]
PT (s)	10.9 (10.6–11.6)[17]
PTT (s)	20 (18.6–22.1)[17]
Fibrinogen (mg/dL)	107.4 (90–163.5)[17]
Antithrombin (%)	96 (69.3–115.3)[17]

Alanine aminotransferase

Alanine aminotransferase (ALT), also known as serum glutamic-pyruvic transaminase, is an enzyme found in the cytoplasm of hepatocytes released in cases of cellular injury in domestic animals.[18] It has been shown valuable in the assessment of hepatic damage in the ferret. The half-life of ALT in dogs is reported as 45 to 60 hours and 5 hours in rabbits. It is likely longer in ferrets.[7] Most ferrets with liver disease present with ALT greater than 275 IU/L.[6] In cases of liver necrosis, however, increases of ALT levels are minimal, whereas increases of biliary enzymes levels as a result of biliary stasis are severe.

Aspartate aminotransferase

Aspartate aminotransferase (AST) is present in similar amounts in liver and muscle and thus is less specific than ALT. The half-life of AST in dogs is longer than ALT.[18] No data about the half-life are available in ferrets. AST has the same properties as ALT.

Alkaline phosphatases

Alkaline phosphatases (ALPs) are isoenzymes that perform the same function (hydrolyzing monophosphates at an alkaline pH) in many if not all body tissues. Cells from liver, bones, kidneys, intestinal mucosa, and placenta have the highest activity.[18] In the ferret liver, membranes bordering the bile canaliculus produce ALPs.[7] Bile stasis, bile duct obstruction, and lipidosis produce increased ALP synthesis.

γ-Glutamyl transpeptidase

γ-Glutamyl transferase (GGT) is an enzyme found mainly in the kidney but also in the liver, spleen, and intestines. In dogs and cats, because of its poor specificity of liver tissue, its main interest is joint interpretation with ALP because ALP is also found in bone and steroid-induced isoenzyme.[18] GGT is supposedly more sensitive than ALP for detection of extrahepatic cholestasis, cholangiohepatitis, and cirrhosis.

Bilirubin

Bilirubin is a product of heme breakdown, produced by the hepatocytes and excreted into the intestines through the biliary tree of the ferret. Thus, serum bilirubin levels are an indication of both hepatocellular and biliary tree function.[18] Ferrets rarely present with hyperbilirubinemia or icterus because of their high renal bilirubin excretion.

Bile acid

Synthesis of bile acid is the primary pathway for catabolism of cholesterol, involving multiple enzymatic reactions in the liver.[18] Additionally, the liver removes bile acid from the hepatic portal vein. Bile acid level assesses the excretory capacity of the liver. Bile acid levels rise in cases of biliary obstruction and in many forms of hepatic disease.[19]

Ammonia

Ammonia is a product of protein catabolism. Elevation is seen when the liver does not remove the ammonia from the portal blood in some pathologic situations, such as a shunt. This test has limited value in ferrets because vascular shunt has never been reported in ferrets.[6]

Cholesterol

Because liver is involved in lipid metabolism, hypercholesterolemia is associated with increased hepatic synthesis, decreased biliary excretion of cholesterol, or both in cats and dogs.[20] High cholesterol values have been reported with cholelithiasis.[21]

Protein

Liver is the main organ involved in protein synthesis. The main categories of serum proteins are albumin, α-globulins (including acute phase protein), β-globulins (including fibrinogen, IgM, and IgA), and γ-globulins (including IgG). The liver is the exclusive site of synthesis of albumin. Albumin levels are typically low in cases of the severe liver disease; however, total protein level may not be affected because globulinemia usually increases. Albumin levels can be affected by various protein-losing conditions but synthesis can be affected by severe liver disease.[19] Decreased albumin and increased globulin levels result in a modification of the albumin/globulin ratio.[19] Liver diseases are usually associated with decreased albumin/globulin ratio.

Serum electrophoresis allows differentiating different protein phases. In the acute inflammatory phase, when IgM are produced, a β peak alone is seen, suggesting an acute hepatitis. Then an increased production of γ-globulin due to the presence of multiple antibodies is seen, and, in severe chronic hepatopathy, an increase of β-globulin and γ-globulin is expected (related to immunoglobulin production).[19] An α_2-microglobulin peak is also sometimes observed in cases of chronic hepatitis and cases of lymphoma. In cases of liver cirrhosis, a so-called β-γ bridge can be observed. Aleutian disease (AD) and *Coronavirus* have been associated with hypergammablobulinemia and polyclonal peaks, and their role has been suggested in chronic hepatopathy.[1,22,23]

Coagulation protein

The liver is involved in various clotting pathways and is the exclusive site of synthesis for factors I (fibrinogen), II (prothrombin), V, VII, IX, X, and XI and antithrombin. Prolonged prothrombin time is an indicator of hepatic dysfunction. In some severe cases, elevation of partial thromboplastin time (PTT) is also observed. Dysfibrinogenemia, an interferent with fibrin polymerization, has also been reported in severe liver disease. Moreover, liver disease is known to decrease absorption of fat-soluble substances in the gut, decreasing absorption of vitamin K.[18] Reference ranges for coagulation factors have been determined in ferret species.[17]

Urinalysis

Bilirubinuria

Only the conjugated water-soluble form of bilirubin is excreted in the urine. Traces of bilirubinuria can be detectable in normal ferrets, but true bilirubinuria is present in cases of suppurative hepatitis or biliary obstruction.[5,9,24]

Biliverdinuria

Green urine is a common finding in *Coronavirus* infection.[22,25] Although the physiologic mechanism of this finding has not been fully elucidated, microhemorrhage into tissues and extravascular destruction of erythrocytes related to vascularitis is hypothesized.[22]

Hematology

Nonspecific modification of hematology profile can be associated with liver disease. Leukocytosis can be seen in cases of severe cholangiohepatitis, suppurative hepatitis, or *Coronavirus* infection.[5,11,25] Lymphocyte ratio or lymphocytosis can reflect lymphoma.[7] Relative neutrophilia is seen with EHBO.[9] Very severe neutrophilic leukocytosis (>55,000 cells/mm^3) has been reported with hemangiosarcoma.[14]

Peritoneal Effusion

Peritoneal effusion is observed when damages are seen in the liver capillaries causing leakage of fluid in the abdominal cavity. The condition worsens because hypoalbuminemia is often present concomitantly. Abdominocenthesis allows diagnostic samples. The fluid is primarily clear but chronic inflammation of the peritoneum can raise the cellularity of a sample, making the fluid serohemorraghic. Cellularity is usually low. Density is usually between 1.005 and 1.020. As discussed previously, such clinical situations have not been reported in ferrets but can be expected in cases of liver failure. Hemoperitoneum fluid has been observed in case of neoplasia.[14] Bile peritonitis has been reported with a yellow fluid with bile pigment.[11] Serous abdominal effusion has also been reported with *Coronavirus* infection, as in cats affected by feline infectious peritonitis.[25]

DIAGNOSTIC IMAGING

Diagnostic imaging allows direct visualization of the liver and the biliary tree. Ultrasonographic exploration is a noninvasive tool to screen for liver disease. Ultrasound probes with a frequency of 7.5 MHz are suitable but those with 10 MHz to 13 MHz have better resolution.[26,27]

In ferrets, the structure of the thorax can make visualization with the ultrasound probe difficult. Ultrasonographic appearance is nonspecific in ferrets and similar to cats and dogs.[27]

Normal Appearance

Few specific descriptions have been reported in ferrets. The ferret liver parenchyma is usually uniformly hypoechoic, with a coarser echostructure than the spleen, similar to what is visualized in small carnivores (**Fig. 2**).[26,28]

The gallbladder appears anechoic with a pear-shaped structure. Size variation is important and volume alone cannot be used as a sign of biliary obstruction. Gallbladder sludge is usually nonsignificant. The afferent vascular flow enters mainly via the portal vein. The efferent flow follows the hepatic vein into the caudal vena cava. The wall of portal veins usually appears hyperechoic compared with hepatic veins.

Pathologic Findings

Liver parenchyma

There are no specific descriptions of liver parenchyma in ferrets to the authors' knowledge. Diffuse alteration of the echogenicity of the parenchyma can be observed. Abnormalities are listed in **Table 2**.[29] Hepatomegaly can be demonstrated when the edge of the liver are round shaped.[5] Usually lipidosis is characterized by a diffuse increase of parenchymal echogenicity (**Fig. 3**). In cats, cholangiohepatitis can be

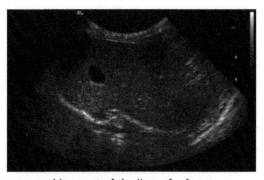

Fig. 2. Normal ultrasonographic aspect of the liver of a ferret.

Table 2
Diagnostic differentials for diffuse alterations in hepatic parenchymal echogenicity

Diffuse Hyperechogenicity	Diffuse Hypoechogenicity	Mixed Echogenicity
Steroid hepatopathy	Passive congestion	Steroid hepatopathy associated with benign hyperplasia
Chronic hepatitis	Acute hepatitis or cholangiohepatitits	Hepatitis
Lymphoma	Lymphoma	Lymphoma
Fibrosis		Neoplasia and metastasis
Cirrhosis		Necrosis
Vacuolar hepatopathies		
Lipidosis		

Data from D'Anjou MA. Liver. In: Penninck D, D'Anjou MA, editors. Atlas of Animal ultrasonography. Ames (IA): Blackwell Publishing Ltd; 2008. p. 226.

observed with a decrease of parenchymal echogenicity and increased visibility of portal vasculature. Chronic hepatitis, fibrosis, and ultimately cirrhosis are characterized with a small or normal by diffuse hyperechogenicity with a small or normal-sized liver (**Fig. 4**). Focal lesions, such as nodular hyperplasia, hepatic cyst, neoplasia, and abscess, can be visualized (**Fig. 5**).

Biliary tract
Obstruction of the biliary tract is well observed by ultrasonography. As discussed previously, distension of the gallbladder cannot be the sole criteria for gallbladder obstruction. In ferrets, when the gallbladder is distended, it may separate the 2 lobes but it never extends through the liver to contact the diaphragm as it does in dogs.[2] Thickening of the biliary tract and the gallbladder wall can be observed (**Figs. 6** and **7**).[9] In carnivores, usually the cystic duct dilates and becomes more tortuous, which has been reported in ferrets with EHBO and cholelithiasis.[9,21]

Nodules or neoplasia can arise next to the bile duct. A diffuse thickening of the gallbladder can be observed in cases of cholecystitis. An accumulation of mucus in the lumen of the gallbladder can cause distension, wall necrosis, and obstruction (**Fig. 8**).

Neoplasia
Various types of hepatic tumors and metastasis are described in ferrets (**Fig. 9**). Focal change can be observed by ultrasound, such as biliary cyst adenomas (**Fig. 10**).[5]

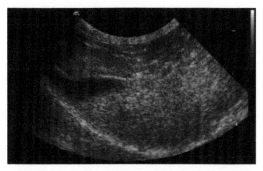

Fig. 3. Diffuse hyperechogenicity in the liver parenchyma of a ferret consistent with hepatic lipidosis.

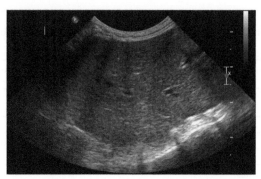

Fig. 4. Diffuse hyperechogenicity and increase visibility of hepatic vein consistent with chronic hepatitis.

Hepatic congestion

Hepatic congestion is usually seen with right-sided cardiopathy, with increased pressure of the cranial vena cava and thus increased pressure in the hepatic vein. The liver is typically enlarged and appears diffusely hypoechoic.[28] In cases of severe congestion, some investigators report that the liver can appear almost cystic.[27]

CYTOLOGY

Smears prepared from liver aspirates include blood and hepatocytes distributed singly and in clusters. Hepatocytes are polyhedral cells that have an oval nucleus, granular chromatin, a single small nucleolus, and a moderate amount of blue-gray cytoplasm. Macrophages are frequently present in small numbers.[30] Liver cytology is not the gold standard for accurate diagnosis.[31] Because cytology does not reflect hepatic architecture, its major indications are fine-needle aspirate of a focal lesion, such as neoplasia and hepatic lipidosis.[5] Increased numbers of lymphocytes in liver fine-needle aspirate can indicate lymphosarcoma.[30] It is not recommended in diffuse parenchymal disease, such as lymphocytic hepatitis.[5] Cytologic criteria have been developed in dogs and the same criteria can be extrapolated in ferrets (**Box 1**).[32]

HISTOPATHOLOGY

Most diagnosis of liver disease relies on histologic descriptions. Every effort should be made to approach a standardized description, as described in canine medicine.[33] Biopsy sample can be obtained preferably by surgery or with true-cut needles.

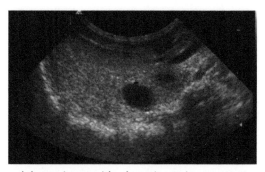

Fig. 5. Hypoechoic nodule consistent with a hepatic cyst in an asymptomatic ferret. Hepatic cysts are common findings.

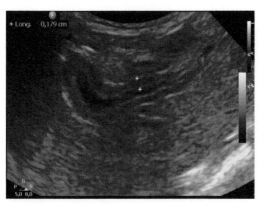

Fig. 6. Hyperechogenicity and thickening of the biliary tract in a ferret with severe cholecystitis.

LIVER DISEASE
Inflammatory Liver Disease

Pathogenesis of hepatitis is poorly understood and causes of most cases remain unknown in dogs and cats. Ferrets have been studied as a model of hepatitis, with speculation of a close liver metabolism to dogs.[34]

In case of hepatitis, inflammation is characterized by infiltration of inflammatory cells with edema and congestion around hepatocytes, bile ducts, or blood vessels defining hepatitis, cholangitis or vasculitis, respectively.

In the first acute inflammation phase, cellular change occurs, including apoptosis, necrosis, and possibly regeneration.[34] Regeneration can take place at this stage if the supportive reticulum is intact and fills the gap integrally. Portal inflammation may involve all or some portal fields. Cells involved are mostly lymphocytes (**Fig. 11**). This portal inflammation may be accompanied by bile extravasation, granulomas, purulent exudate, destruction of bile duct, ductular reaction, or fibrosis (**Fig. 12**).

Secondly, an influx of inflammatory cells can be observed leading to chronic hepatitis. In areas where the reticulum is changed, healing can only occur by scarring and the process leads to fibrosis. The severity of the disease is determined by the quantity of inflammation, the extent of hepatocellular apoptosis and necrosis, and the pattern

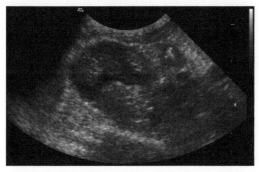

Fig. 7. Hyperechogenicity and thickening of the gallbladder with a biliary sludge in the lumen observed in a ferret with EHBO.

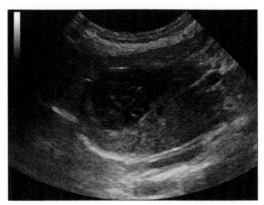

Fig. 8. Accumulation of biliary content in the gallbladder and hyperechoic striation pattern consistent with a mucocele in a ferret presented for jaundice.

of fibrosis.[35] If scarring tissue is produced extensively, vascular changes and structure distorsion occur, leading to cirrhosis.

Cirrhosis is defined as a diffuse process characterized by fibrosis of the liver and conversion of normal liver architecture into abnormal nodules and portal-central vascular anastomosis. This end result of chronic damage to the liver seems uncommon in ferrets.[5] Serum chemistries are compatible with liver damage (elevation of ALT and GGT) and loss of function (elevation of bilirubin). Ultrasound may detect changes in size and consistency of the liver suggestive of cirrhosis. A definitive diagnosis is made via biopsy. Histopathology shows bridging fibrosis with areas of regeneration but overall loss of healthy hepatocytes.

Lymphocytic hepatitis
Lymphocytic hepatitis is common in pet ferrets and potentially underdiagnosed because it is subclinical. Moreover, clinical signs are difficult to distinguish from gastrointestinal disease because both are usually present. Most patients are over 1.5 years old when diagnosed.[5] This disease can be discovered incidentally during routine blood panel. Some investigators state that mild lymphocytic portal infiltrate is normal in this species.[1] Lymphocytic hepatitis is usually associated with digestive conditions (inflammatory bowel disease or chronic inflammation caused by

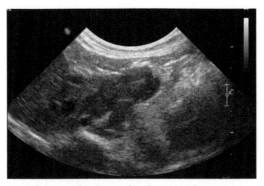

Fig. 9. Heterogenous nodule on the liver of a ferret with concurrent adrenal carcinoma consistent with metastasis.

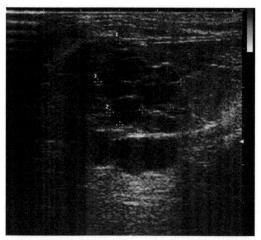

Fig. 10. Multiple hypoechoic nodule consistent with a biliary cystadenoma in a ferret.

Box 1
Cytologic findings consistent with liver disease

Acute and nonspecific reactive hepatitis

- Presence of moderate reactive nuclear patterns (more pronounced chromatin, prominent nucleoli)
- Increased numbers of inflammatory cells, excluding lymphocytes
- Absence of increased numbers of bile duct cell clusters
- Increased numbers of mast cells also indicative of nonspecific reactive hepatitis

Cirrhosis

- Chronic hepatitis criteria
- Intracellular bile accumulation
- Increased numbers of bile duct cell clusters

Lymphoma

- Presence of large numbers of lymphoblasts with a minimum of 5% of all cells found

Carcinoma (primary or metastatic)

- Clusters of epithelial cells with several cytologic characteristics of malignancy intermixed with normal hepatocytes
- Liver cells presenting a high nucleus/cytoplasm ratio, large cell diameters, increased numbers of nucleoli per nuclei, small numbers of cytoplasmic vacuoles
- Frequently, small numbers of lymphocytes

Extrahepatic cholestasis

- Excessive extracellular bile pigment in the form of biliary casts
- Increased numbers of nucleoli within hepatocytes
- Decreased hepatic cell size
- Low numbers of lymphocytes.

Data from Stockhaus C, Van Den Ingh T, Rothuizen J, et al. A multistep approach in the cytologic evaluation of liver biopsy samples of dogs with hepatic diseases. Vet Pathol 2004;41:461–70.

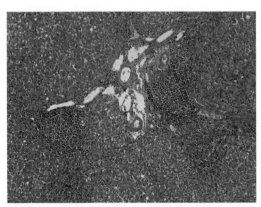

Fig. 11. Photomicrograph of a lymphocytic hepatitis. Portal areas are diffusely severely infiltrated by lymphocytes and few plasma cells forming large lymphoid nodules. Hematoxylin-eosin staining (original magnification ×10). (*Courtesy of* VetDiagnostics, A. Nicollier, DVM, Dipl ECVP, Lyon.)

Coronavirus infection), suggesting an ascending inflammatory process from the lower digestive tract, and biliary inflammation is often noted.[5] Biochemistry change include elevation of ALT (200–500 IU/L) and GGT.[5] An index of ALT values between 200 IU/L and 700 IU/L has been reported as suggesting mild to severe lymphocytic hepatitis.[5] Definite diagnosis is confirmed with liver biopsy sampling intestinal tract and lymph node in the same procedure are recommended. Other diagnostic procedures include ultrasound-guided biopsy.[5]

Suppurative hepatitis

In suppurative hepatitis, clinical signs are usually more obvious and ferrets affected show more profound lethargy than in case of lymphocytic hepatitis. Fever, anorexia, vomition or diarrhea, icterus are usually present. Suppurative hepatitis shares the same cause as lymphocytic hepatitis; thus, underlying disease must be investigated.[5]

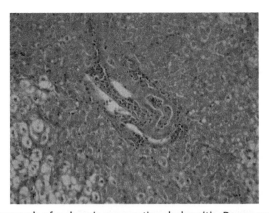

Fig. 12. Photomicrograph of a chronic suppurative cholangitis. Degenerated inflammatory cells are observed in the lumen of bile ducts. The portal area is mildly infiltrated by lymphocytes and plasma cells. Hematoxylin-eosin staining (original magnification ×20). (*Courtesy of* VetDiagnostics, A. Nicollier.)

There is probably underlying lymphocytic gastroenteritis present in most cases, leading to intestinal bacterial overgrowth, ascending biliary inflammation, and lymphocytic hepatitis, all of which predispose patients to bacterial cholangiohepatitis. Suppurative hepatitis has been associated with disseminated idiopathic myofasciitis.[36] Granulomatous hepatitis has been seen in *Coronavirus* infection and *Mycobacterium* infection.[25,37] Severe elevation of ALT of more than 1000 IU/L, with lesser elevations of GGT, AST, and ALP, are described. Bilirubin is also elevated.[5]

Infectious and toxic hepatitis

Several etiologic agents have been identified in cases of liver disease, causing liver inflammation.

Bacterial disease

Helicobacter The ferret is an animal model for *Helicobacter* infection because *H mustelae* shares several characteristics with the human *H pylori*.[38,39] Some species of *Helicobacter* are so-called enterohepatic species but, although *H mustelae* is well known in gastric disease, its pathogenicity in liver disease remains undescribed.[38] One retrospective study of hepatobiliary disease in a ferret colony showed presence of bacteria related to *H cholecystus* in hepatic biopsy, suggesting a potential cause of cholangiohepatitis.[40] Isolation of *Helicobacter* DNA in affected tissue and relationship with liver disease are controversial. In dogs, *Helicobacter* DNA has been detected in liver tissue affected with primary biliary cirrhosis and primary sclerosing cholangitis. In the same study, however, *Helicobacter* DNA was also detected in the control group; thus, statistical evidence of pathogenicity was not proved.[41] Equally in humans, incidence of *Helicobacter* spp is slightly raising the risk of cholelithiasis and benign liver disease but pathogenicity remains difficult to establish.[42]

Campylobacter *Campylobacter jejuni* is a pathogen that is associated with diarrhea and enterocolitis in several species. Experimental infection of young ferrets with *C jejuni* caused diarrhea and severe inflammatory response. During the acute phase, the bacteria were isolated in the liver but did not trigger any inflammatory response or histologic change.[43] A similar case reported an intracellular campylobacter-like organism related to *Desfulvibrio* spp, which was isolated in liver tissue of a ferret affected with proliferative colitis. Liver changes included inflammatory infiltrate.[44]

Mycobacterium Ferrets may be naturally or experimentally infected by bovine, avian, and human mycobacteria. Sporadic cases are described in pet ferrets and are common in the wild population of ferrets in New Zealand.[45] *M avium* and *M celatum* have been isolated in liver tissue in ferrets affected with disseminated mycobacteriosis.[6,46–48] Experimental infections with *M bovis* occasionally involve liver.[49] Characteristic granulomatous lesions have been observed in affected liver tissue.[47] Mycobacteriosis remains a major differential to consider with hepatic abscess in ferrets.

Sepsis Septicemia and hematogenous spread of bacteria can affect liver secondarily. *Escherichia coli* hepatitis and enteritis have been associated with in a colony of black-footed ferrets.[50] A *Corynebacterium mustelae* sp Nov has been isolated from liver, lung, and kidney in a 3-year-old ferret with lethal sepsis.[51]

Parasitic disease

Toxoplasma *Toxoplasma gondii* is a protozoal parasite that infects ferrets, but there is only a single report of toxoplasma-like infection in ferrets.[52] Areas of necrosis in the liver and toxoplasma-like organisms were isolated. The black-footed ferret, a related species, has demonstrated clinical toxoplasmosis. Lesions include pneumonia, encephalitis, myocarditis, myositis, and acute to chronic hepatitis.[53]

Fungal disease

Cryptococcus There are several reports of disseminated *Cryptococcosis* in ferrets.[54–56] When they developed generalized *Cryptococcosis*, clinical signs and findings are limited to lower respiratory tract disease with pneumonia, pleurisy, and mediastinal lymph node involvement or infection in a segment of intestine with subsequent spread to mesenteric lymph nodes. *C bacillisporus* (formerly *C neoformans* var *grubii*) accounted for the infections in ferrets. Liver involvement is rare and has only been reported once; respiratory and neurologic signs were predominant.[54]

Pneumocystis carinii *Pneumocystis carinii* is a fungal organism causing pneumonia in ferrets and in immunocompromised humans. Research has been focusing on studying experimental infection with *P carinii* in immunosuppressed ferrets. In experimental conditions, inducing extrapulmonary *P carinii* infection in the liver was successful in a minority of individuals, however this finding has not been reported in pet ferret.[57]

Viral disease

Distemper Ferret distemper, due to the same morbillivirus that causes distemper in dogs, is one of the most important diseases of the species. Clinical signs are similar to those seen in dogs: weight loss, anorexia, hyperkeratosis of the nasal planum and footpads, and oculonasal discharge. The diagnosis may be confirmed by microscopic examination of necropsy tissues; numerous viral inclusions and syncitia are seen in a wide range of tissues, including the liver and gallbladder.[58] Fluorescent antibody tests can be run on peripheral blood, mucous membrane scrapings, or conjunctival swabs, and vaccines do not interfere with these tests. Biopsy samples of footpad skin can be examined microscopically for the characteristic viral inclusions.

Influenza Influenza viruses are part of the family of orthomyxovirus and ferrets are highly susceptible. Ferrets are an experimental model in influenza research, especially because of their susceptibility to influenza A and B from human strains. Experimental infection of different strains of influenza induced severe pneumonia and fever, and some strains have a degree of liver involvement, including severe portal hepatitis.[59–61]

Coronavirus Infectious hepatitis and enteritis of ferrets have been reported under the names, *epizootic catarrhal enteritis* and *green slime disease*. A type 1 coronavirus has been identified as a causative agent.[37] It is highly contagious with transmission from direct contact. Outbreaks of the disease have been reported anecdotally at ferret shows, in pet shops, and in multiferret homes.[7] Young ferrets seem to experience a milder form of the disease; older ferrets are severely affected. A significant hepatitis and enteritis cause the signs of the disease: profuse, green, mucoid diarrhea, depression, dehydratation, anorexia, weight loss, and death.[7]

AST levels greater than 700 U/L in ferrets are suggestive of this disease. Polyclonal gammopathy is also observed. Ultrasound features include peritonitis, abdominal adenomegaly, splenomegaly, and nephromegaly. No change in the liver ultrasound structure was seen in a study of 11 ferrets.[62]

Diagnosis is confirmed with biopsy of the liver showing varying degrees of hepatic destruction and the gastrointestinal tract showing pyogranulomatous inflammation.[7] White foci and white nodules can be seen on affected tissue.[22,25] Postmortem, pyogranulomatous lesions are seen in the parenchyma of various tissues: spleen, kidney, liver, and lymph nodes.[22,25] Reverse transcription–polymerase chain reaction assays were developed to screen for ferret coronavirus. Fecal swabs or sample are preferred.[22] Coronavirus serology is also available and demonstrates past exposure to the virus. These tests alone cannot confirm a systemic *Coronavirus* infection.[22]

Aleutian disease AD is a parvovirus associated with neurologic dysfunction in ferrets.[23,63] Pathogenesis of AD in ferrets is controversial; many individuals remain asymptomatic.[23,64] A case report of AD in a ferret with liver involvement was described.[63] Histologic findings included plasmocytic infiltrates in various organs, mainly kidney but also in the liver. Lymphocytic and plasmocytic infiltrates in periportal areas and proliferations of the bile ducts were seen.[63] Experimental infection by mink AD and ferret AD showed a high prevalence of periportal lymphoid cell infiltration.[65] Some investigators report that AD may cause mild periportal lymphocytic infiltrate in asymptomatic ferrets.[1]

AD is typically difficult to investigate because asymptomatic carriage is common.[64] Hyperproteinemia and hypergammaglobulinemia can be present but are inconstant.[63,66] Serology testing demonstrates past exposure but positive titer is frequent in asymptomatic ferrets.[23]

Hepatitis E Hepatitis E can cause liver inflammation in humans, potentially causing death in pregnant women. The role of pet animals has been investigated, suggesting a potential relationship and a carriage of the virus.[67] Fecal testing and polymerase chain reaction screening in pet ferrets in the Netherlands have shown evidence of a ferret hepatitis E virus.[68] Clinical importance has not been reported but should be kept in mind in cases of hepatitis due to the potential zoonotic threat.

Toxic hepatitis

Few reports of toxic hepatitis have been reported in ferrets. Acetaminophen toxicity has been reported in ferrets.[69] Overdose potentially causes acute hepatic necrosis, methemoglobinemia, and renal failure. Toxicity of aflatoxin remains to be proved in ferrets. In one study, ferrets fed with a toxic ration of groundnut meal did not show any significant histopathologic change.[70]

Copper Toxicosis

Copper toxicosis was diagnosed in 2 sibling ferrets on the basis of high hepatic copper concentrations and histologic changes in hepatic tissue. Clinical signs in these 2 ferrets were mostly nonspecific and included severe central nervous system depression, icterus in 1 ferret, hypothermia, and lethargia. A genetic copper toxicosis in these 2 ferrets was suggested because they were siblings with the same phenotypic coat color and because no environmental source of copper was identified.[8]

Hepatic Lipidosis and Vacuolar Hepatopathy

Hepatic lipidosis

Liver has a key role in metabolizing fatty acid in exporting lipids and lipoproteins. Lipid accumulation in the liver occurs because the intake of fatty acid rises in the diet. But mustelids, including ferrets, have a metabolic ability to mobilize rapidly visceral fat and polyunsaturated fatty acid, predisposing them to liver steatosis.[71] For those reasons, ferrets are an experimental model of fatty liver syndrome.[71,72] In experimental conditions, 5 days of food deprivation after being fed a high-fat diet induced liver steatosis.[71] Obese ferrets and ferrets fed an inappropriate high-fat diet are predisposed to this condition, although healthy ferrets in general do not seem sensitive to lipidosis, according to some investigators.[5]

Any cause of sudden weight loss, anorexia, or any debilitating disease can be related to hepatic lipidosis. Hepatic lipidosis has been associated with various causes of dysorexia: chronic gastric disease, megaesophagus,[73] diabetes mellitus,[74,75] pregnancy toxemia,[76] and *Coronavirus* infection.[5,77]

Many cases of lipidosis are subclinical.[5] Serum chemistries may be normal or may show mild elevation of ALT, ALP, and GGT.[5] The liver looks generally brown to yellow and swollen. Definite diagnosis can be achieved by ultrasound-guided or surgical biopsies of liver and histologic analysis. Screening for concurrent disease is recommended because this is usually a secondary condition. Steroid usage or endocrine conditions may predispose to this disease.[5] Histolopathology shows diffuse lipid vacuolation of the hepatocytes (**Fig. 13**).

Vacuolar hepatitis

Most cases of vacuolar hepatitis are subclinical. Clinical signs are vague: lethargy, malaise, and dysorexia. It is a common histopathologic finding with increased vacuolization of hepatocytes.[5] Hormone impregnation is a potential cause, with high estradiol level secondary to adrenal gland disease.[5] Corticosteroid administration can also be incriminated although steroid hepatopathy is reported as rare in ferrets by some investigators.[5,6]

Biliary Tract Disease

Cholecystitis

Cholecystitis is an inflammation of gallbladder, most often due to lithiasis or biliary sludge. In a case report, a ferret presented for acute abdominal pain was diagnosed with a severe cholangiohepatitis and a cholecystitis leading to a ruptured gallbladder (**Fig. 14**). Visualization of gas bubbles in ultrasound was diagnostic of emphysematous cholecystitis due to presence of gas-producing bacteria. *Pseudomonas aeruginosa* was isolated from bile culture. *Escherichia coli* and *Clostridum perfringens*, frequently isolated bacteria in dogs, have been seen in ferrets (Minh HUYNH, DVM, 2012, personal communication). Ultrasound-guided cholecystocenthesis can be recommended in order to submit a bile sample for bacteriology. Chemical bile peritonitis was seen and cytologic examination of the abdominal effusion showed biliary yellowish pigments or a basophile acellular characteristic substance.[11]

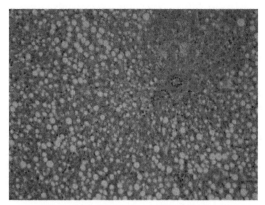

Fig. 13. Photomicrograph of moderate hepatic lipidosis showing a diffuse vacuolation of the hepatocytes. Hematoxylin-eosin staining (original magnification ×10). (*Courtesy of* Vet-Diagnostics, A. Nicollier.)

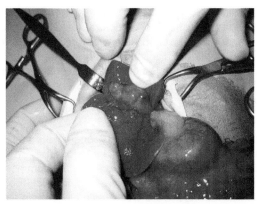

Fig. 14. Surgery—inflammatory gallbladder associated with abnormal distension in a ferret with cholecystitis.

Extrahepatic bile duct obstruction

EHBO associated with cholangiohepatitis has been reported in 2 ferrets (**Fig. 15**).[9] Severe elevation of ALT (>1000 IU/L) and bilirubin (>60 μmol/L) was observed in both ferrets with EHBO with mild elevation of AST and ALP. Bilirubinuria were seen in both cases. A protein plug was detected and removed in both cases. Gallbladder has not been removed in both ferrets, so histologic confirmation of gallbladder mucocele has not been established. Cultures of the biliary tract contents were negative for bacteria. Another report of EHBO was seen postmortem in a cystic mucinous hyperplasia of the gallbladder mucosa.[10]

Cholelithiasis has been reported associated with cholestasis.[21] Total obstruction was not observed but sediment accumulation had a role in cholestasis. Severe elevation apply to 5 measurements were also observed in ALT (>1000IU/L), GGT (97IU/L), bilirubin (6.2 mg/dL), ALP (361 IU/L), and cholesterol (458 mg/dL). Flocculent material was seen in the bile. Marked hyperplasia of the epithelium of the common bile duct was observed. Neutrophilic inflammation and hepatic necrosis was seen. No bacterial growth was seen.

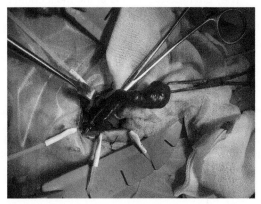

Fig. 15. Surgery—EHBO in a ferret with severe distension of the gallbladder and the biliary tract.

The obstruction of biliary tract may be functional (altered gall bladder wall contractility or thickening of the biliary tract) or structural (result of a cholelith or mucous plug).[9] Pancreatic disease is one of the most common causes of canine EHBO, whereas tumors and inflammatory disease of the biliary tract, pancreas, or both are the most common causes in cats.[78] Pancreatitis is a rare condition in ferrets[6] even if it is common to find hypoechoic appearance of pancreas during ultrasound, but individuals with this condition usually show no symptoms.

Coccidiosis

Probably the most common parasites seen in young ferrets are coccidia. They are protozoal parasites that multiply inside the cells. Infections may be subclinical or associated with moderate to severe diarrhea. *Isospora* spp are common species reported in pets, but *Eimeria* spp have been found in free-ranging black-footed ferrets. A case of biliary coccidiosis was reported in a 9-week-old male ferret in a research colony.[79] Hepatic coccidiosis should be considered in young ferrets showing signs of decreased hepatic function and blockage of bile ducts. At necropsy, the liver appears enlarged with nodular abcesses and distended bile ducts. The gallbladder may also be distended. Developing stages are observed on histopathologic examination of tissues. Characteristic oocysts may be seen in fresh bile.[79]

Neoplasia

The liver is a common site for primary and metastatic neoplasia in the ferret. In a review of 1525 neoplasms, 25 primary neoplasms and 71 metastatic neoplasms were seen. It is the most affected gastrointestinal organ. In a survey of 155 tumors, 17 were hepatic tumors.[1,3,80] Lymphoma, adenocarcinoma, hepatobiliary adenomas, and biliary adenocarcinomas are reported most frequently. Susceptibility of mustelids to hepatotoxins and hepatocarcinogens has been incriminated to explain the high incidence of hepatic tumors.[81–83]

Hepatic cysts and cystadenomas

Hepatic cysts can be incidentally found in one or more hepatic lobes and are reported as common in pet ferrets. They are variable, from small and focal to large and numerous.[5] Hepatic cysts have to be distinguished from the biliary cystadenoma. Ultrasound monitoring for mass growth and evidence of biochemistry modification is strongly recommended.[84] Biliary cystadenomas are the most common primary liver tumors in ferrets.[13,85] They are reported as one of the most common tumors, with an incidence of 20% in captive black-footed ferrets.[86] Although they are histologically benign, they can have an aggressive behavior. They may grow and replace large portions of hepatic parenchyma in multiple lobes and could result in loss of hepatic function,[5] leading to hepatic failure.[13,84] Mild to moderate increases in ALT and GGT can be seen in some cases.[5]

Hepatoma

Hepatomas are benign hepatocellular neoplasms, which can produce clinical disease, either by damaging the hepatic tissue or by altering the hepatic function.[5] In humans they are reported to cause hypoglycemia.[87] Clinical signs may include weight loss and lethargy. A report indicated a severe elevation of ALT of 1050 IU/L without elevation of AST or GGT with hypoglycemia.[5]

Hepatic carcinoma

One case of peliod hepatocellular carcinoma was diagnosed in a ferret.[88] The left medial liver lobe was affected with a 12-cm diameter mass. The mass had rubbery-to-soft consistency and had completely effaced normal hepatic parenchyma. Immunohisto-chemical analysis was necessary to differentiate hepatocellular neoplasia from vascular neoplasm, such as hemangiosarcoma.[88] Concurrent adrenocortical hyper-plasia was observed in this case and the investigatord speculated about a possible association.[88] Hepatic carcinoma generally results in increased concentration of hepatic enzyme.[13]

Hepatocellular and biliary adenocarcinomas are malignant aggressive tumors that may involve one or more lobes and have metastatic potential.[5] Serum chemistry in a report included elevated ALT (>4000 IU/L) with mildly elevated AST (>500 IU/l) and GGT (>100 IU/L), normal ALP, and hypoglycemia. Cholangiocarcinoma was seen in a ferret colony with *Helicobacter* involvement.[40]

Hemangiosarcoma

Incidence of hepatic hemangiosarcoma is variable, according to the literature. Hepatic hemangiosarcoma seems rare in ferrets in a retrospective study.[13] Cases from a ferret colony were reported, however, with up to 22% incidence of hepatic hemangiosar-coma.[89] Its macroscopic appearance can be a mass involving several lobes or a bleeding mass. Few case reports of hepatic hemangiosarcoma in ferrets exist and may have a similar biologic behavior to hemangiosarcoma in other species. Its behavior is highly malignant, and metastasis to other lobes is common.[14]

Lymphoma

Lymphoma is considered the most common malignant neoplasm of ferrets, and the disease spectrum involves peripheral and visceral lymph nodes, including hepatic nodes.[6] Clinically, hepatomegaly is often seen with other typical signs of lymphoma (weight loss, anorexia, lethargy, adenomegaly without fever, lymphocytosis, dyspnea, and pleural effusion in cases of concurrent mediastinal lymphoma).[5] Juvenile ferrets more often acutely have a lymphoblastic form, whereas, from 5 years, older ferrets often suffer from multicenter or isolated lymphoma but are typically affected with a chronic lymphocytic form of lymphoma. Lymphoblastic lymphoma has been re-ported with hepatic involvment.[40,90] Lymphoma has been associated with mycobacterial infection and granulomatous lesion in a ferret.[47] Concurrent liver

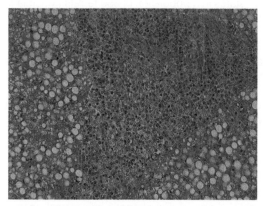

Fig. 16. Photomicrograph of hepatic lymphoma. Portal areas are diffusely severely infil-trated by large round blastic cells showing nuclear atypia. Numerous mitoses are observed. Hematoxylin-eosin staining (original magnification ×20). (*Courtesy of* VetDiagnostics, A. Nicollier.)

eosinophilic infiltrate and granulomas have been seen with a Hodgkin-like lymphoma in ferrets, suggesting that T-cell lymphoma can induce hypereosinophilic syndrome.[91]

The diagnosis may not be possible by cytologic examination of aspirates unless infiltration of neoplastic cells is diffuse enough. Hepatic biopsy and histopathology are the gold standard for diagnosing lymphoma in ferrets (**Fig. 16**).[30]

Hepatic metastasis

The most common neoplastic processes seen in ferret livers are metastatic masses from other sites, mainly adrenal cortical adenocarcinomas and lymphomas. Both of these neoplasms tend to produce pale multiple masses when they involve the liver; some right adrenal neoplasias invade the caudate liver lobe locally without general metastasis.

In one retrospective study, among 71 metastatic neoplasms recorded, there were 48 malignant lymphomas, 11 cases of metastatic adrenocortical carcinoma, 10 cases of adenocarcinoma of unspecified origin, 1 malignant mast cell tumor, and 1 metastatic pancreatic exocrine adenocarcinoma.[13]

SUMMARY

Hepatic diseases in ferrets are common but symptoms are often subclinical. Concurrent digestive disease and systemic signs are often observed. Clinical pathology and diagnostic imaging are useful tools to screen such conditions. Histopathology is necessary to have an accurate diagnosis. Inflammatory hepatitis, hepatic lipidosis, and hepatic neoplasia are the most common diseases encountered in this species. Because liver disease can be part of a systemic disease, screening for concurrent disease and additional examination must be interpreted accordingly.

REFERENCES

1. Fox JG. Biology and diseases of the ferret. Philadelphia: Lea & Febiger; 1988.
2. Poddar S. Gross and microscopic anatomy of the biliary tract of the ferret. Acta Anat (Basel) 1977;97:121–31.
3. Andrews PL, Illman O, Mellersh A. Some observations of anatomical abnormalities and disease states in a population of 350 ferrets (Mustela furo L.). Z Versuchstierkd 1979;21:346–53.
4. Shavila J, Ioannides C, King LJ, et al. Effect of high fat diet on liver microsomal oxygenations in ferret. Xenobiotica 1994;24:1063–76.
5. Burgess M. Ferret gastrointestinal and hepatic diseases. In: Lewington J, editor. Ferret husbandry, medicine and surgery. 2nd edition. Philadelphia: Saunders Elsevier; 2007. p. 203–23.
6. Hoefer HL, Fox JG, Bell JA. Gastrointestinal diseases. In: Quesenberry KE, Carpenter JW, editors. Ferrets, rabbits and rodents: clinical medicine and surgery. 3rd edition. St. Louis (MO): Saunders; 2012. p. 27–61.
7. Jenkins RJ. Rabbit and ferret liver and gastrointestinal testing. In: Fudge A, editor. Philadelphia: WB Saunders Company; 2000. p. 291–304.
8. Fox JG, Zeman DH, Mortimer JD. Copper toxicosis in sibling ferrets. J Am Vet Med Assoc 1994;205:1154–6.
9. Hauptman K, Jekl V, Knotek Z. Extrahepatic biliary tract obstruction in two ferrets (Mustela putorius furo). J Small Anim Pract 2011;52:371–5.
10. Reindel JF, Evans MG. Cystic mucinous hyperplasia in the gallbladder of a ferret. J Comp Pathol 1987;97:601–4.

11. Huynh M. Ruptured gallbladder in a ferret. Seattle: Proc Annu Conf Assoc Avian Vet 2011. p. 361.
12. Rothuizen J. General principles in the treatment of liver disease. In: Ettinger SJ, Feldman EC, editors. Textbook of veterinary internal medicine. 2nd edition. St. Louis (MO): Elsevier Saunders; 2005. p. 1435–42.
13. Williams BH, Weiss CA. Neoplasia. In: Quesenberry KE, Carpenter JW, editors. Ferrets, rabbits and rodents: clinical medicine and surgery. 2nd edition. St. Louis (MO): 2004. p. 91–106.
14. Darby C, Ntavlourou V. Hepatic hemangiosarcoma in two ferrets (Mustela putorius furo). Vet Clin North Am Exot Anim Pract 2006;9:689–94.
15. Hein J, Spreyer F, Sauter-Louis C, et al. Reference ranges for laboratory parameters in ferrets. Vet Rec 2012;171(9):218.
16. Morrissey JK. Ferrets. In: Carpenter JW, Marion CJ, editors. Exotic animal formulary. 3rd edition. St. Louis (MO): Elsevier saunders; 2012. p. 582–3.
17. Benson KG, Paul-Murphy J, Hart AP, et al. Coagulation values in normal ferrets (Mustela putorius furo) using selected methods and reagents. Vet Clin Pathol 2008;37:286–8.
18. Hoffman WE, Solter PF. Diagnostic enzymology of domestic animals. In: Kaneko JJ, Harvey JW, Bruss ML, editors. San Diego (CA): Academic press; 2008. p. 351–78.
19. Tennant BC, Center SA. Hepatic function. In: Kaneko JJ, Harvey JW, Bruss ML, editors. Clinical biochemistry of domestic animals. 6th edition. San Diego (CA): Academic press; 2008. p. 379.
20. Webster CR. History, clinical signs, and physical findings in hepatobiliary disease. In: Ettinger SJ, Feldman EC, editors. Textbook of veterinary internal medicine. St. Louis (MO): Elsevier Saunders; 2004. p. 1422–34.
21. Hall BA, Ketz-Riley CJ. Cholestasis and cholelithiasis in a domestic ferret (Mustela putorius furo). J Vet Diagn Invest 2011;23:836–9.
22. Murray J, Kiupel M, Maes R. Ferret coronavirus-associated diseases. Vet Clin North Am Exot Anim Pract 2010;13:543–60.
23. Welchman Dde B, Oxenham M, Done SH. Aleutian disease in domestic ferrets: diagnostic findings and survey results. Vet Rec 1993;132:479–84.
24. Eshar D, Wyre NR, Brown DC. Urine specific gravity values in clinically healthy young pet ferrets (Mustela furo). J Small Anim Pract 2012;53:115–9.
25. Garner MM, Ramsell K, Morera N, et al. Clinicopathologic features of a systemic coronavirus-associated disease resembling feline infectious peritonitis in the domestic ferret (Mustela putorius). Vet Pathol 2008;45:236–46.
26. Krautwald-Junghanns ME, Pees M, Reese S, et al. Diagnostic imaging of exotic pets. Hannover (Lower Saxony): Schlutersche; 2011.
27. Johnson-Delaney CA. Ultrasonography in ferret practice. In: Lewington J, editor. Ferret husbandry, medicine and surgery. 2nd edition. Philadelphia: Saunders Elsevier; 2007. p. 203–23.
28. Penninck D, D'Anjou MA. Atlas of animal ultrasonography. Ames (IA): Blackwell Publishing Ltd; 2008.
29. D'Anjou MA. Liver. In: Penninck D, D'Anjou MA, editors. Atlas of animal ultrasonography. Ames (IA): Blackwell Publishing Ltd; 2008. p. 217–62.
30. Rakich PM, Latimer KS. Cytologic diagnosis of diseases of ferrets. Vet Clin North Am Exot Anim Pract 2007;10:61–78, vi.
31. Cohen M, Bohling MW, Wright JC, et al. Evaluation of sensitivity and specificity of cytologic examination: 269 cases (1999-2000). J Am Vet Med Assoc 2003;222: 964–7.

32. Stockhaus C, Van Den Ingh T, Rothuizen J, et al. A multistep approach in the cytologic evaluation of liver biopsy samples of dogs with hepatic diseases. Vet Pathol 2004;41:461–70.
33. WSAVA Liver Standardization group. Standards for clinical and histological diagnosis of canine and feline liver diseases. Philadelphia: Saunders Elsevier; 2006.
34. Boomkens SY, Penning LC, Egberink HF, et al. Hepatitis with special reference to dogs. A review on the pathogenesis and infectious etiologies, including unpublished results of recent own studies. Vet Q 2004;26:107–14.
35. Sterczer A, Gaal T, Perge E, et al. Chronic hepatitis in the dog—a review. Vet Q 2001;23:148–52.
36. Garner MM, Ramsell K, Schoemaker NJ, et al. Myofasciitis in the domestic ferret. Vet Pathol 2007;44:25–38.
37. Martinez J, Reinacher M, Perpinan D, et al. Identification of Group 1 coronavirus antigen in multisystemic granulomatous lesions in ferrets (Mustela putorius furo). J Comp Pathol 2008;138:54–8.
38. Solnick JV, Schauer DB. Emergence of diverse Helicobacter species in the pathogenesis of gastric and enterohepatic diseases. Clin Microbiol Rev 2001;14: 59–97.
39. Dubois A. Animal models of Helicobacter infection. Lab Anim Sci 1998;48: 596–603.
40. Garcia A, Erdman SE, Xu S, et al. Hepatobiliary inflammation, neoplasia, and argyrophilic bacteria in a ferret colony. Vet Pathol 2002;39:173–9.
41. Boomkens SY, de Rave S, Pot RG, et al. The role of Helicobacter spp. in the pathogenesis of primary biliary cirrhosis and primary sclerosing cholangitis. FEMS Immunol Med Microbiol 2005;44:221–5.
42. Pandey M. Helicobacter species are associated with possible increase in risk of biliary lithiasis and benign biliary diseases. World J Surg Oncol 2007;5:94.
43. Nemelka KW, Brown AW, Wallace SM, et al. Immune response to and histopathology of Campylobacter jejuni infection in ferrets (Mustela putorius furo). Comp Med 2009;59:363–71.
44. Fox JG, Dewhirst FE, Fraser GJ, et al. Intracellular Campylobacter-like organism from ferrets and hamsters with proliferative bowel disease is a Desulfovibrio sp. J Clin Microbiol 1994;32:1229–37.
45. Pollock C. Mycobacterial Infection in the Ferret. Vet Clin North Am Exot Anim Pract 2012;15:121–9.
46. Schultheiss PC, Dolginow SZ. Granulomatous enteritis caused by Mycobacterium avium in a ferret. J Am Vet Med Assoc 1994;204:1217–8.
47. Saunders GK, Thomsen BV. Lymphoma and Mycobacterium avium infection in a ferret (Mustela putorius furo). J Vet Diagn Invest 2006;18:513–5.
48. Valheim M, Djonne B, Heiene R, et al. Disseminated mycobacterium celatum (type 3) infection in a domestic ferret (Mustela putorius furo). Vet Pathol 2001; 38:460–3.
49. McCallan L, Corbett D, Andersen PL, et al. A new experimental infection model in ferrets based on aerosolised mycobacterium bovis. Vet Med Int 2011;2011: 981410.
50. Bradley GA, Orr K, Reggiardo C, et al. Enterotoxigenic Escherichia coli infection in captive black-footed ferrets. J Wildl Dis 2001;37:617–20.
51. Funke G, Frodl R, Bernard KA. Corynebacterium mustelae sp. nov., isolated from a ferret with lethal sepsis. Int J Syst Evol Microbiol 2010;60:871–3.
52. Thornton RN, Cook TG. A congenital Toxoplasma-like disease in ferrets (Mustela putorius furo). N Z Vet J 1986;34:31–3.

53. Burns R, Williams ES, O'Toole D, et al. Toxoplasma gondii infections in captive black-footed ferrets (Mustela nigripes), 1992-1998: clinical signs, serology, pathology, and prevention. J Wildl Dis 2003;39:787–97.

54. Malik R, Alderton B, Finlaison D, et al. Cryptococcosis in ferrets: a diverse spectrum of clinical disease. Aust Vet J 2002;80:749–55.

55. Eshar D, Mayer J, Parry NM, et al. Disseminated, histologically confirmed Cryptococcus spp infection in a domestic ferret. J Am Vet Med Assoc 2010;236:770–4.

56. Morera N, Juan-Salles C, Torres JM, et al. Cryptococcus gattii infection in a Spanish pet ferret (Mustela putorius furo) and asymptomatic carriage in ferrets and humans from its environment. Med Mycol 2011;49:779–84.

57. Oz HS, Hughes WT, Vargas SL. Search for extrapulmonary Pneumocystis carinii in an animal model. J Parasitol 1996;82:357–9.

58. Evermann JF, Leathers CW, Gorham JR, et al. Pathogenesis of two strains of lion (Panthera leo) morbillivirus in ferrets (Mustela putorius furo). Vet Pathol 2001;38:311–6.

59. Lipatov AS, Kwon YK, Pantin-Jackwood MJ, et al. Pathogenesis of H5N1 influenza virus infections in mice and ferret models differs according to respiratory tract or digestive system exposure. J Infect Dis 2009;199:717–25.

60. Shinya K, Makino A, Tanaka H, et al. Systemic dissemination of H5N1 influenza A viruses in ferrets and hamsters after direct intragastric inoculation. J Virol 2011; 85:4673–8.

61. Humbert Smith J, Nagy T, Driskell E, et al. Comparative Pathology of Ferrets infected with H1N1 Influenza A Viruses Isolated from Different Hosts. J Virol 2011;85:7572–81.

62. Dominguez E, Novellas R, Moya A, et al. Abdominal radiographic and ultrasonographic findings in ferrets (Mustela putorius furo) with systemic coronavirus infection. Vet Rec 2011;169:231.

63. Une Y, Wakimoto Y, Nakano Y, et al. Spontaneous Aleutian disease in a ferret. J Vet Med Sci 2000;62:553–5.

64. Pennick KE, Stevenson MA, Latimer KS, et al. Persistent viral shedding during asymptomatic Aleutian mink disease parvoviral infection in a ferret. J Vet Diagn Invest 2005;17:594–7.

65. Porter HG, Porter DD, Larsen AE. Aleutian disease in ferrets. Infect Immun 1982; 36:379–86.

66. Kenyon AJ, Howard E, Buko L. Hypergammaglobulinemia in ferrets with lymphoproliferative lesions (Aleutian disease). Am J Vet Res 1967;28:1167–72.

67. Kuniholm MH, Purcell RH, McQuillan GM, et al. Epidemiology of Hepatitis E virus in the United States: result of the third national health and nutrition examination survey, 1988-1994. J Infect Dis 2009;200:48–56.

68. Raj VS, Smits SL, Pas SD, et al. Novel hepatitis e virus in ferrets, the Netherlands. Emerg Infect Dis 2012;18:1369–70.

69. Dunayer E. Toxicology of ferrets. Vet Clin North Am Exot Anim Pract 2008;11: 301–14, vi–vii.

70. Platonow N, Beauregard M. Feeding of ferrets with the raw meat and liver of chickens chronically poisoned with toxic groundnut meal. Can J Comp Med Vet Sci 1965;29:63–5.

71. Nieminen P, Mustonen AM, Karja V, et al. Fatty acid composition and development of hepatic lipidosis during food deprivation—mustelids as a potential animal model for liver steatosis. Exp Biol Med (Maywood) 2009;234:278–86.

72. Mustonen AM, Puukka M, Rouvinen-Watt K, et al. Response to fasting in an unnaturally obese carnivore, the captive European polecat Mustela putorius. Exp Biol Med (Maywood) 2009;234:1287–95.

73. Blanco MC, Fox JG, Rosenthal K, et al. Megaoesophagus in nine ferrets. J Am Vet Med Assoc 1994;205:444–7.
74. Benoit-Biancamano MO, Morin M, Langlois I. Histopathologic lesions of diabetes mellitus in a domestic ferret. Can Vet J 2005;46:895–7.
75. Phair KA, Carpenter JW, Schermerhorn T, et al. Diabetic ketoacidosis with concurrent pancreatitis, pancreatic beta islet cell tumor, and adrenal disease in an obese ferret (Mustela putorius furo). J Am Assoc Lab Anim Sci 2011;50: 531–5.
76. Batchelder MA, Bell JA, Erdman SE, et al. Pregnancy toxemia in the European ferret (Mustela putorius furo). Lab Anim Sci 1999;49:372–9.
77. Williams BH, Kiupel M, West KH, et al. Coronavirus-associated Epizootic Catarrhal Enteritis in Ferrets. J Am Vet Med Assoc 2000;217:526–30.
78. Pike FS, Berg J, King NW, et al. Gallbladder mucocele in dogs: 30 cases (2000-2002). J Am Vet Med Assoc 2004;224:1615–22.
79. Williams BH, Chimes MJ, Gardiner CH. Biliary coccidiosis in a ferret (Mustela putorius furo). Vet Pathol 1996;33:437–9.
80. Chesterman FC, Pomerance A. Spontaneous neoplasms in ferrets and polecats. J Pathol Bacteriol 1965;89:529–33.
81. Carter RL, Percival WH, Roe FJ. Exceptional sensitivity of mink to the hepatotoxic effects of dimethylnitrosamine. J Pathol 1969;97:79–88.
82. Koppang N, Helgebostad A. Vascular changes and liver tumours induced in mink by high levels of nitrite in feed. IARC Sci Publ 1987;(84):256–60.
83. Koppang N, Rimeslatten H. Toxic and carcinogenic effects of nitrosodimethyl-amine in mink. IARC Sci Publ 1976;(14):443–52.
84. Antinoff N, Williams BH. Neoplasia. In: Quesenberry KE, Carpenter JW, editors. Ferrets, rabbits and rodents: clinical medicine and surgery. 3rd edition. St. Louis (MO): 2012. p.103–21.
85. Fox JG, Li X, Murphy JC. Serous biliary cystadenoma in ferrets (Mustela putorius furo). Contemp Top Lab Anim Sci 1996;35:78–9.
86. Lair S, Barker IK, Mehren KG, et al. Epidemiology of neoplasia in captive black-footed ferrets (Mustela nigripes), 1986-1996. J Zoo Wildl Med 2002;33:204–13.
87. Tietge UJ, Schofl C, Ocran KW, et al. Hepatoma with severe non-islet cell tumor hypoglycemia. Am J Gastroenterol 1998;93:997–1000.
88. Jones Y, Wise A, Maes R, et al. Peliod hepatocellular carcinoma in a domesticated ferret (Mustela putorius furo). J Vet Diagn Invest 2006;18:228–31.
89. Cross BM. Hepatic vascular neoplasms in a colony of ferrets. Vet Pathol 1987;24: 94–6.
90. Batchelder MA, Erdman SE, Li X, et al. A cluster of cases of juvenile mediastinal lymphoma in a ferret colony. Lab Anim Sci 1996;46:271–4.
91. Blomme EA, Foy SH, Chappell KH, et al. Hypereosinophilic syndrome with Hodgkin's-like lymphoma in a ferret. J Comp Pathol 1999;120:211–7.

Diagnosis of Renal Disease in Rabbits

Frances Margaret Harcourt-Brown, BVSc, FRCVS, RCVS

KEYWORDS

- Rabbit • Kidney • Renal failure • Calcification • Azotemia • Radiography
- *Encephalitozoon cuniculi* • *Osteosclerosis*

KEY POINTS

- Acute renal failure is a potential complication of any disease that causes stress or shock in rabbits. It may coexist with gut stasis.
- Chronic renal failure (CRF) is manifested by weight loss and lethargy in rabbits. They cannot vomit and often eat well despite poor renal function. Most rabbits with CRF are seropositive for *Encephalitozoon cuniculi*.
- Impaired calcium excretion is a feature of CRF and can lead to ectopic calcification of many tissues, including the aorta, kidneys, and bones.
- Nephrolithiasis is common and can cause postrenal acute renal failure by obstructing the ureters.
- Radiography is an essential part of the diagnosis of renal disease in rabbits.

INTRODUCTION

In any species, the function of the kidney is to

- Filter the blood, detoxify and eliminate waste products
- Conserve essential body constituents
- Regulate water and electrolyte balance
- Maintain acid-base balance
- Hormone production

Renal function is achieved by several complex metabolic activities that require an effective mechanism for the blood to be filtered. This occurs in the nephron, which is a structural and functional unit composed of a glomerulus, proximal convoluted tubule, loop of Henle, distal convoluted tubule, and collecting duct (**Fig. 1**). Molecules are actively or passively transported between the fluid within the renal tubule and the blood by a variety of biochemical processes (**Fig. 2**). Although the kidneys represent

Crab Lane Veterinary Surgery, 30 Crab Lane, Bilton, Harrogate, North Yorkshire HG1 3BE, UK
E-mail address: fhbvet@aol.com

Vet Clin Exot Anim 16 (2013) 145–174
http://dx.doi.org/10.1016/j.cvex.2012.10.004
1094-9194/13/$ – see front matter © 2013 Elsevier Inc. All rights reserved.

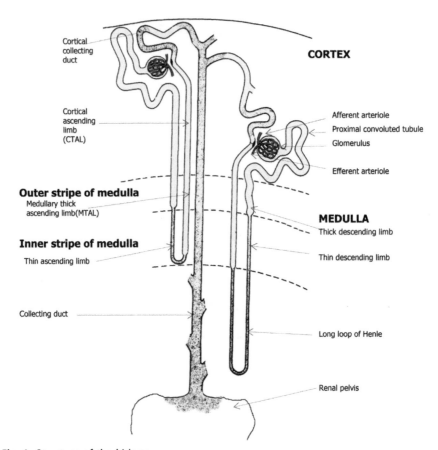

Cortical collecting duct

CORTEX

Cortical ascending limb (CTAL)

Afferent arteriole

Proximal convoluted tubule

Glomerulus

Efferent arteriole

Outer stripe of medulla
Medullary thick ascending limb(MTAL)

MEDULLA
Thick descending limb

Inner stripe of medulla

Thin ascending limb

Thin descending limb

Collecting duct

Long loop of Henle

Renal pelvis

Fig. 1. Structure of the kidney.

a small percentage of the body's mass, 15% to 20% of the cardiac output circulates in a rapidly dividing system of vessels; 70% of the blood goes to the renal cortex[1] where the glomeruli are situated. Within the kidney, the renal artery divides and subdivides into vessels that enter the glomeruli as afferent arterioles. In the glomerulus the afferent arterioles divides into many capillaries (approximately 50) that drain into efferent arterioles, which enter a network of peritubular capillaries that run adjacent to the tubules before draining into the renal cortical vein.

HORMONAL ACTIVITY IN THE KIDNEY

In the kidney, there are receptors for antidiuretic hormone, parathyroid hormone (PTH), aldosterone, prostaglandins, and other hormones, such as cortisol and insulin.[1]

Renin is formed in the kidney by the juxtamedullary apparatus and is regulated by several mechanisms, such as the sympathetic nervous system, sodium depletion, and alterations in blood pressure. Renal hypotension stimulates renin release mediated by prostaglandins. Renin activates conversion of angiotensin I to angiotensin II under the influence of angiotensin-converting enzymes. Angiotensin II is a potent vasoconstrictor that also stimulates aldosterone release. Aldosterone increases tubular secretion of potassium.

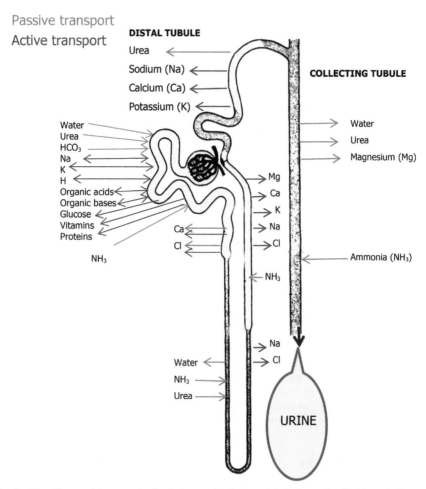

Fig. 2. Direction and transport of substances in the renal tubule and collecting duct.

Vitamin D is activated in the kidney. It is the site of the final step in vitamin D metabolism when cholecalciferol (25[OH]D) is converted to calcitriol (1,25[OH]$_2$D), which is its biologically active form. Conversion of 25[OH]D to 1,25(OH)$_2$D is stimulated by PTH, which is released in response to falling blood calcium or phosphorus concentrations. The main action of 1,25(OH)$_2$D is to maintain calcium homeostasis by stimulating the synthesis of carrier proteins to transport calcium across the intestinal mucosa. 1,25(OH)$_2$D also increases phosphorus absorption.

Erthrypoietin is metabolized in the kidney from erythropoietinogen, which is synthesized in the liver. Erythropoietin acts on stem cells in the bone marrow to produce erythrocytes.

RENAL ANATOMY

As in other species, rabbit kidneys are retroperitoneal and are situated on either side of the aorta and vena cava. The entire ventral surface is covered by peritoneum. Both kidneys have a fibrous capsule and are embedded in adipose tissue. The gross appearance of rabbit kidneys is similar to cat kidneys in size and shape. They have a reddish brown color, with a smooth surface and a simple structure. The size of the kidneys varies with the size of the rabbit, but they are approximately 3 cm long, 2 cm wide, and 10 cm thick. Nerves, blood vessels, and ureters enter and exit at the hilus, where there is a sinus within the kidney, which contains the funnel-shaped renal pelvis and a variable amount of fat plus branches of the renal artery, renal veins, renal nerves, and lymphatics that extend into the parenchyma of the kidney.

STRUCTURE OF THE KIDNEY

As in other species, the parenchyma of the kidney is composed of a cortex surrounding an internal medulla. The cortex is pale with red dots, which are the glomeruli. The medulla has 2 distinct stripes, the outer and inner zones, which can be identified on a longitudinally sectioned kidney (**Fig. 3**). The loops of the nephron, the medullary collecting ducts, and capillaries can be seen as radial striations in the medullas.

Although rabbit nephrons have the same basic structure as those of other species (see **Fig. 1**), the rabbit is the only known mammal in which the tubules can be separated from kidney slices with the tubular epithelium intact, which is why rabbit kidneys are used for many in vitro studies of renal function. The nephrons terminate into collecting tubules, which open into the renal calyces. The calyces have a submucosal circular layer of muscle fibers that contract approximately 12 times per minute to propel urine into the renal pelvis, which collects urine from the collecting ducts. In some other species, the medulla is separated into conical masses that culminate in papillae that protrude into the renal pelvis. This does not occur in the rabbit. Instead the kidney is unipapillate with extensive evaginations of the pelvis into the medullary tissue.[2] The walls are of the renal pelvis have a thin muscular layer and urine is expelled into the ureter, in which contractions of the smooth muscle occur approximately every 10 seconds to stimulates the passage of urine through the ureters to the bladder.

GLOMERULAR FILTRATION

The glomerulus acts as a filtration barrier with a membrane that passes electrolytes and small molecules (eg, glucose) but retains large molecules, such as proteins and blood cells.

The glomerular filtration rate (GFR) is the quantity of glomerular filtrate formed in all the nephrons in both kidneys. More than 99% of this filtrate is reabsorbed. The remainder is urine.

Many factors influence GFR, including oncotic and hydrostatic pressures. Oncotic pressure regulation is complex and is regulated by neuroendocrine feedback mechanisms that alter absorption and secretion of electrolytes between blood and filtrate along the course of the nephron. Transfer may be active or passive and each section of the tubule has different enzyme systems that activate absorption of electrolytes from or secretion the filtrate, which ultimately forms urine (see **Fig. 2**). Hormones, such as PTH, can stimulate active transfer of electrolytes.

Hydrostatic pressure in the kidney is affected by systemic arterial blood pressure, although it is also regulated within the kidney by several humoral (prostaglandins and angiotensin II) and neural mechanisms. The renal nerves are made up of predominantly adrenergic fibers that are vasoconstrictory. In rabbits, vasoconstriction from adrenergic stimulation makes renal blood flow variable and unstable.[3] Stress from unpleasant handling procedures has been shown to cause oliguria in rabbits.[4]

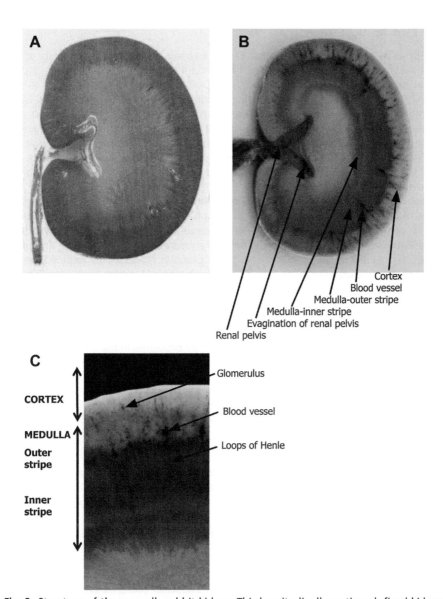

Fig. 3. Structure of the normally rabbit kidney. This longitudinally sectioned, fixed kidney from a wild rabbit shows the normal structure. (*A*) A scanned section that has been stained with hematoxylin and eosin. (*B*) Shows the cut surface of the sectioned kidney and (*C*) shows an enlarged view of part of the sectioned kidney.

Angiograms taken during periods of forced apnea in rabbits showed total cessation of blood flow to the kidneys.[5]

Unlike humans and dogs, in which all the glomeruli are present at birth, in rabbits the number of glomeruli increase after birth and ectopic glomeruli are present in the adult kidney.[2] There is a wide variation in the number of glomeruli that are active at any one time and diuresis increases the number of active glomeruli rather than GFR. As much as a 16-fold increase in water diuresis is possible without significant change in GFR.[6]

ACID-BASE REGULATION

Acid-base balance is the state of equilibrium between the acidity and alkalinity of the body that is essential to maintain normal tissue metabolism, and the kidneys play a vital role in maintaining that equilibrium. Carbonic anhydrase, produced in the renal tubular epithelial cells, is an important enzyme in maintaining acid-base balance because it catalyzes the breakdown of carbonic acid to hydrogen and bicarbonate ions. Ammonia produced in the kidney by glutamine deamination is also important. It is produced in response to a fall in plasma pH or a decreased concentration of bicarbonate. Ammonia acts as part of the buffering system in the renal tubule by combining with hydrogen ions before being excreted in the urine as ammonium ions.

Rabbits are susceptible to acid-base disorders. Renal reabsorption of bicarbonate by the renal tubule is not as efficient as in most other mammals. Carbonic anhydrase is absent from the thick ascending limb of the renal tubule of rabbits[6,7] in contrast to humans, monkeys, and rats, in which carbonic anhydrase is present in large amounts. In rabbits, glutamine deamination only takes place in response to reduced serum bicarbonate concentrations but not a drop in plasma pH, which compromises the rabbit's response to metabolic acidosis. In other species, there are alternative biochemical pathways that result in ammonia synthesis but these pathways seem to be absent in the rabbit.[6] Respiratory control of blood pH is perpetuated in acidotic rabbits.[8]

In addition to correcting acidosis, the rabbit has problems in the renal response to alkalosis. A large bicarbonate load can reach the kidney of rabbits as a result of bacterial fermentation in the gut and from tissue metabolism of acetate. In other species, bicarbonate is neutralized by the products of ureagenesis and alkalosis is avoided, but in rabbits, insufficient ammonium may be available from tissue metabolism to neutralize bicarbonate, especially during periods of protein deficit.[6]

CALCIUM METABOLISM IN RABBITS

Rabbits have evolved a calcium metabolism that can meet a high demand (**Fig. 4**). All the teeth of rabbits continually erupt and grow at a rate of 2 mm/wk to 2.5 mm/wk, which requires a constant supply of large amounts of calcium for the formation of new dental tissue. Female rabbits produce large litters and can be pregnant and lactating simultaneously, which requires calcium for the developing fetuses and growing kits. In rabbits, passive diffusion of calcium across the intestinal wall rather than active vitamin D–dependent transport is the main method of calcium absorption from the gut, so there is no feedback mechanism. Calcium is absorbed according to difference in calcium concentration between intestinal contents and blood rather than metabolic need. A consequence of passive absorption is that calcium uptake from the gut is proportional to dietary calcium content[9] and, perhaps because of efficient passive absorption from the gut, total serum calcium concentrations of rabbits are 30% to 50% higher than in other domestic mammals and vary over a wide range. Studies in laboratory rabbits showed a variation of 2.89–3.92 mmol/l.[10]

Instead of regulating calcium input from the gut, rabbits regulate calcium output into the urine to maintain calcium homeostasis and the kidneys play a major role. The rabbit kidney is capable of increasing the excretion of calcium into the urine considerably[11] and calcium balance is regulated by excreting or conserving calcium according to metabolic need, mediated by PTH and $1,25(OH)_2D$.[12] Tubular reabsorption of calcium increases during periods of calcium deprivation[13] and decreases during periods of high calcium intake.[14]

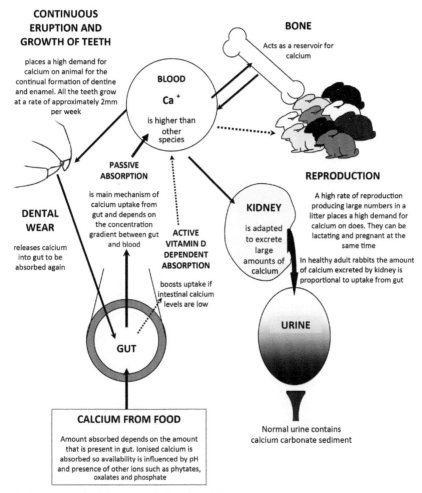

Fig. 4. Summary of calcium metabolism in rabbits.

DISEASES THAT AFFECT RENAL FUNCTION IN RABBITS

Kidney abscesses, pyelonephritis, pyelitis, and amyloidosis are infrequent as naturally occurring diseases in rabbits.[15,16] Other conditions are more common.

Congenital Defects

Although they are rare, congenital defects, such as renal agenesis aplasia or renal cysts, have been described in rabbits.[17,18]

Neoplasia

Renal neoplasia is occasionally encountered in rabbits. The condition may be primary or secondary (**Figs. 5** and **6**). Malignant neoplasms, such as lymphoma and renal carcinomas, occur. A benign tumor, an embryonal nephroma, is a reportedly common tumor of laboratory rabbits.[19] The tumors can be an incidental postmortem finding and do not affect renal function. They appear as whitish, sharply circumscribed nodules of tissue projecting above the cortical surface.

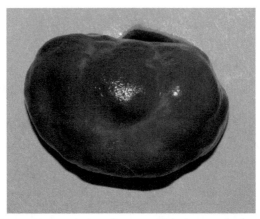

Fig. 5. Renal lymphoma: this is a kidney from a rabbit that was euthanized with an intestinal lymphoma involving the cecum. Histopathologically, it proved to be a lymphoma.

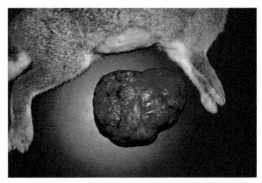

Fig. 6. Large neoplastic kidney: the mass in this figure was an enlarged kidney that was removed from an 18-month-old neutered male wild cross rabbit showing signs of weight loss and lethargy. Exploratory laparotomy was performed to investigate the large palpable abdominal mass. The rabbit died soon after surgery. Could this picture be moved so it is in the section about neoplasia. At the moment it looks as if the picture has something to do with E. Cuniculi, which it doesn't.

Fatty Infiltration of the Kidney

Fatty infiltration of the kidney is an endpoint of gut stasis in rabbits. Once gut motility is reduced and food does not move through the digestive tract, absorption of carbohydrates from the small intestine is reduced and volatile fatty acid synthesis and absorption from the cecum fall so the rabbit goes into a negative energy balance. This stimulates the mobilization of free fatty acids from adipose tissue that are transported to the liver to be metabolized as an energy source using β-oxidation, which causes ketone body production and metabolic acidosis. The free fatty acids infiltrate the liver and kidneys, causing fatty degeneration and organ failure.

Encephalitozoon cuniculi

E cuniculi infection is common in pet rabbits and the parasite has a predilection to renal tissue. Affected rabbits often have obviously pitted, scarred kidneys on gross postmortem examination (**Fig. 7**). Histologically, early lesions show focal to segmental granulomatous interstitial nephritis. Lesions may be present at all levels of the renal

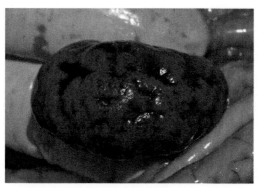

Fig. 7. Scarred kidney due to encephalitozoonosis. This kidney shows the typical appearance of chronic (or previous) infection with *E cuniculi*. There are multiple pitted areas of the cortex. The rabbit showed no signs of renal disease and died from other causes.

tubule, usually with minimal involvement of the glomeruli, and spores may be seen in the tissue or free within the collecting tubules. In longstanding cases, interstitial fibrosis, collapse of the parenchyma, and mononuclear infiltration are typical changes in renal tissue. The parasite is often eliminated from the kidney tissue by this stage[20] although it may be detectable in other tissues.[21] The parasite also has a predilection to central nervous system tissue, and ataxia, with or without bladder atony and urinary incontinence, is another clinical sign linked with *E cuniculi*.

Calcification of the Kidney (Nephrocalcinosis)

Calcification of the kidney is usually seen in association with ectopic calcification of other tissues, especially arteries, arterioles, myocardium, and bone. It is associated with hypercalcemia or hyperphosphatemia (especially both) and precipitation occurs when the calcium/phosphate solubility product is exceeded in extracellular fluid. The mineral that is initially deposited is amorphous calcium phosphate but hydroxyapatite is formed soon after.[22] In the kidney, calcification occurs in the cortical and corticomedullary tubules and mineralization of the renal cortex can be seen radiographically (**Fig. 8**), ultrasonographically, and on gross postmortem examination of the kidneys

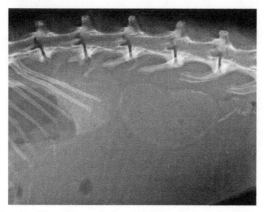

Fig. 8. Nephrocalcinosis: this radiograph shows bilateral cortical mineralization in a 6-year-old female neutered rabbit. She was thin and cachexic. The kidneys are enlarged and there were mineral deposits in the mesometrium.

(**Fig. 9**). The kidneys appear mottled and misshapen (**Fig. 10**). Histopathology is more sensitive than visual examination for detecting mineral deposits in the tissue.

Causes of calcification of the kidney

- CRF is an important cause of renal calcification, but calcification of the kidney also causes CRF so it can be difficult to know which condition came first. In pet rabbits, CRF seems to be the main cause of calcification of the kidney.[21] Clinical cases are usually seropositive to E cuniculi and it is probable, but impossible to prove, that in most cases, the parasite initiated the renal pathology and ultimately caused CRF and calcification.
- Vitamin D toxicity causes increased intestinal absorption of calcium and phosphorus, which can precipitate in the renal cortex. Rabbits seem susceptible to vitamin D toxicity and there are reports of renal calcification (and ectopic calcification of other tissues) in colonies of rabbits that have accidentally received high doses of vitamin D in their feed.[23,24]

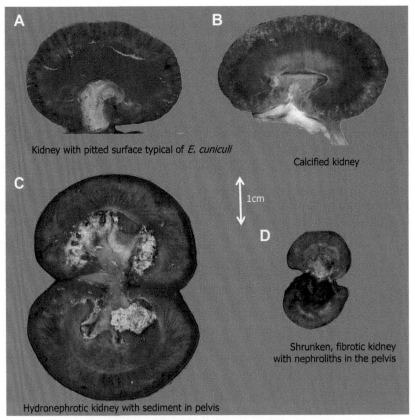

Kidney with pitted surface typical of E. cuniculi

Calcified kidney

1cm

Shrunken, fibrotic kidney with nephroliths in the pelvis

Hydronephrotic kidney with sediment in pelvis

Fig. 9. Sectioned kidneys showing common pathology. These kidneys were harvested during postmortem examination and sectioned longitudinally before being immersed in water and scanned to show detail of the changes that have taken place. Kidney A is a sectioned, scarred kidney that is typical of chronic inflammation associated with Encephalitozoon cunicul. Kidney B is a sectioned kidney that was affected by nephrocalcinosis. The cortex is calcified. Kidneys C and D were the right and left kidneys from the rabbit whose radiograph is shown in **Fig. 20**.

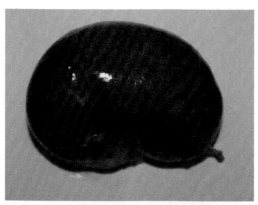

Fig. 10. End-stage CRF: this small fibrotic kidney was from a rabbit showing all the signs of terminal renal failure. She was thin but eating well. She was presented for treatment because she was lame. Radiography showed ectopic calcification of the kidney and aorta, with dystrophic calcification in the arthritic joints. Her skeleton showed generalized osteosclerosis. Her skull radiograph is shown in **Fig. 26** and her eye is shown in **Fig. 19**. Her blood results were total blood calcium of 5.04 mmol/L, phosphate 2.7 mmol/L, urea 24.4 mmol/L, and creatinine 310 μmol/L.

- High dietary calcium. Many urinary tract diseases, including calcification of the kidneys, are often attributed to high dietary calcium levels although this is not proved. A tendency for renal calcification has been induced in laboratory rabbits by force-feeding them high dietary calcium levels (4.03%).[25] Calcium levels in the diets of pet rabbits (approximately 0.5%–1.2%) are not high enough, however, to cause renal calcification. A more recent study[26] failed to induce ectopic calcification by feeding high dietary calcium to rabbits, so there must be other contributory factors, such as impaired renal function, reduced water intake, and calcium:phosphorus imbalance.
- High dietary phosphorus has been cited as a caused or calcification of the renal cortex and corticomedullary region in laboratory rabbits.[27] Restricting dietary phosphorus prevented the condition. No details of the vitamin D content of the laboratory rabbits were included in these reports.
- Other causes: renal calcification has been induced in laboratory rabbits by administering phosphate, vitamin D, oxalate, or furosemide before unilateral nephrectomy.[28]

Nephrolithiasis

Kidney stones are common in pet rabbits. Nephrolithiasis is a different condition from nephrocalcinosis although both conditions involve calcium deposits within the kidney. The type and distribution of the mineral are different. Nephrocalcinosis occurs in the cortex and corticomedullary region whereas nephroliths accumulate in the renal pelvis (**Fig. 11**). Calcium phosphate is the mineral that is deposited in ectopic calcification but, in rabbits, nephroliths are usually composed of calcium carbonate.

Nephroliths may be present in one or both kidneys (**Figs. 12** and **13**) and their texture varies from an aggregate of gritty material and sludge to discrete stones (see **Figs. 9** and **11**). The condition is progressive, with stones building up in the renal pelvis until it becomes dilated. Nephroliths can pass out of the kidney and become lodged in the renal pelvis (**Fig. 14**) or ureter.

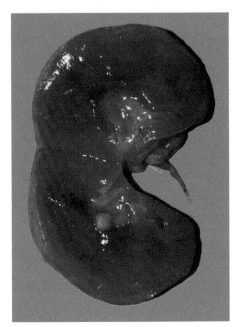

Fig. 11. Single nephroliths in the renal pelvis: this kidney is from a 7-year-old neutered wild rabbit that was hand reared and kept as a pet. She had previously shown neurologic signs and was known to be seropositive for encephalitozoonosis. She had started to lose weight and was diagnosed with renal failure a year before she was euthanized because of posterior paresis. The kidney stone was an incidental finding during postmortem examination. It was not on radiographs taken when the rabbit was first diagnosed with CRF.

Rabbits are naturally predisposed to stone formation because of the presence of large amounts of calcium in the urine, but the cause of nephrolithiasis is poorly understood. Kidney stones are aggregates of crystals mixed with a protein matrix and it is not clear why precipitation takes place in some individuals. Hyalurolan, a glycosaminoglycan that

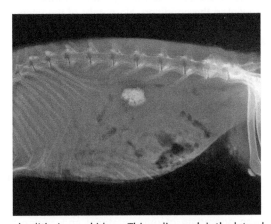

Fig. 12. Multiple nephroliths in one kidney. This radiograph is the lateral abdominal view of a mature entire male rabbit was presented for treatment because he was incontinent and had lost weight. There is urine in the fur on the ventral abdomen. Although this rabbit was a potential candidate for nephrectomy, the owners declined and he was euthanized.

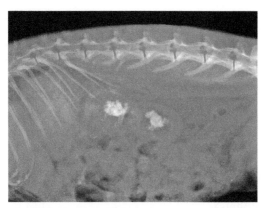

Fig. 13. Bilateral nephrolithiasis. These kidney stones were seen on an abdominal radiograph of a 5-year-old neutered male rabbit that was taken because the rabbit temporarily stopped eating. He was overweight and showed no other clinical signs. Blood urea and creatinine were within the reference range. The rabbit was lost to follow-up.

is abundant in the renal medulla but absent from the medulla, has been implicated in experimental renal stone formation in rabbits.[29] It has sponge-like properties and is important in water regulation and providing structural support for the nephron. Crystal binding to hyaluralon leads to crystal retention and hyaluralon production is increased during renal inflammation or disease.[30] Water intake may also play a part in stone formation. Flow of urine through the kidney flushes crystals into the ureter. Any factor that decreases urine flow, such as mechanical obstruction, dehydration, or inadequate water intake, predisposes to stone formation. Many rabbits eat a dry diet of hay and concentrated food rather than a natural diet of moist plant material and are provided with sipper bottles to drink from. They would drink more from water bowls.[31]

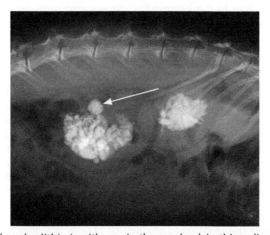

Fig. 14. Advanced nephrolithiasis with one in the renal pelvis: this radiograph of a mature neutered female rabbit that had previously shown neurologic signs and was seropositive for encephalitozoonosis. Bilateral nephrolithiasis had been monitored radiographically and by serial blood samples for 18 months during which the rabbit was apparently healthy until she suddenly became totally anorexic and moribund, presumably due to the large nephrolith (*arrow*) that obstructed the entrance to the ureter and resulted in acute hydronephrosis.

Ureteral obstruction predisposes to nephrolithiasis and laboratory studies have shown that even temporary obstruction of the upper urinary tract results in the rapid formation of kidney stones.[32] Other studies have shown that stones rapidly form in the remaining kidney of unilaterally nephrectomized rabbits if infarcts are induced by the ligation of the renal blood supply.[33] This might explain the link between E cuniculi and nephrolithiasis. Rabbits with kidney stones are usually seropositive for E cuniculi[21] and show histopathologic signs of chronic interstitial granulomatous inflammation and fibrosis. It is possible that fibrosis and inflammation within the kidneys stimulates hyalurolan production and reduces GFR. Inflammatory cells also act as nidi for stone formation. Once crystals have started to form within the renal pelvis, they obstruct urine flow and increase the tendency for stone formation, so a vicious circle is formed.

RENAL FAILURE IN RABBITS
Acute Renal Failure

Acute renal failure occurs when kidney function is abruptly reduced by disease or physiologic event. It is not a primary condition but a secondary one. The severity of the condition ranges from reversible mild elevations in urea and creatinine levels to irreversible electrolyte imbalances, oliguria, and death. There are 3 types of acute renal failure.

Prerenal acute renal failure

Prerenal acute renal failure occurs when renal perfusion is reduced (eg, due to shock, hemorrhage, dehydration, or reduced cardiac output). Rabbits cannot vomit, so dehydration from actual fluid loss only occurs in rabbits with enteritis, although it can occur in rabbits with gut stasis because of inadequate fluid intake and redistribution of fluid within the gastrointestinal tract. Dehydration can also be caused by mismanagement (ie, water deprivation due to faulty sipper bottles, frozen water, or owner oversight in replenishing the bowl).

In rabbits, stress readily causes temporary vasoconstriction of the renal arterioles and reduces blood flow to the kidneys.[34,35] Stress also reduces gut motility so gut stasis and acute renal failure may be seen together. In these situations, azotemia is reversible and resolves if fluids and electrolytes are given before renal ischemia or fatty infiltration occurs.

Renal acute renal failure

Renal acute renal failure is due to acute structural damage to the kidney. It may be caused by exposure to nephrotoxins, such as parenteral gentamicin,[36] fatty infiltration of the kidney, or severe renal ischemia. Acute renal failure is potentially fatal complication of any severe life-threatening disease in rabbits (eg, enterotoxemia or severe gastric dilation[21]) that causes hypovolemia or severe prolonged shock. Reduction in GFR due to renal ischemia seems to be mediated neurally rather than by angiotensin II.[37] Occasionally, renal infarcts may be seen (**Fig. 15**) on gross examination of the kidneys.

Postrenal acute renal failure

Postrenal acute renal failure is due to obstruction of urine flow through the ureters and lower urinary tract. Obstruction may within the ureter or urethra and hydronephrosis is the result. Some rabbits survive the initial pain and stress of hydronephrosis, especially if it is unilateral. Others die from shock. Ureteral obstruction is usually due to nephroliths passing out of the kidney but can also be caused by adhesions or fat necrosis in the mesometrium after ligation of blood vessels during ovariohysterectomy. The ureters

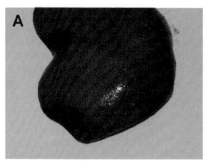
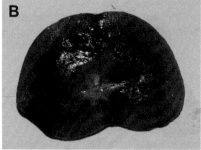

Fig. 15. Kidney infarct: this kidney was from an adult female rabbit that was suffering from posterior paresis and cystitis. She rapidly became moribund and died despite treatment. Histopathology showed acute papillary necrosis associated with renal ischemia. (*A*) shows the gross appearance of the whole kidney. (*B*) shows a longitudinal section that reveals the extent of the infarct.

are close to the vaginal artery (**Fig. 16**). Inguinal bladder herniation is another potential cause of urethral obstruction.

Chronic Renal Failure

CRF occurs when kidney function is impaired for a period of more than 2 to 4 weeks and is characterized by irreversible renal structural lesions. It is a progressive disease although the time course is variable. Rabbits can live for years with impaired renal function. The inciting cause of CRF may never be known as secondary changes, such as inflammation, fibrosis, and mineralization, occur and mask evidence of the original disease. CRF is divided into the following stages.

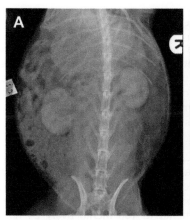
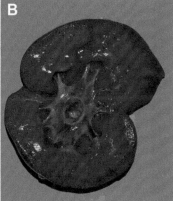

Fig. 16. Bilateral hydronephrosis due to obstruction of the ureters as a complication of ovariohysterectomy. The radiograph (*A*) shows a dorsoventral view of a 1-year-old female rabbit that had undergone recent ovariohysterectomy. She was referred because of recurrent abdominal pain and anorexia since the operation. The radiographs show that both kidneys are enlarged and were painful. Exploratory laparotomy revealed adhesions at the entrance of both ureters to the bladder. They were encapsulated in necrotic fat. Both ureters were dilated although there obstruction was only partial in the right ureter. The rabbit was euthanized and postmortem examination confirmed hydronephrosis (*B*). Correct placement of the ligatures around the uterine artery is essential during ovariohysterectomy. It is safe to place them near the cervices.

Early stages

One of the first signs of loss of functional nephrons in other species is a decreased ability to concentrate urine so polydipsia and polyuria develop and compensatory mechanisms take place to maintain renal function as nephrons are lost. In dogs and cats, single nephrons can adapt to increase GFR and an increase in glomerular blood pressure occurs.[38] In rabbits, not all the nephrons are active, so increasing the number of active glomeruli may be a compensatory mechanism in the early stages of CRF and would why clinical signs of early renal disease are often absent.

Advanced stages

As renal failure progresses, the ability to excrete toxins is impaired and clinical signs of uremia develop. Blood urea and creatinine rise although, in rabbits, there has to be 50% to 75% loss of renal function before this occurs.[39]

End stage

End-stage renal disease occurs when renal function is severely impaired. Because the rabbit kidney is important in calcium regulation, it is derangements in calcium metabolism that cause most of the clinical signs that are associated with end-stage renal disease. Ectopic mineralization is common.[40] High blood calcium levels are a feature of uremic rabbits both clinically[21] and in experimental studies.[33,41–43] The hypercalcemia is due to continued intestinal absorption of calcium and impaired renal excretion. Laboratory studies have shown that aortic mineralization is seen with a 20% increase in blood calcium levels. Calcium phosphate is laid down initially with hydroxyapatite crystals appearing after 196 days.[44] An increase in bone density (osteosclerosis) is common with end-stage renal disease in rabbits (**Fig. 17**), which is the opposite of many other species that develop osteopenia due to insufficient calcium uptake from the gut due to impaired vitamin D synthesis by diseased kidneys.

DIAGNOSIS OF RENAL DISEASE IN RABBITS

In other species, clinical signs of uremia include depressed appetite, depression, nausea, vomiting, mucosal ulcers, weight loss, anemia, and arterial hypertension. Many of these signs are not obvious in uremic rabbits and, in many cases, renal disease is diagnosed in association with other diseases, such as myiasis, posterior paresis, or abscesses.[15,21] There are some clinical signs, however, that may alert the clinician to the possibility that renal disease may be present.

Clinical Examination

Polydypsia/polyuria can be a sign of renal disease in rabbits but is not consistent. Some rabbits drink a lot of water but never show evidence of renal disease. Others have obvious renal pathology but are not polydypsic. Polydypsia is a sign that owners easily miss. Rabbits normally drink 50 mL/kg to 100 mL/kg every 24 hours and produce 50 mL/kg/d to 75 mL/kg/d of urine,[45] although these quantities are variable. The composition and water content of the diet affect the quantity of water that is drunk. Rabbits that eat fresh greens may not drink at all.[46] Dry foods (eg, hay, muesli mixes, nuggets, and pellets) absorb water in the intestinal tract and, therefore, increase thirst. Conditions that prevent a rabbit eating (eg, food deprivation or dental disease) can result in an increase in thirst, with rabbits drinking up to 650% more water.[6]

Oliguria occurs when urine production is less than 7 mL/kg/d and is a poor prognostic sign associated with acute renal failure.

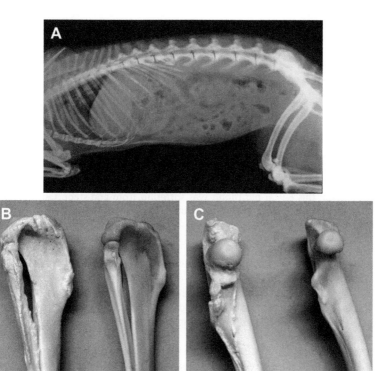

Fig. 17. Osteosclerosis. (*A*) The skeleton of a rabbit with advanced renal failure and generalized osteosclerosis. The bones are radiodense with a blurred outline sue to mineral deposits on the surfaces. (*B, C*) Prepared tibiofibulars and femurs from an osteosclerotic rabbit (*left*) and a normal rabbit (*right*). Histologically the bones show thickening of the cortex and replacement of the metaphyseal cancellous bone by increased lamellar bone. The bone deposited on the cortical surface contains nubbins of cartilage.

Anorexia is associated with the some of the conditions that cause acute renal failure. Inappetance, in conjunction with reduced or absent fecal output, is a feature of gut stasis that may coexist with prerenal azotemia. Left untreated, rabbits with gut stasis progress to hepatic lipidosis, ketoacidosis, fatty infiltration of the kidneys, liver and kidney failure, and death. In the terminal stages, the rabbits are totally anorexic, ataxic, and hypothermic with muscular weakness.

Sudden and complete loss of appetite, hiding behavior, and unresponsiveness to external stimuli are associated with acute abdominal pain, which may be due to the passage of ureteral stones, hydronephrosis, or both[47] or other life-threatening abdominal conditions, such as intestinal obstruction. These rabbits are at risk of acute renal failure.

A good appetite is usually seen in rabbits with CRF until late stages. Nausea is a feature of CRF in other species and is a reason for loss of appetite in humans. Rabbits cannot vomit, so it is unlikely that they experience nausea, which may explain their good appetite during CRF.

Marked weight loss is a feature of CRF both clinically and in laboratory studies.[33,40,48] Affected rabbits eat well but may lose 30% to 40% of their normal body weight and appear cachexic (**Fig. 18**).

Abdominal palpation is an important part of clinical examination of rabbits and can indicate renal disease. The left kidney is not as firmly attached as the right kidney

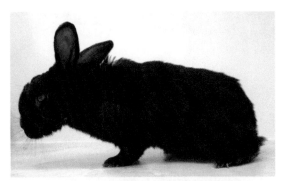

Fig. 18. Cachexia: this 8-year-old rabbit was suffering from end-stage CRF. He shows the typical appearance of a rabbit with the disease. He is emaciated and reluctant to move, presumably due to bone pain from osteosclerosis. He was eating well. He has a cataract in the left eye, which was not due to the CRF but may have been linked by *E cuniculi* infection.

and is usually palpated easily, unless the rabbit is obese or ascitic. The caudal pole of the right kidney usually is felt behind the ribs on the right side of the abdomen. Palpation of the kidneys may reveal pain, renomegaly or decreased kidney size. Occasionally crepitus associated with the presence of kidney stones may be felt. Renomegaly is usually due to neoplasia or hydronephrosis. Small, fibrotic kidneys are a feature of end-stage CRF.

Locomotor problems, such as reluctance to move, ataxia, hindlimb weakness, shifting lameness, hunched posture, and spontaneous fractures, can be associated with osteosclerosis that is associated with cases of end-stage renal failure. Radiography is diagnostic (see **Fig. 18**).

Signs of cardiorespiratory disease, such as tachypnea or syncope, may be seen in rabbits with bronchial or aortic calcification.

Corneal dystrophy is sometimes seen in rabbits with end-stage renal failure **(Fig. 19)**. It seems to be associated with derangements in lipid metabolism and dystrophic calcification.

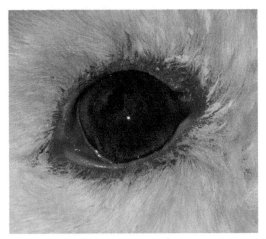

Fig. 19. Corneal dystrophy: corneal dystrophy is not uncommon in rabbits with end-stage CRF. The surface of the cornea is pitted with a gritty appearance. Histologically, there was mild hyalinization and fibrosis with areas of lymphocytic inflammation.

Imaging

Abdominal radiography is mandatory all cases of suspected renal failure. Many changes, such as renomegaly or small kidneys, may be seen (**Figs. 20–26**). Calcium is an excellent contrast medium, so nephroliths or dystrophic or ectopic mineralization that is often seen in rabbits with renal failure is often obvious on radiographs. A methodical approach is required to examine the radiographs (**Box 1**).

Intravenous pyelography is useful for assessing renal function and evaluating the renal pelvis and ureters. It is contraindicated in acute renal failure because precipitation of the agent in the renal tubules can be nephrotoxic. The most useful indication for intravenous pyelography in rabbits is for those in which unilateral nephrectomy is under consideration, perhaps due to stones or hydronephrosis (see **Fig. 21**). It is reassuring to know the remaining kidney is structurally normal and excreting urine. A patient needs to be well hydrated before infusion of an iodinated contrast medium and may need sedation for intravenous fluids to be given at a rate of 10 mL/kg/h. The contrast agent is either given as a bolus (850 mg iodine/kg) or and an infusion (1200 mg iodine/kg) over 15 to 30 minutes. Radiographs are taken 2 to 5 minutes after infusion and then at regular intervals.

Ultrasound examination is useful to examine the renal parenchyma and to show renal cysts or hydronephrosis. The fibrous capsule of the kidney should be visible and a thin hyperechoic line. The renal cortex has a granulated appearance and hyperechoic in comparison with the medulla. Hydronephrosis can be identified by anechoic pelvic dilation. Dilated ureters may also be identifiable. Nephrocalcinosis can be seen as a typical corticomedullary ring.[50] Nephroliths may cast acoustic shadows.

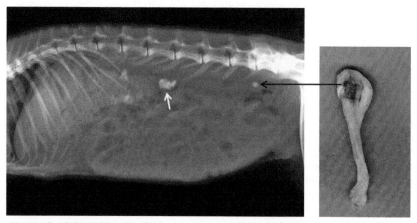

Fig. 20. Nephrolithiasis, hydronephrosis, renomegaly, renal atrophy (or agenesis), and ureterolithiasis. This lateral radiograph of a 4-year-old male neutered (MN) dwarf lop rabbit shows many abnormalities. The rabbit was presented moribund and died shortly after admission. He had suddenly become anorexic, presumably due to the passage of a nephrolith out of the right kidney and into the renal pelvis. The right kidney is enlarged and has mineralized deposits in the medulla or dilated renal pelvis. There is ureteral stone (*black arrow*) which was in the right ureter. The left kidney is tiny, fibrotic, and full of stones (*white arrow*) it not known if this kidney was small from birth (renal aplasia) or its small size was due to fibrosis. The relative size and gross appearance of the sectioned kidneys are shown in **Fig. 9.** The postmortem appearance of the ureter and stone is shown alongside. The section of ureter was placed in water to be scanned.

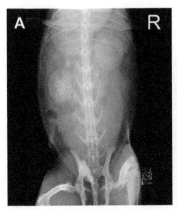
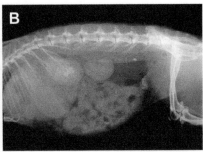

Fig. 21. Intravenous pyelography: these radiographs show a ventrodorsal view (*A*) and lateral view (*B*) of the abdomen of a 6-year-old rabbit with anorexia and abdominal pain. A ureteral stone and hydronephrosis of the right kidney were seen on plain radiographs. After intravenous infusion of iohexol, the left kidney was seen to be functional and radiographically normal. A blood sample indicated no elevation in kidney parameters, so the right kidney and ureter were removed and the rabbit lived for several more years.

Clinical Pathology

References ranges and conversion factors are given in **Tables 1** and **2**. Interpretation of clinical pathology results relating to renal disease is summarized in **Table 3**. Blood pH, ketones, and electrolytes are important in assessing renal function and prognosis. An analyzer that measures these parameters (eg, i-STAT) is useful. In general, the diagnosis of renal disease by changes in clinical pathology is similar to that of other species although there are some differences in rabbits. These changes are discussed.

Blood urea and creatinine

As in other species, blood urea and creatinine are the most commonly used markers of renal disease but may be insensitive.[51] Severe renal pathology may be present in rabbits with marginally elevated urea and creatinine levels[21] but urea and creatinine levels can be high in rabbits without renal pathology. Rabbits have a limited capacity to concentrate urea and a greater volume of urine is required when urea load increases,[6] so prerenal azotemia develops readily during periods of dehydration. Urea and creatinine levels may reach high levels in rabbits with gut stasis and can be greater than in rabbits with significant renal pathology.[15]

Many factors influence blood urea concentrations in rabbits and small fluctuations are difficult to interpret. High-protein diets increase blood urea levels and they may fall during periods during periods of catabolism because urea is metabolized by the cecal microflora synthesis.[52]

Blood calcium

Blood calcium levels in rabbits vary over a wide range and are dependent on dietary intake. This physiologic variation in serum calcium concentrations makes interpretation of blood results difficult. Reference ranges differ between sources and total serum calcium concentrations are correlated with serum albumin.[53] Despite these problems, serum calcium is an important parameter in the diagnosis of renal disease. It is usually at the high end or above the laboratory reference range in cases of CRF.

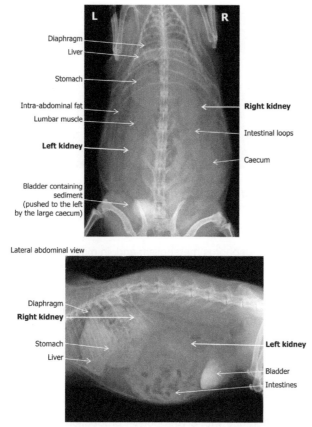

Fig. 22. Normal position of the kidneys on abdominal radiographs. Ventro dorsal view (*Top*). Lateral view (*bottom*). The rabbit is overweight so the intra-abdominal fat contrasts with the organs.

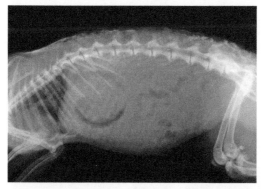

Fig. 23. Dystrophic calcification: this radiograph shows a 9-year-old entire dwarf lop male rabbit presented for treatment of a skin condition. He was suffering from cheyletiellosis but the skin was also inflamed, presumably due to a hypersensitivity reaction. Radiography showed not only dystrophic calcification in the inflamed skin but also mild osteosclerosis and aortic calcification. A blood sample indicated raised urea, creatinine, calcium, and phosphorus. The rabbit was euthanized.

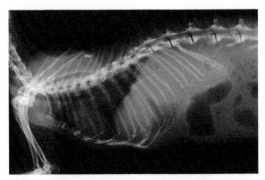

Fig. 24. Aortic calcification: calcification of the aorta shows on radiographs as 2 parallel lines in the craniodorsal abdomen that extend into the thoracic cavity and curve around the base of the heart. The lines stop at the atrioventricular border.

Inorganic phosphorus

Renal function affects phosphorus metabolism and, in most species, hyperphosphatemia is a feature of CRF due to impaired excretion by the kidneys and stimulates PTH release (renal secondary hyperparathyroidism).

In rabbits, hypophosphatemia can be seen in association with naturally occurring renal disease.[21,54] Experimental studies have shown a resistance to renal secondary hyperparathyroidism,[33,48] although the response is dependent on the calcium and phosphate content of the diet. Hyperphosphatemia in conjunction with high blood calcium levels is a poor prognostic sign in rabbits, especially if urea and creatinine are also raised because this signifies advanced renal failure with a high probability of ectopic mineralization that affects organ function.[21]

Anemia

Anemia is due to interference with erythropoietin production in other species and is often present in rabbits with CRF. It is a nonspecific sign, however, of any chronic illness in rabbits and is not specific to renal disease.[53]

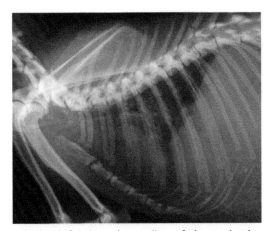

Fig. 25. Tracheobronchial calcification: the outline of the tracheobronchial tree can be enhanced by ectopic calcification so that it is obvious on thoracic radiographs. The rabbit in this radiograph also showed increased bone density. These radiographic signs should alert the clinician to the probability of underlying kidney disease.

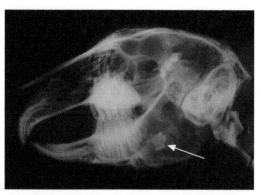

Fig. 26. Osteosclerosis and calcification of the hyoid bone: this lateral skull radiograph shows good contrast between the bone and soft tissue although the cortical lines are thick and slightly blurred. There is a diamond-shaped area of increased mineralization in the masseteric fossa (*arrow*), which is the osteosclerotic hyoid bone.

Encephalitozoon cuniculi serology

It is always useful to know if a rabbit with renal disease, especially CRF, is seropositive or seronegative for *E cuniculi* although the significance of titers is not clear. The titer levels do not correspond with severity of tissue damage. Measurement of both IgG and IgM titers can give a better prognostic indicator than IgG alone because a high

---

Box 1
Examination of radiographs for signs of renal disease

1. Look at whole radiographic area for signs of ectopic calcification, which may be associated with underlying renal disease (see **Fig. 23**)

2. Identify both kidneys and assess their position. The position of the kidneys is variable because they may be displaced by fat or the by the cecum, which varies in size and shape throughout the day. The right kidney is cranial to the left and sits close to the costal arch in the region of T13-L1. It is in the region of L3–L5. In overweight rabbits, the retroperitoneal and perirenal fat can alter the position of the kidneys, so the left kidney may be found in the midabdomen (see **Fig. 22**). Radiographically, renal length is reportedly 1.25 to 1.75 times the length of the second lumbar vertebra,[49] although, anecdotally, a range of 1.5 to 2.0 is normal

3. Look for signs of renal cortical calcification (see **Fig. 8**).

4. Look for nephroliths in the renal pelvis of both kidneys and assess their consistency. Is the appearance homogenous indicating presence of sediment or are there discrete stones?

5. Examine the path of the ureters from kidney to bladder for presence of stones.

6. Examine bladder and urethra from presence of excessive amounts of sludge or uroliths. Sediment is voided from the bladder during urination or manual expression. Sludge remains in the bladder after urination or manual expression.

7. Examine the craniodorsal abdomen and thorax for evidence of aortic mineralization (see **Fig. 24**).

8. Examine the lungs for evidence of bronchial calcification (see **Fig. 25**).

9. Examine the skeleton for evidence of osteosclerosis (see **Fig. 17**). A good radiograph with clear contrast between hard and soft tissue is often suspicious of renal disease. If skull radiographs are available, examine the mandible for the diamond shape of the hyoid bone, which shows clearly if ectopic mineralization is present (see **Fig. 26**).

Table 1
Reference ranges for laboratory tests in rabbits

Parameter	Reference Range
Hematology	
Erythrocytes	$4-7 \times 10^{12}$/L
Hemoglobin	10–15 g/dL
PCV	31%–40%
MCV	60–75 μm^3
MCH	19–23 pg
MCHC	34.5 g/dL
Reticulocytes	2%–4%
Platelets	$250-600 \times 10^3$/L
White cells	$6.3-12 \times 10^9$/L
Neutrophils	$1.5-4 \times 10^9$/L (30%–50%)
Lymphocytes	$2.5-7 \times 10^9$/L (30%–60%)
Monocytes	$<0.7 \times 10^9$/L (0%–7%)
Eosinophils	$<0.5 \times 10^9$/L (0%–5%)
Basophils	$<0.8 \times 10^9$/L (0%–8%)
Biochemistry	
Albumin	27–50 g/L
ALP	12–96 IU/L
ALT	45–80 IU/L
AST	5–130 IU/L
Bilirubin	3.4–8.5 μmol/L
Bile acids	>40 μmol/L
Calcium (total)	3.2–3.7 mmol/L
Calcium (ionized)	1.71 (+0.11) mmol/L
Cholesterol	0.3–3.00 mmol/L
Creatinine	20–225 μmol/L
CPK	50–200 IU/L
Gamma GT	0–7.0 IU/L
Globulin	15–27 g/L
Glucose	4.2–7.8 mmol/L
Phosphate (inorganic)	1.0–2.0 mmol/L
Potassium	3.5–5.6 mmol/L
Sodium	138–150 mmol/L
Total protein	54–75 g/L
Urea	6.14–8.38 mmol/L
Physiologic parameters	
Arterial blood pH	7.2–7.5
GFR	3.5 + 1.5 mL/mm/kg
HCO_3	12–24 mmol/L
Pco_2	20–46 torr
Urinanalysis	
Color	Red, orange, brown, or yellow
Specific gravity	1.003–1.036 (fixed range 1.008–1.012)

(continued on next page)

Table 1 (continued)	
Parameter	**Reference Range**
pH	8–9
Protein	Trace is normal
Cells	Small numbers of erythrocytes and leukocytes are normal
Glucose	Trace can be normal
Crystals	Large amount of calcium carbonate and small amount of struvite or oxalate are normal

Abbreviations: ALP, Alkaline phosphatase; ALT, Alanine aminotransferase; AST, Aspartate amino-transferase; CPK, Creatine phosphokinase; GFR, Glomerular filtration rate; GT, Glutamylytransferase; MCH, Mean corpuscular haemoglobin; MCHC, Mean corpuscular haemoglobin concentration; MCV, Mean corpuscular volume; PCV, Packed cell volume.
Data from Refs.[3,45,57]

IgM signifies active infection.[54] A negative titer means that the rabbit has either never been exposed or has eliminated the infection completely so treatment is not necessary.

Urinanalyis
Urinalysis is helpful in the diagnosis of renal disease. Normal rabbit urine may vary in color from red to brown to orange to yellow. It contains mucus from mucus-secreting glands in the renal pelvis, which means there is a small amount of protein in the urine. Small amounts of ammonium magnesium phosphate crystals are a normal finding.[55] The pH of normal rabbit urine is strongly alkaline (8–9) due to the herbivorous diet and the urine is often cloudy or turbid due to the presence of calcium sediment. In general, clear urine is not a good sign. It may be due to renal or metabolic disease or due to urine retention, so only the urinary supernatant is expressed during urination, leaving the sediment in the bladder. The amount of sediment depends on

Table 2 Conversion factors for biochemical data			
Parameter	**SI Unit**	**Conventional Unit**	**Multiply by**
Albumin	g/L	g/dL	0.1
Bile acids	μmol/L	μg/mL	0.39
Bilirubin	μmol/L	mg/dL	0.058
Calcium	mmol/L	mg/dL	4
Cholesterol	mmol/L	mg/dL	38.67
Creatinine	μmol/L	mg/dL	0.011
Globulin	g/L	g/dL	0.1
Glucose	mmol/L	mg/dL	18
Phosphate	mmol/L	mg/dL	3.1
Potassium	mmol/L	mg/dL	3.9
Sodium	mmol/L	mg/dL	2.3
Total protein	g/L	g/dL	0.1
Triglycerides	mmol/L	mg/dL	88.6
Urea	mmol/L	mg/dL	6

Table 3
Significant parameters for laboratory assessment of renal function

Acute Renal Failure	
Urine	
Urine volume	Decreased in severe acute renal failure—poor prognosis
Urine pH	Increased in rabbits with ketoacidosis—poor prognosis
Urine specific gravity	Specific gravity outside fixed range of 1.008–1.012 indicates active renal function.
Hematuria, proteinuria	May indicate cause of renal disease (eg, trauma, stones, or infection)
Blood	
Total protein	Increased in cases of dehydration
Hematocrit	Increased in cases of dehydration; decreased in cases of severe hemorrhage, which might affect renal function
Potassium:	High in cases of acute renal failure, especially postrenal; life threatening
Blood pH	Outside normal range of 7.2–7.5 indicates life-threatening acid-base disorders.
Ketones	Presence of ketones indicates ketoacidosis—poor prognosis
Total protein	High in cases of dehydration
Urea/creatinine	Can be very high but reversible if acute renal failure is prerenal
Chronic Renal Failure	
Urine	
Urine volume	Increase indicates CRF but CRF may be present if urine output is normal.
Sediment in urine	Clear urine occurs in end-stage renal failure when kidneys cease to excrete calcium; poor prognostic sign.
Specific gravity	Specific gravity outside fixed range of 1.008–1.012 indicates some renal function.
Blood	
Hematocrit	Anemia may be due to CRF or chronic disease.
Blood urea	May be high end of normal or above normal range with CRF; marked increases are significant.
Creatinine	May be high end of normal or above normal range with CRF; marked increases are significant.
Calcium	Usually high end or above normal range
Inorganic phosphorous	Hypophosphatemia in early stages of CRF Hyperphosphatemia in late stages or in rabbits on low-calcium, high-phosphorus diets. Hyperphosphatemia in conjunction with raised calcium, urea, and creatinine is diagnostic for CRF.
Potassium	Low or normal
Total protein	May be high in cases of chronic dehydration with end-stage CRF or low if protein-losing glomerulonephropathy or cachexia is present.

- The pH of the urine: the lower the pH, the more sediment there is. Clear urine is excreted during periods of ketoacidosis. Neutral or acidic urine is a poor prognostic sign in rabbits.

- The amount of calcium absorbed from the digestive tract: anorexic rabbits or those on calcium-deficient diet excrete clear urine. Rabbits on a high-calcium diet excrete urine with more sediment.
- The rabbit's calcium requirement: rabbits with a high calcium demand, such as pregnant, lactating, or growing rabbits, excrete clear urine.
- The concentration of the urine: diuresis and increased output of dilute urine dilute the sediment. Impaired renal function results in clear urine.
- Urine retention: rabbits that do not empty their bladder frequently and entirely can have a build-up of sediment in the urine. Inactivity, obesity, neurologic problems, or any diseases that make urination or adopting the position to urinate painful can lead to urine retention.

In comparison with dogs and cats, rabbits have limited ability to concentrate the urine. The specific gravity is 1.003 to 1.036 with a fixed range of 1.008 to 1.012.[56] Urine needs to be spun to remove sediment before measuring specific gravity, which should be performed with a refractometer rather than a test strip. Specific gravity outside the fixed range indicates that the kidneys can concentrate or dilute urine. Specific gravity within the fixed range in a rabbit that is azotemic and dehydrated indicates renal failure. A trace of glucose may be present in the urine, especially if the rabbit has been recently stressed.

SUMMARY

Renal disease is common in pet rabbits and definitive diagnosis can be difficult. Blood sample results are less useful than in other species but radiography is useful and is indicated for all cases in which renal disease is suspected.

REFERENCES

1. Ruckesbuch Y, Phaneuf LP, Dunlop R. The urinary system. In: Physiology of small and large animals. Philadelphia: Decker; 1991. p. 146–51.
2. Cruise LJ, Brewer NR. Anatomy. In: Manning PJ, Ringler DH, Newcomer CE, editors. The biology of the laboratory rabbit. 2nd edition. San Diego (CA): Academic Press; 1994. p. 47–61.
3. Pearson WP. The renal circulation of conscious rabbits. Comp Biochem Physiol A Comp Physiol 1987;87:515–9.
4. Brod J, Sirota JH. Effects of emotional disturbance on water diuresis and renal blood flow in the rabbit. Am J Physiol 1949;157:31–9.
5. Anschuetz RA, Speigel PK, Forster RP. Angiographic demonstration of total renal shutdown during apneic 'diving' in the rabbit. Comp Biochem Physiol A Comp Physiol 1971;40:109–12.
6. Brewer NR, Cruise LJ. Physiology. In: Manning PJ, Ringler DH, Newcomer CE, editors. The biology of the laboratory rabbit. 2nd edition. San Diego (CA): Academic Press; 1994. p. 63–71.
7. Dobyan DC, Magill LS, Friedman PA, et al. Carbonic anhydrase histochemistry in rabbit and mouse kidneys. Anat Rec 1982;204:185–97.
8. Kiwull-SchÖne H, Kalhoff H, Manz F, et al. Minimal-invasive approach to study pulmonary, metabolic and renal responsed to alimentary acid-base changes in conscious rabbits. Eur J Nutr 2001;40:255–9.
9. Cheeke PR, Amberg JW. Comparative calcium excretion by rats and rabbits. J Anim Sci 1973;37:450.

10. Buss SL, Bourdeau JE. Calcium balance in laboratory rabbits. Miner Electrolyte Metab 1984;10:127–32.
11. Whiting SJ, Quamme GA. Effects of dietary calcium on renal calcium, magnesium and phosphate excretion by the rabbit. Miner Electrolyte Metab 1984;10:217–21.
12. Bourdeau JE, Bouillon R, Zikos D, et al. Renal responses to calcium deprivation in young rabbits. Miner Electrolyte Metab 1988;14:150–7.
13. Bourdeau JE, Lau K. Regulation of cystosolic free calcium concentration in the rabbit connecting tubule: a calcium absorbing renal epithelium. J Lab Clin Med 1992;119:650–62.
14. Kennedy A. The urinary excretion of calcium by normal rabbits. J Comp Pathol 1965;75:69–74.
15. Hinton M. Prerenal uraemia in the rabbit. Vet Rec 1980;107:532.
16. Hinton M, Lucke VM. Histological findings in amyloidosis of rabbits. J Comp Pathol 1982;92:285–94.
17. Lindsay JR, Fox RR. Inherited diseases and variations. In: Manning PJ, Ringler DH, Newcomer CE, editors. The biology of the laboratory rabbit. 2nd edition. San Diego (CA): Academic Press; 1994. p. 293–313.
18. Maurer KJ, Marini KP, Fox JG, et al. Polycystic kidney syndrome in New Zealand White rabbits resembling human polycystic kidney disease. Kidney Int 2004;65:482–9.
19. Weisbroth SH. Neoplastic diseases. In: Manning PJ, Ringler DH, Newcomer CE, editors. The biology of the laboratory rabbit. 2nd edition. San Diego (CA): Academic Press; 1994. p. 259–92.
20. Percy DH, Barthold SW. Rabbit. In: Pathology of laboratory rodents and rabbits. 3rd edition. Oxford (United Kingdom): Blackwell Publishing; 2007. p. 253–308.
21. Harcourt-Brown FM. Radiographic signs of renal disease in rabbits. Vet Rec 2007;160:787–94.
22. Whyte MP. Extraskeletal (ectopic) calcification and ossification. In: Favus MJ, editor. Primer on the metabolic bone diseases and disorders of mineral metabolism. Philadelphia: Lippincott-Raven; 1996. p. 422–3.
23. Stevenson RG, Palmer NC, Finley GG. Hypervitaminosis D in rabbits. Can Vet J 1976;17:54–7.
24. Zimmerman TE, Giddens WE, DiGiacomo RF, et al. Soft tissue mineralization in rabbits fed a diet containing excess vitamin D. Lab Anim Sci 1990;40:212–5.
25. Kamphues VJ, Carstensen P, Schroeder D, et al. Effect of increasing calcium and Vitamin D supply on calcium metabolism in rabbits. J Anim Physiol Anim Nutr (Berl) 1986;50:191–208.
26. Clauss M, Burger B, Leisegang A, et al. Influence of diet on calcium metabolism, soft tissue calcification and urinary sludge in rabbits (Oryctolagus cuniculus). J Anim Physiol Anim Nutr (Berl) 2011;96:798–807.
27. Ritskes-Hoitinga J, Skott O, Urhenholt TR, et al. Nephrocalcinosis in rabbits-a case study. Scand J Lab Anim Sci 2004;3:143–8.
28. Cramer B, Husa L, Pushanathan C. Pattern and permanence of phosphate induced nephrocalcinosis in rabbits. Pediatr Radiol 1998;28:14–9.
29. Wakatsuki A, Nishio S, Iwata H, et al. Possible role of hyaluronate in experimental renal stone formation in rabbits. J Urol 1985;133:319–23.
30. Verkoelen VF. Crystal retention in renal stone disease: a crucial role for the glycosamine hyaluralon. J Am Soc Nephrol 2006;17:1673–87.
31. Tschudin A, Clauss M, Codron D. Preference of rabbits from drinking from open dishes versus nipple drinkers. Vet Rec 2011;168:190.

32. Itatani H, Yoshioka T, Namiki M, et al. Experimental model of calcium-containing renal stone formation in a rabbit. Invest Urol 1979;17:234–40.
33. Eddy AA, Falk RJ, Sibley RK. Subtotal nephrectomy in the rabbit: a model of chronic hypercalcaemia, nephrolithiasis and obstructive nephropathy. J Lab Clin Med 1986;107:508–16.
34. Kaplan BL, Smith HW. Excretion of inulin, creatinine, xylose and urea in the normal rabbit. Am J Physiol 1935;113:354–60.
35. Korner PI. Renal blood flow, glomerular filtration rate, renal PAH extraction ratio and the role of the renal vasomotor nerves in the unanesthetized rabbit. Circ Res 1963;12:353–60.
36. Enriquez JL, Schydlower M, O'Hair KC, et al. Effect of vitamin b6 supplementation on gentamicin nephrotoxicity in rabbits. Vet Hum Toxicol 1992; 34:32–5.
37. Kim SJ, Lim YT, Kim BS. Mechanism of reduced GFR in rabbits with ischaemic acute renal failure. Ren Fail 2000;22:129–41.
38. Chandler ML. Pathophysiology of chronic renal failure. UK Vet 2002;7:4–11.
39. Campbell TW. Clinical chemistry of mammals: laboratory animals and other species. In: Thrall MA, editor. Veterinary haematology and clinical chemistry. Philadelphia: Lippincott, Williams and Wilkins; 2004. p. 463–78.
40. Tvedegaard E. Arterial disease in chronic renal failure. An experimental study in the rabbit. Acta Pathol Microbiol Immunol Scand A 1987;95:3–28.
41. Tvedegaard E, Nielsen M, Kamstrup O. Osteosclerosis of the femoral head in long term uraemic rabbits. Acta Pathol Microbiol Immunol Scand A 1982;90: 235–9.
42. Tvedegaard E. Absorption of calcium, magnesium and phosphate during chronic renal failure and the effect of vitamin D in rabbits. Z Versuchstierkd 1985;27: 163–8.
43. Bas S, Aguilera-Tejero E, Estepa JC, et al. The influence of acute and chronic hypercalcaemia on the parathyroid response to hypocalcaemia in rabbits. Eur J Endocrinol 2002;146:411–8.
44. Rokita E, Cichocki T, Divoux S, et al. Calcification of the aortic wall in hypercalcaemic rabbits. Exp Toxicol Pathol 1992;44:310–616.
45. Gillett CS. Selected drug dosages and clinical reference data. In: Manning PJ, Ringler DH, Newcomer CE, editors. The biology of the laboratory rabbit. 2nd edition. San Diego (CA): Academic Press; 1994. p. 468–71.
46. Cheeke PR. Water functions and requirements. In: Rabbit feeding and nutrition. Orlando (FL): Academic Press; 1987. p. 154–60.
47. Harcourt-Brown FM, Harcourt-Brown SF. Clinical value of blood glucose measurement in pet rabbits. Vet Rec 2012;170:674.
48. Bas S, Bas A, Estepa JC, et al. Parathyroid gland function in the uremic rabbit. Domest Anim Endocrinol 2004;26:99–110.
49. Hinton MH, Gibbs C. Radiological examination of the rabbit: II the abdomen. J Small Anim Pract 1982;23:687–96.
50. Cramer B, Husa L, Pushanathan C. Nephrocalcinosis in rabbits- correlation of ultrasound, computed tomography, pathology and renal function. Pediatr Radiol 1998;28:9–13.
51. Loeb WF. Clinical biochemistry of laboratory rodents and rabbits. In: Kaneko JJ, Harvey JW, Bruss ML, editors. Clinical biochemistry of domestic animals. San Diego (CA): Academic Press; 1997. p. 845–54.
52. Fekete S. Recent findings and future perspectives of digestive physiology in rabbits: a review. Acta Vet Hung 1989;37:265–79.

53. Harcourt-Brown FM, Baker SJ. Parathyroid hormone, haematological and biochemical parameters in relation to dental disease and husbandry in pet rabbits. J Small Anim Pract 2001;42:130–6.
54. Jeklova E, Jekl V, Kovarcik K, et al. Usefulness of detection of specific IgM and IgG antibodies for diagnosis of clinical encephalitozoonosis in pet rabbits. Vet Parasitol 2010;170:143–8.
55. Flatt RE, Carpenter AB. Identification of crystalline material in urine of rabbits. Am J Vet Res 1971;32:655–8.
56. Jenkins JR. Clinical pathology. In: Meredith A, Flecknell PA, editors. BSAVA manual of rabbit medicine and surgery. 2nd edition. Gloucester (United Kingdom): British Small Animal Veterinary Association; 2006. p. 45–51.
57. Harcourt-Brown FM. Clinical pathology. In: Textbook of rabbit medicine. Oxford (United Kingdom): Butterworth Heinemann; 2002. p. 140–64.

Point-of-Care Blood Gas and Electrolyte Analysis in Rabbits

María Ardiaca, LV (veterinarian)*, Cristina Bonvehí, LV (veterinarian),
Andrés Montesinos, LV (veterinarian)

KEYWORDS

- Blood gas • Rabbit • Acidosis • Alkalosis • Electrolytes

KEY POINTS

- The use of point-of-care blood gas analyzers allows rapid turnaround time of results, improvement of diagnostics, and immediate therapeutic management with potential improvement in outcome.
- Point-of-care analysis allows reduction of preanalytical error caused by sample deterioration during transportation to laboratory facilities.
- Despite the extensive use of rabbits as laboratory animals and numerous studies focused on acid-base disorders in this species, little information with potential clinical application for pet rabbits is available.

Point-of-care blood gas analyzers gained relevance in clinical practice because of their capacity to offer complete information about gas exchange in the lungs, acid-base, and electrolytic state of the patient. Blood gas analyzers directly measure pH, partial pressure of oxygen (Po_2), partial pressure of carbon dioxide (Pco_2), electrolytes, and metabolites on arterial, venous, or capillary blood samples. Measured results may be used to derive additional calculated parameters such as bicarbonate (HCO_3), total CO_2 (TCO_2), O_2 saturation ($satO_2$), anion gap (AnGap), or base excess (BE). However, some of the calculated values are derived using formulas or normograms that are accurate for human plasma but their validity for veterinary species is not always proved.

In critically ill patients or those recovering from general anesthesia, clinical status can change quickly. The use of point-of-care blood gas analyzers allows rapid turnaround of results, improvement of diagnostics, and immediate therapeutic management with potential improvement in outcome. Another important advantage is the absence of interference from factors such as peripheral vasoconstriction or inadequacy of the pulmonary ventilation/perfusion ratio, which can affect noninvasive methods such as pulsoximetry or capnography in ill patients. The point-of-care analysis also allows reduction of preanalytical error caused by sample deterioration during transportation to laboratory facilities.[1–10]

Centro Veterinario Los Sauces, C/Santa Engracia, 63, Madrid 28010, Spain
* Corresponding author.
E-mail addresses: cvsauces@terra.es; cvsauces@cvsauces.com

Vet Clin Exot Anim 16 (2013) 175–195
http://dx.doi.org/10.1016/j.cvex.2012.10.005
1094-9194/13/$ – see front matter © 2013 Elsevier Inc. All rights reserved.

Despite the extensive use of rabbits as laboratory animals and numerous studies focused on acid-base disorders in this species, little information with potential clinical application for pet rabbits is available.

The authors have experience with the use of the i-STAT handheld analyzer and disposable cartridges (Abbot Point of Care Inc, Abbott Park, IL, USA). This system is easy to handle (minimizing the need for staff training), requires low levels of maintenance, and has minimal downtime. The technique requires a small sample volume (0.1 mL of whole blood) and provides quick results (about 130 seconds).[11,12] This article outlines a practical approach for the use of blood gas analysis in pet rabbits using the i-STAT analyzer. Excellent reviews on the topic are available in the scientific literature for readers interested in gaining more profound knowledge of blood gas analysis.[1-10]

SAMPLE COLLECTION

A venous sample is preferred to evaluate the acid-base balance, whereas an arterial sample is required to fully evaluate the respiratory status.[1-3,7] The sample must be collected anaerobically and the processing must be as quick as possible. It is necessary to allow cartridges to reach room temperature.[11,12]

The amount of anticoagulant can be critical because of its dilution effect. To reduce this source of preanalytical error, the procedure needs to be as standardized as possible. The use of 1-mL blood gas–specific syringes with dry lithium heparin might be preferable for arterial samples. Some brands provide only self-filling syringes, which are not suitable; syringes that allow negative pressure application should be used. Arterial samples from small patients are more difficult to draw and so they tend to be smaller than venous samples. The use of blood gas–specific syringes reduces the risk of sample dilution by anticoagulant and air mixture, which can affect the accuracy of the results.[1,3,13]

Alternatively, a liquid form of lithium heparin can be used. The following technique is used by the authors and represents a modification of a previously published technique for dogs in an attempt to solve the problem of the smaller patient size of the rabbit.[13] The sampling is conducted as follows: (1) fill a regular 1-mL syringe with anticoagulant, (2) expel the anticoagulant by depressing the plunger completely, (3) change the needle to the one that will be used for sampling, (4) aspirate 1 mL of air and rapidly expel the air and the rest of the anticoagulant through the needle, (5) repeat the air aspiration and expulsion twice more or until the anticoagulant is almost no longer visible, (6) fill the syringe with at least 0.5 mL of arterial or venous blood, (7) release the negative pressure completely before pulling the syringe out, and (8) process the sample immediately.

Venous Sampling

Venous samples can be collected from the lateral saphenous or jugular vein using a 1-mL syringe and a 25-G or 27-G needle. The authors prefer to reserve the marginal ear and cephalic veins for catheter placement. Adequate sampling from these veins is more difficult because of their lesser diameter.[14]

Arterial Sampling

Arterial samples can be collected from the central ear artery (**Fig. 1**). Arterial puncture is painful to the patient. An ointment containing lidocaine or other topical anesthetic, applied 5 to 10 minutes before the sampling, reduces the pain considerably during the puncture and prevents the rabbit from moving its head. The site is then aseptically

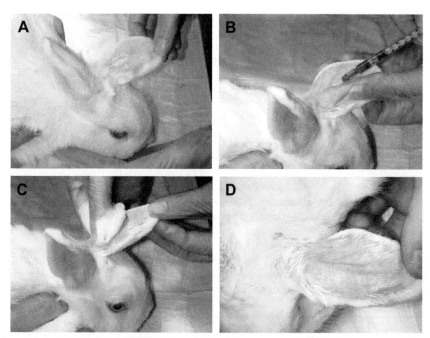

Fig. 1. Arterial sampling technique in rabbits. (*A*) Apply topical anesthetic ointment over the central ear artery for 5 to 10 minutes. (*B*) Prepare the area aseptically and draw the sample. (*C*) Apply pressure for 30 to 60 seconds. (*D*) Make sure no hematoma formation is visible before returning the rabbit to the cage.

prepared. Shaving is not necessary, but might be advisable for better visualization of the artery in dark-haired rabbits. The authors use a 1-mL heparinized syringe and a 30-G needle for this technique. Mild negative pressure is necessary. Once an appropriate blood volume is collected, all the negative pressure must be released from the plunger before the needle is pulled out. Suction during needle extraction causes the air to enter violently through the sample, causing hemolysis and a possible alteration in results. After extraction, compression must be applied for 30 to 60 seconds to reduce the risk of hematoma formation from the artery. Although the risk of pinnae necrosis after central ear artery puncture is frequently mentioned, the authors have not observed this side effect using the technique described. With properly applied pressure, the risk of hematoma formation is minimal with this technique. Sampling can be challenging in dwarf breeds with small pinnae, but it is possible, nevertheless.

With the use of a point-of-care analyzer, it is expected that samples are analyzed immediately. If this is the case, they do not need additional care. It is advisable that all the air bubbles are expelled within 30 seconds after collection of the sample. Exposition of the sample to air leads to escape of CO_2, causing decreased P_{CO_2} (partial pressure of carbon dioxide), increased pH, and low results for calculated HCO_3^- and TCO_2. Increase in the P_{O_2} can be expected after 30 minutes. Delayed processing also leads to increment in CO_2 and decreased pH, because of metabolic processes that continue to happen in the blood sample. The results for calculated HCO_3^- and TCO_2 are consequently high. If immediate processing is not possible, the samples should be stored anaerobically and under refrigeration.[1,15]

Some xenobiotics can influence the results using the i-STAT analyzer. For example, EC8+ cartridges are not recommended by the manufacturer for patients that receive propofol, whereas G3+, CG4+, CG8+, EG6+, and EG7+ are free of interference at therapeutic doses in humans.

STEPS TO INTERPRET BLOOD GAS ANALYSIS RESULTS

Before interpreting the results, a reference interval and a reference point must be established.[1,3,5,7,10] It is common practice to work with reference intervals for most chemistry and hematology variables, derived from a healthy population. For the purposes of evaluation of pH, Pco_2, HCO_3^-, TCO_2, BE extracellular fluid (BE_{ecf}), and AnGap, an easier approach is to establish a single reference point for comparison (ie, pH is higher or lower than 7.4).[1] The reference values can vary among different instruments and populations. Results obtained by the authors from healthy pet rabbits with the use of EC8+ and CG8+ cartridges for the i-STAT analyzer are presented in **Tables 1** and **2**. All the physiologic values mentioned in this article relate to these results, unless otherwise mentioned. The values obtained for healthy pet rabbits are consistent with some previously published data for conscious and anesthetized laboratory rabbits.[16–19]

In arterial samples, it must first be determined if the sample is truly arterial. As in other mammalian species, arterial samples from rabbits are visually distinct from venous samples, presenting a more vivid red color and flowing into the syringe

Table 1
Results from venous samples from healthy rabbits (n = 45) analyzed with i-STAT EC8+

Parameter	95% Reference Interval	Proposed Reference Point	Total Range (Lowest and Highest Value Registered)	Arithmetic Mean[a]	Standard Deviation[a]
pH	7.245–7.533[b]	7.4	7.205–7.527	7.389	0.074
Pco_2 (mm Hg)	28.9–52.9[b]	40	29.2–56.0	40.9	6.1
HCO_3^- (mmol/L)[d]	17.0–32.5[c]	24.7	16.9–31.6	NA	NA
TCO_2 (mmol/L)[d]	18–34[c]	26	18–33	NA	NA
BE_{ecf} (mmol/L)[d]	−10–8[c]	1	−10–8	NA	NA
Na (mmol/L)	136–147[b]		138–147	141	2.6
K (mmol/L)	3.4–5.7[b]		3.4–5.8	4.7	0.6
Cl (mmol/L)	93–113[c]		93–113	NA	NA
AnGap (mmol/L)	11–26[c]	17	11–26	NA	NA
Hematocrit (%)	29–46[b]		27–46	37	4.3
Hemoglobin (g/dL)	9.8–15.5[b]		9.2–15.6	12.7	1.5
Blood urea nitrogen (mg/dL)	9–33[b]		9–39	21	6.2
Glu (mg/dL)	93–245[c]		93–251	NA	NA

Abbreviations: NA, not available; RI, Reference Interval.
[a] Arithmetic mean and standard deviation are displayed only for results following a normal distribution.
Method of calculation of 95% RI:
[b] Parametric robust method.
[c] Nonparametric percentile method.
[d] Results automatically calculated by I-Stat system.

Table 2
Results from arterial samples from healthy rabbits (n = 20) analyzed with GC8+ cartridges for the i-STAT analyzer (reference interval was not calculated to avoid misleading results due to small sample size)

Parameter	Total Range (Lowest and Highest Value Registered)	Proposed Reference Point
pH	7.387–7.532	
Pco_2 (mm Hg)	29.2–56.0	
Po_2 (mm Hg)	65–84	
$pH_{corrected}$[a]	7.358–7.502	7.4
$pco_{2corrected}$ (mm Hg)[a]	29.1–36.8	33
$Po_{2corrected}$ (mm Hg)[a]	75–101	
$satO_2$ (%)	93–96	>92%
HCO_3^-[b]	17.5–27.6	22.3
TCO_2 (mmol/L)[b]	18–29	23
BE_{ecf}	−7–5	0
Na (mmol/L)	136–142	
K (mmol/L)	3.5–5.1	
Ionized calcium (mmol/L)	1.67–1.85	
Hematocrit (%)	23–42	
Hemoglobin (g/dL)	7.8–14.3	
Glu (mg/dL)	106–205	

[a] Corrected results: pH, Pco_2, and Po_2 are temperature-dependent results and are measured at 37°C; the temperature correction algorithm incorporated in the analyzer display corrected results at the patient's temperature (38.4–40.2°C in these rabbits). All the rabbits were breathing room air.
[b] Results automatically calculated by I-Stat system.

more readily (**Fig. 2**). Once the analysis is performed, a value of oxygen saturation more than 92% ($satO_2$ >92%) proves that the sample comes from an artery. However, in severe respiratory dysfunction, arterial samples can show saturation values less than 92%.[1–4,7,10]

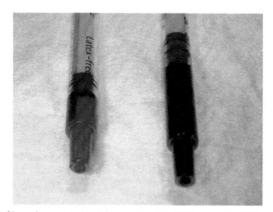

Fig. 2. Arterial (*left*) and venous (*right*) samples from the same rabbit are shown. Arterial samples usually present a more vivid red color and enter the syringe more readily during extraction.

Identify if Acidemia or Alkalemia is Present

The blood pH represents the balance between acids and alkalis present in an organism. It is measured by blood gas analyzers and is directly proportional to the ratio of HCO_3^-/P_{CO_2}.

Neutral pH (eudremia) is considered to be 7.4 in humans and dogs.[1,2] In our experience, the reference point in rabbits is similar. The midpoint value for the pH obtained from 44 healthy rabbits is 7.395, being the 95% confidence interval (CI) for the median pH 7366 to 7417. We therefore consider it safe to assume 7.4 as a reference point for pH in arterial and venous samples from pet rabbits.

Acidemia is not synonymous with acidosis, nor is alkalemia synonymous with alkalosis. Under normal conditions, plasma pH in rabbits varies slightly around 7.4 (see **Tables 1** and **2**). Hence, the presence of acidemia (pH <7.4) or alkalemia (pH >7.4) might be physiologic. On the other hand, the neutral pH does not necessarily imply the absence of acid-base disorders (ie, concurrent respiratory alkalosis and metabolic acidosis can cancel each other out, giving a normal pH). The terms acidosis and alkalosis are used to name the pathologic conditions with alterations in P_{CO_2}, HCO_3^-, or BE levels.[1]

Identify Markers of Respiratory or Nonrespiratory (Metabolic) Acid-Base Disorder

P_{CO_2}

P_{CO_2} is used to evaluate the ventilation and the respiratory component of the acid-base status. It is measured directly by all the blood gas analyzers. A reference point for the P_{CO_2} in rabbits using the i-STAT system is 40 mm Hg in venous samples (EC8+ cartridges) and 33 mm Hg in arterial samples (GC8+ cartridges). Disorders that occur with changes in P_{CO_2} are termed respiratory acidosis (increased P_{CO_2}) or respiratory alkalosis (decreased P_{CO_2}). CO_2 is a volatile acid that is produced by cellular metabolism and is exhaled in the lungs. Hypoventilation leads to accumulation of CO_2 in blood (increased P_{CO_2}) and a decrease in the pH value. Hyperventilation increases the elimination of CO_2 (decreased P_{CO_2}) and leads to an increase in pH value.[1–6,10]

Many neurologic, muscular, respiratory, or extrarespiratory conditions can lead to hypoventilation or hyperventilation and subsequently to a respiratory acid-base disorder. Trauma, fatigue, cardiac or renal insufficiency with edema formation, respiratory infections, respiratory obstructions, abdominal or thoracic pain, ascites, pleural effusions, sedation, or anesthesia are common causes of hypoventilation in rabbits. Any disease that compromises neurologic control of respiration, breathing mechanics, or proper air flow through the airway can lead to hypoventilation. In contrast, fear, anxiety, hypoxemia (caused by certain respiratory or cardiac diseases), or anemia can lead to increased respiratory rate and hyperventilation. Hyperventilation requires a considerable muscular effort and cannot be maintained for a prolonged period. Therefore, muscular fatigue caused by hyperventilation leads to hypoventilation and acidosis. Iatrogenic respiratory alkalosis can be produced by overzealous artificial ventilation.[1–7]

HCO_3^- and BE_{ecf}

The HCO_3^- and base excess (BE_{ecf}) reflect the nonrespiratory component of acid-base balance. HCO_3^- is the most abundant plasma buffer and can bind to excess free H^+.[1,3,7,9]

Low HCO_3^- indicates metabolic acidosis caused by excess of endogenous acid production (ie, lactic acidosis, ketoacidosis), decreased acid excretion (renal failure), or excess loss of HCO_3^- (ie, gastrointestinal loss through diarrhea, renal tubular acidosis). Blood gas analysis does not provide information regarding the underlying cause of the misbalance, but can help in the diagnosis. Any disease causing alterations in cellular metabolism, hormonal disorders, or renal or hepatic insufficiency can be a metabolic source of acid-base disorders. Overdose of exogenous acids, such as acetylsalicylic acid or ethylene glycol, can be a cause of metabolic acidosis.[1,3,5,7]

High HCO_3^- indicates metabolic alkalosis and it may be caused by pyloric obstruction, gastric stasis, or antacid treatments. Vomiting is a common cause of metabolic alkalosis in humans and carnivores. Being practically absent in rabbits, vomiting cannot be considered as a cause of acid-base disorder in this species. Iatrogenic metabolic alkalosis can be induced by excessive administration of HCO_3^- containing fluids or use of loop diuretics (hypochloremic alkalosis).[1,3-7]

The HCO_3^- concentration is calculated by the i-STAT analyzer from the pH and P_{CO_2}:

$$\log HCO_3^- = pH + \log P_{CO_2} - 7.608$$

The formula is derived from the Henderson-Hasselbalch equation and its application is independent of the species. However, as can be deduced from the formula, the calculated HCO_3^- value is not completely independent from the respiratory component (P_{CO_2}). The use of the BE_{ecf} concept is an attempt to isolate the metabolic component eliminating the influence of respiratory activity:

$$BE_{ecf} = HCO_3^- - 24.8 + 16.2 \left(pH - 7.4\right)$$

The BE_{ecf} value represents the total quantity of acid and base that would be required to titrate the average intracellular fluid (plasma plus interstitial fluid) to an arterial plasma pH of 7.40 at P_{CO_2} of 40 mm Hg at 37°C. Several formulas have been proposed, and the i-STAT analyzer uses the one derived from the Siggaard-Andersen normogram. Because the midpoints for HCO_3 and pH in rabbits are close to those in humans, most of the formulas using HCO_3 and pH values might be applicable for rabbits. Excess concentration of base in the average extracellular fluid remains virtually constant during acute changes in the P_{CO_2} and reflects only a nonrespiratory component of pH disturbances. Low values of BE indicate metabolic acidosis, whereas high values indicate metabolic alkalosis.[1,3-7,9]

There are other buffers in the organism, such as hemoglobin (Hb), phosphates, certain proteins, and carbonates. These substances are responsible for an immediate response to acid-base disturbances, but they rapidly reach their maximum capacity. Renal function has the most prominent role regulating the amount of acid and base in the blood through complex modulatory mechanisms of urinary excretion of H^+ and HCO_3^-. However, adaptation of kidney function needs more time to develop.[1,3,7]

HCO_3 and BE_{ecf} were found to follow a bimodal distribution in clinically healthy rabbits. A possible explanation for this phenomenon is that the HCO_3 levels follow the fluctuation in lactate levels observed in rabbits. Lactate concentration increases during the hard feces phase and decreases during the soft feces phase.[20] It is plausible that HCO_3 partially buffers the excess of protons from lactic acid or adjusts to preserve the electroneutrality. The midpoint (median) of HCO_3 for healthy rabbits is 24.9 mmol/L in venous samples. The midpoint for HCO_3 in human medicine with the i-STAT analyzer is 24.8 mmol/L in venous samples.

Evaluate the Compensatory Response

In general, the respiratory system attempts to compensate the metabolic acid-base disorders and vice versa. The compensatory response is parallel to the primary disorder (ie, Pco_2 and HCO_3^- change in the same direction) in an attempt to keep the pH stable. For example, when metabolic acidosis is present ($\downarrow HCO_3^-$), the respiratory center is stimulated and hyperventilation occurs ($\downarrow Pco_2$). Hyperventilation eliminates excess acid in the form of CO_2. In metabolic alkalosis ($\uparrow HCO_3^-$), hypoventilation preserves CO_2 ($\uparrow Pco_2$). With a normal respiratory function, the maximum compensation is quickly achieved because of the volatile nature of CO_2. However, as mentioned earlier, it cannot be maintained for long. In humans and dogs, the maximum respiratory compensatory response is believed to be about 7 to 9 mm Hg.[1–3,7]

When a respiratory disorder is present, the intracellular buffering mechanisms activate first. A chronic respiratory process produces a more significant compensatory response that is primarily caused by renal adaptation, which takes a longer time to develop (typically 2–5 days). Renal adaptation is established through increased or decreased acid (H^+) or base (HCO_3^-) excretion. Thus, the nonrespiratory compensatory response is slower than respiratory compensation.[1–3,7]

The compensatory response mitigates the pH changes, but it is rarely sufficient to return the pH to a normal value. However, normal pH can be achieved in mild derangements or as a result of mixed acid-base disorder.[1,3,7]

An adequate compensatory response helps to rule out disorders of the compensatory system. In many cases, dysfunction of several systems is present and compensation is inadequate or absent. If this is the case, a complex or mixed acid-base disorder is diagnosed.[1,3,7]

The degree of compensatory response varies among species.[2] We were not able to find consistent references for a compensatory response in rabbits. Although many studies have been performed, most of them were based on in vitro experiments. They prove that acid-base disturbances in rabbits result in changes in HCO_3 and proton secretion, but lack clinical application.[21–25] Few data collected from the literature suggest that compensatory response in rabbits can match the values presented in **Table 3**.[22–24]

Table 3
Compensatory responses in rabbits with primary acid-base disturbances. Note that these data come from experimental studies, because the compensatory responses in rabbits were not studied for clinical application. Compensatory responses in dogs are displayed for comparison

Primary Disorder	Change in Primary Analyte[22–24]	Change in Compensatory Analyte (Rabbits)	Change in Compensatory Analyte (Dogs)[2]
Nonrespiratory acidosis	$\downarrow$1 mEq HCO_3^-[23] $\downarrow$1 mmol/L BE[24]	$\downarrow$1 mm Hg Pco_2[23] $\downarrow$0.62 mm Hg Pco_2[24]	$\downarrow$0.7 mm Hg Pco_2 NA
Nonrespiratory alkalosis	1 mEq HCO_3^- $\uparrow$1 mmol/L BE	$\uparrow$0.4 mm Hg Pco_2 $\uparrow$0.62 mm Hg Pco_2	$\uparrow$0.7 mm Hg Pco_2 NA
Acute respiratory acidosis	$\uparrow$1 mm Hg Pco_2	NA	$\uparrow$0.15 mEq HCO_3^-
Chronic respiratory acidosis (50–56 h)	$\uparrow$1 mm Hg Pco_2[22]	$\uparrow$ 0.25 mEq/L HCO_3^-[22]	$\uparrow$0.35 mEq HCO_3^-
Acute respiratory alkalosis	$\downarrow$1 mm Hg Pco_2	NA	$\downarrow$0.25 mEq HCO_3^-
Chronic respiratory alkalosis	$\downarrow$1 mm Hg Pco_2	NA	$\downarrow$0.55 mEq HCO_3^-

Abbreviation: NA, not available.

Example: adult 2-year-old female rabbit is presented with anorexia

The venous blood gas analysis shows the following results:

pH: 7.293
P_{CO_2}: 29.7 mm Hg
HCO_3^-: 14.4 mEq/L
BE: −12 mmol/L

Acidemia is present and nonrespiratory acidosis is diagnosed based on low HCO_3^- and BE values. The P_{CO_2} value is low, indicating respiratory alkalosis, which would produce alkalemia. Therefore, hyperventilation in this case is compensatory and is not the primary derangement. A decrease of 1 mm Hg in P_{CO_2} is expected for every 1 mEq/L decrease in HCO_3^-. The midpoints for HCO_3^- and P_{CO_2} are used for the calculation:

Decrease in HCO_3^- from midpoint = 24.9 − 14.4 = 10.5 mEq/L
Expected decrease in P_{CO_2} = 1 × 10.5 = 10.5 mm Hg
Expected P_{CO_2} value = 40 − 10.5 = 29.5 mm Hg

The measured P_{CO_2} value is 29.7 mm Hg, closely matching the expected value. In this case, the compensatory response (hyperventilation) can be considered adequate, and pH is maintained within reference limits. If the value is very different (more than 1–2 mEq/L or 1–2 mm Hg) than expected, a dysfunction of both systems and a concurrent respiratory and nonrespiratory disorder is diagnosed. However, the precise diagnostic decision in rabbits is not possible because of lack of scientific data.

Using the BE approach in the previous example:

Decrease in BE from midpoint: 1 − (−12) = 13 mmol/L
Expected decrease in P_{CO_2}: 0.62 × 13 = 8 mm Hg
Expected P_{CO_2} value = 40 − 8 = 32 mm Hg

The expected value is 2.2 mm Hg higher than the measured value, indicating that a possible mild respiratory alkalosis is present.

Example: a 5-month-old male rabbit is presented with severe dyspnea and nasal discharge, which has been progressive over the last 2 days

The venous blood gas analysis shows the following results:

pH: 7.297
P_{CO_2}: 67.9 mm Hg
HCO_3^-: 33.2 mEq/L
BE: 7

Acidemia is present and primary respiratory acidosis is diagnosed. A high HCO_3^- result cannot be responsible for the acidemia and represents the compensatory response.

Increase in P_{CO_2} from midpoint = 67.9 − 24.9 = 25.4 mm Hg
Expected increase in HCO_3^- = 0.25 × 25.4 = 6.4 mEq/L
Expected HCO_3^- value = 24.9 + 6.4 = 31.3 mEq/L

The actual HCO_3^- is close to the expected value, showing an adequate metabolic compensation of respiratory acidosis. Note the positive BE as a result of compensation of primary respiratory acidosis.

Understanding the compensatory response in acid-base disorders, it is easy to realize that if P_{CO_2} and HCO_3^- are changing in the opposite directions (one is increased and the other decreased), a mixed acid-base disorder is diagnosed. In such cases, it is probably not worth trying to clarify whether the primary acid-base disorder is respiratory or nonrespiratory. Both need treatment, and careful monitoring of the patient and serial blood gas analysis provide information about the effectiveness of therapy.[1,3,7]

It is generally assumed that overcompensation does not occur.[1-3,7] However, because of slower kidney response, a postcompensation syndrome may arise. This is the case with posthypercapnic alkalosis. During chronic hypercapnia, the kidneys respond, reducing HCO_3^- excretion. Subsequently, HCO_3^- starts to accumulate in the blood after 48 hours. When treating the primary respiratory dysfunction, if respiratory function is restored quickly (eg, in respiratory obstruction), the excess HCO_3^- may show itself in the form of metabolic alkalosis. This kind of condition is mild and resolves rapidly and spontaneously.

Evaluate the AnGap

The AnGap is the measure of difference between cations and anions: AnGap = $[Na^+] + [K^+] - [Cl^-] - [HCO_3^-]$ in plasma (using the EC8+ cartridge).[1,3-5,7,10] The value represents the amount of other ions that are not measured (calcium, sulfates, phosphates, lactate, ketoacids, protein). Physiologically, it is not possible to have an anion defect, therefore the value of the AnGap is always positive.[1,3,7,10] It provides additional information in classifying the type of acid-base disorder. Because the number of unmeasured cations is small and relatively constant, increases in AnGap frequently reflect conditions that increase unmeasured anions (most commonly lactic acidosis, uremic acidosis, ketoacidosis, or exogenous toxins that produce acidic metabolites).[1,3,7,26,27]

A high AnGap is most commonly associated with an increase in the organic acid load of the organism and low HCO_3 values. AnGap may be normal in conditions typically associated with an increased gap acidosis if concurrent hypoalbuminemia, hyperchloremia, or mixed acid-base disorders are present.[3,7,28] A normal AnGap metabolic acidosis can be found in small bowel diarrhea, use of carbonic anhydrase inhibitors and parenteral amino acid solutions, chronic respiratory alkalosis, dilutional acidosis, renal tubular acidosis, and atypical hypoadrenocorticism.[28]

Uremic acidosis results from reduced renal excretion of phosphates, sulfates, and organic acids, and may be more severe in acute renal failure. Ketoacidosis can occur when energy demands are not met by carbohydrate metabolism, as in anorexia, starvation, and pregnancy toxemia.[26,29] The normal digestive function of the rabbit produces absorption of acetic, butyric, and propionic acids in the gut.[20] The role of these anions and lactate in the acid-base balance of the rabbit is not fully understood.

Lactate levels are higher in rabbits compared with humans, dogs, or horses. In addition, the lactate levels fluctuate during the day, being higher during the hard feces phase and lower during the soft feces phase. We observed that HCO_3^- is significantly higher among samples with pathologically low lactate levels (lactate <2.5 mmol/L). According to our experience with healthy rabbits, lactate represents around 40% of the AnGap. Several cases of high AnGap acidosis were observed in our patients with normal lactate and chloride levels. This finding suggests that other acids, such as ketoacids or phosphates, were responsible for acidosis in those patients.

Pseudohyponatremia, frequently found in rabbits as a result of hyperglycemia, can have a slightly acidifying effect because of a compensatory decrease in HCO_3 to maintain electroneutrality.[1] This situation could predispose the rabbit to acid-base disorder, limiting the buffering ability. Some xenobiotics (acetylsalicylic acid, carbenicillin, toxics) can be responsible for increased anion concentration and therefore a high AnGap.[1,3,7,10]

A low AnGap is most commonly associated with alkalemia and a positive value of BE_{ecf} in ill rabbits treated in our center. Respiratory acidosis, hyponatremia, and uremia were identified in samples with low AnGap acidemia in our center.

Normal AnGap acidosis is not consistently associated with hyperchloremia in rabbits in our experience. Nor it is associated with lower HCO_3 levels as would be expected in other species. In human medicine, the normal AnGap acidosis is typically associated with HCO_3 loss and consequent increase in chloride levels. Induced hyperchloremia is known to provoke high AnGap acidosis in rabbits.[30] However, in ill rabbits presented at our center, we systematically find the HCO_3 levels significantly higher (although decreased compared with normal levels) in patients with normal AnGap acidosis compared with those with high AnGap acidosis (analysis of variance [ANOVA], $P<.001$). However, the HCO_3 gap is significantly lower among the rabbits with normal AnGap acidosis, being predominantly a negative value. Chloride and sodium levels are not significantly different between both groups (ANOVA, $P = 0.427$). Hyponatremia is identified in approximately 50% of rabbits with high and normal AnGap acidosis. BE_{ecf} is significantly lower in high AnGap acidosis (ANOVA, $P<.001$). These facts suggest the complex nature of acid-base disorders in rabbits and show that the mechanisms of acid-base balance are not understood in this species. Electrolytes can play an important role, as previously suggested.[30] Further research is needed. In some cases of high AnGap acidosis with positive HCO_3 gap, concurrent metabolic alkalosis can be suspected (gastrointestinal stasis or obstruction syndrome, refeeding alkalosis, diuretic therapy, hypokalemia, hyperaldosteronism, or hypercalcemia can be responsible). The high AnGap acidosis with negative HCO_3 gap in rabbits could be caused by increased organic acid load and concurrent HCO_3 loss (renal tubular acidosis, diarrhea). Although normal AnGap acidosis can be caused by hyperchloremia, it can also be caused by increased organic acid load with less pronounced or absent bicarbonate loss and concurrent hyponatremia. Hypoalbuminemia might be responsible for normal AnGap values in acidotic rabbits in some cases.

Evaluating the Oxygenation of the Patient (Arterial Samples)

SatO2 and CaO2

The $satO_2$ provides information on the amount of O_2 binding to Hb, but it does not indicate total blood oxygen content.[1,3–5,7] For example, Hb of an anemic patient can be fully saturated ($satO_2$ can be 98%–100%) and still the patient has hypoxemia. The arterial oxygenation content (Cao_2) indicates the actual oxygen content available for tissues:

$$Cao_2 = (Hb \times 1.34 \times satO_2/100) + (Pao_2 \times 0.003)$$

This calculation is especially useful in anemic patients that have normal $satO_2$ and Pao_2 (partial pressure of oxygen, arterial), but reduced Cao_2 until transfusion is completed. Normal Cao_2 values in the arterial blood of 15 healthy rabbits were found to range from 10 to 19 mL/dL (using a Po_2 value provided by the temperature correction algorithm incorporated in the i-STAT system). Arterial samples from ill rabbits with respiratory symptoms showed Cao_2 values from 6.7 to 16.5 mL/dL.

P/F ratio

It is also important to evaluate the effectiveness of oxygen loading by the lungs into the bloodstream. Two formulas are used when evaluating this factor. Both may need correction at different locations, because the parameters used are dependent on barometric pressure, which changes with altitude. The P/F ratio is the simpler of the two:

$$P/F \text{ ratio} = Po_2/Fio_2$$

Fio_2 is the fraction of inspired oxygen. If the animal is breathing room air, Fio_2 may be assumed to be 0.21 at lower altitudes. If animal is not breathing room air, Fio_2 can be measured using an oximeter (preferred) or estimated following the guidelines in the **Table 4**. Observing the variation of the Fio_2 in **Table 4**, it is easy to understand that the estimation of Fio_2 can lead to erroneous conclusions regarding patient oxygenation, and care must be taken when making clinical decisions. Note that Fio_2 equal to 1 is achieved only during mechanical ventilation with an intratracheal tube.

A P/F ratio of more than 400 is considered to indicate adequate pulmonary function in dogs and humans. A value of less than 200 indicates severe pulmonary dysfunction, whereas a value between 200 and 400 is considered to indicate progressive pulmonary dysfunction as it approaches 200. Values obtained by the authors from arterial samples of 15 healthy rabbits, breathing room air, and using the Po_2 value provided by the temperature correction algorithm range from 357 to 481, with a mean value of 390 (standard deviation = 44). A P/F ratio ranging from 180 to 371 was obtained from rabbits with symptomatic respiratory disease.

ALVEOLAR-ARTERIAL OXYGEN GRADIENT

The second formula to evaluate the upload of oxygen to the bloodstream is the equation of the alveolar-arterial gradient (A-a gradient), which is an attempt to measure the difference between the predicted Po_2 in the alveolus (based on gas physics principles) and the arterial oxygen tension:

$$A\text{-}a = (Fio_2 \times (P_b - P_{H2O}) - (Pco_2/R)) - Pao_2$$

P_b is the barometric pressure at the facility and P_{H2O} is the partial pressure of water vapor (about 52 mm Hg at 39°C). R is the respiratory quotient, which approximates 0.8 in rabbits, but can vary slightly depending on patient status, age, diet, and even position. The A-a gradient must be calculated only in patients breathing room air. Attempting to determine it in a patient that needs oxygen supplementation can be harmful to the animal. In such cases, the use of the P/F ratio is preferred.

The A-a gradient value obtained from 15 healthy rabbits, breathing room air, and using Pco_2 and Po_2 values provided by the temperature correction algorithm ranges from 9 to 35 mm Hg. All but one sample produced an A-a gradient between 21 and 35 mm Hg. The mean barometric pressure in Madrid is 760 mm Hg. These values from rabbits are high compared with those in dogs, cats, or humans. In dogs, cats,

Table 4		
Approximate values of Fio_2 achieved by different oxygen supplementation methods		
Administration Technique	**Recommended Oxygen Flow Rate (L/min)**	**Mean Fio_2 Achieved**
Face mask (loose fit)	2–5	0.4–0.5
Flow-by	2–5	0.25–0.4
Intratracheal tube (with spontaneous breathing)	1	0.4–0.6
Oxygen cage	As needed to maintain Fio_2 at 40%–60%	0.21–0.6
Mechanical ventilation	1–2	1

Data from Irizarry R, Reiss A. Beyond blood gases: making use of additional oxygenation parameters and plasma electrolytes in the emergency room. Compend Contin Educ Vet 2009;31(10):E1–8.

and humans, the normal A-a gradient is less than 10 mm Hg, and values more than 30 are considered to indicate respiratory disease. The difference is partially caused by lower oxygen and carbon dioxide tension in the arterial blood of rabbits, compared with dogs or humans. However, the A-a gradient results obtained from rabbits in our center are also higher than some previously published data for nonanesthetized laboratory rabbits, although they are consistent with others.[25] The A-a gradient from ill rabbits with respiratory symptoms attended in our clinic varied from 15 to 60 mm Hg. Further investigation is needed to prove the clinical application of these formulas in rabbit medicine.

In 1 study, buprenorphine at an approximate dose of 0.02 mg/kg intravenously (IV) or subcutaneously was found to decrease respiratory rate and P_{O_2} and increase P_{CO_2} and the A-a gradient in arterial samples from conscious rabbits.[25] According to the study, these changes were well tolerated by healthy animals. In ill rabbits predisposed to respiratory depression and acidosis, caution should be exercised when considering administration of buprenorphine or other opioids. Controversy is frequent when discussing sedation and opioid analgesia in depressed patients. Our opinion is that the benefit of rational use of anxiety and pain relief provide an important benefit for the patient and justify its application despite potential secondary effects.

ACID-BASE DISORDERS IN PET RABBITS

The analysis of 200 cases of blood gas analysis presented to our center during 2011 to 2012 shows that, in our experience, acid-base disorders are identified in approximately 65% of the samples from ill rabbits. Approximately 40% of the critically ill rabbits present significant acidemia (pH <7.245). Significant alkalemia (pH >7.533) is less common (approximately 3% of patients). Acid-base disorders are identified in 30% of the patients with pH within normal limits.

Primary respiratory acidosis (P_{CO_2} >52.9) is diagnosed in about 48% of acidotic rabbits. Adequate renal compensation of primary respiratory acidosis is rarely found. Subadequate compensation is usually observed, suggesting that the cases were acute or these rabbits had concurrent renal disease with an inability to compensate respiratory acidosis or they had concurrent metabolic disorder. Changes in blood acid-base status due to hypercapnia occur during the first 20 to 60 minutes. In a previous study, blood buffer values obtained from rabbits were not different from those reported for other terrestrial mammals and the whole body buffer capacity was even higher than that reported for man and dog, complying with the high tolerance to CO_2 reported for the rabbit.[21] On the other hand, an acute respiratory disorder is easily identified as illness by the rabbit's owner. Consequently, it is possible that respiratory disorders are diagnosed in the acute phase in many cases. Respiratory acidosis and concurrent metabolic alkalosis were identified in several cases.

Primary metabolic acidosis (HCO_3^- <17) was identified in 52% of the acidotic samples. Approximately 90% of the rabbits showing a low HCO_3 value also have a decreased BE value (BE ≤10). Concurrent metabolic and respiratory acidosis are found in approximately 30% of acidotic patients. Based on the clinical findings and the degree of derangement in P_{CO_2} and HCO_3^- values, we presume that the primary disorder was metabolic in these rabbits. In most cases of metabolic acidosis, a concurrent respiratory alkalosis is diagnosed (50% of cases). A logical explanation is that respiratory alkalosis is caused by stress and fear from handling or hypoxia in ill rabbits. However, these results can also suggest that the calculation for predicted respiratory compensation is underestimating the respiratory adaptation capacity of the rabbit. Primary respiratory alkalosis (with high P_{CO_2} and normal HCO_3^- values) was suspected only in 1 case over the 2-year period. Air mixing with the sample can lead to erroneously low P_{CO_2} values.

Primary metabolic alkalosis ($HCO_3^- > 32.5$) was diagnosed in 9% of cases. Respiratory compensation was suspected in approximately one-third. Five cases of hypochloremic alkalosis were detected.

The blood gas analysis provides little information about the underlying process causing acid-base disturbance. The causes of respiratory acidosis or alkalosis are probably obvious in all cases, but it is challenging to identify the source for metabolic acid-base disorders. Any disease can lead to excessive production of organic acids. Renal and gastrointestinal diseases most frequently cause the HCO_3^- losses. Thus, the most common causes of metabolic acidosis in rabbits are probably renal or hepatic insufficiency, shock, starvation, and diarrhea. Dehydration and hypotension accompanying disease can lead to excessive acid production by tissues and renal insufficiency. Dehydration and hypotension therefore contribute to the establishment and maintenance of acidosis. As mentioned earlier, many ill rabbits have concurrent respiratory and metabolic dysfunction with the inability to adequately compensate the primary acid-base disorder.

Common symptoms of metabolic acidosis in the rabbit are the acidic odor of breath and urine, acidic urinary pH, fever, anorexia, and hypotension (Systolic Arterial Tension <90 mm Hg). Ventricular arrhythmias and decreased consciousness are found in more severe cases. The respiration pattern of the acidotic rabbit is different from the shallow and fast respiration of the simply stressed rabbit. A deep and slow respiration is observed in most cases of acidosis, because changes affect mostly tidal volume and not the respiratory frequency, which might even be decreased (<30 rpm).

Excessively aggressive fluid therapy with crystalloids not containing HCO_3 or HCO_3 precursors is described as a cause of metabolic acidosis as a result of high chloride load in humans and dogs. Hyperchloremic acidosis in rabbits seems to be rare, but the clinician should be aware of the iatrogenic effects of fluid or diuretic therapy.

Certain pathologic conditions of the gastrointestinal tract of the rabbit play an important role, because they can elicit important acid or base losses. The most common cause of gastrointestinal acid loss in humans and carnivores is vomiting. Vomiting is virtually nonexistent in rabbits. However, the gastrointestinal stasis and pseudo-obstruction or obstructionlike syndrome is frequently found. True or foreign body obstruction is rare in rabbits in our experience. However, we frequently see rabbits with severe dehydration of gastrointestinal contents, which causes pseudo-obstruction. Trichobezoars or hair balls are occasionally observed, but in many cases, the dehydrated intestinal contents were found to be vegetable material on necropsies. Gastric bloat syndrome is also frequent. Gastric stasis or pyloric obstruction leads to kidnapping of gastric acid in the stomach, while the alkaline secretions of the intestine keep being absorbed. This situation can be a cause of hypochloremic alkalosis (even although vomiting is absent). Obstruction at a lower level can lead to HCO_3 leaking into the intestinal lumen, causing acidosis. Starvation and free radicals from catabolic processes also contribute to the establishment of acidemia. Subsequently, gastrointestinal stasis in rabbits can lead to metabolic acidosis, alkalosis, or a mixed disorder, depending on the case. If normal respiratory and kidney function are present, compensation mechanisms are activated and can mitigate the pH alterations during the initial phase of the disease. HCO_3 loss through diarrhea is another common cause of metabolic acidosis.

Compensated metabolic alkalosis is normal during pregnancy in rabbits, as it is in humans.[19] Diet also has an important role on acid-base balance in the herbivore rabbit. Alkali-enriched diets are recommended for humans to diminish the net acid load of their usual diet. In contrast, rabbits have to deal with a high dietary alkali impact on acid-base balance.[24,31] Studies have shown that it is not possible to induce a systemic metabolic acidosis in rabbits even by high-dose application of ammonium chloride under normal herbivore nutrition. The resulting renal acidification, which likely is a base-saving response, seems unexpected in view of persisting high alkali intake but may explain systemic acid-base homeostasis. However, previous stress on renal acid-base control by alimentary alkali depletion elicits growing susceptibility to chronic metabolic acidosis in the rabbit.[24,31]

ANALYSIS OF ELECTROLYTES AND METABOLITES

Sodium, potassium, and chloride values are used to calculate the AnGap, as explained earlier. However, these values also might provide important information that might be helpful for diagnostic and prognostic purposes.

Sodium

Sodium is the most abundant extracellular cation in the body and the most responsible for plasmatic osmolality. Hyponatremia becomes pathologic when it leads to a state of hypotonicity, with the tendency of free water to move from the vascular to the intracellular space. The main deleterious effects derive from cerebral edema. Plasma tonicity is calculated using the following formula:

$$Ton = (2 \times Na) \, (mEq/L) + (glucose/18) \, (mg/dL)$$

Based on the results of a study conducted in our center on 150 ill and 44 healthy rabbits (unpublished), 136 to 147 mEq/L seems to be the physiologic range of sodium in pet rabbits when measured in whole blood in lithium heparin with the EC8+ cartridges for the i-STAT analyzer. This reference range is lower than described for dogs and cats,[10] but it is similar to that in humans (as provided by the manufacturer). The normal values for calculated plasma tonicity in the same study were found to be 279 to 301 mOsm/L. The minimum plasma sodium concentration of 135 mEq/L is necessary to maintain plasma tonicity in normoglycemic conditions. Less than this limit, changes in glucose levels (hyperglycemia) seem to be necessary to maintain plasma tonicity within normal limits.

The study shows that low sodium levels are commonly seen in ill pet rabbits in our facility. Approximately 51.3% of the samples presented sodium levels less than 136 mEq/L. True hyponatremia in this study was found to be present in 34% of the samples; the rest were pseudohyponatremic. Significantly higher mortality seems to be associated with sodium levels less than 129 mEq/L in rabbits.

It is essential to differentiate between true hyponatremia (hypotonic hyponatremia) and pseudohyponatremia. Pseudohyponatremia (isotonic or hypertonic) itself has no consequences for the patient's health. The clinician must identify it and avoid treating it. The underlying disease should actually be addressed. In human medicine, complications from pseudohyponatremia have been associated mostly with subsequent medical interventions that were applied unnecessarily, such as diuresis, fluid restriction, and hypertonic saline administration.[32–34] The determination of tonicity gives us information regarding the type of hyponatremia and its cause that cannot be obtained by simply measuring sodium. Pseudohyponatremia in rabbits is mostly caused by hyperglycemia, because sodium levels decrease in response to high glucose levels to maintain tonicity. The incidence of hyperglycemia in ill rabbits seems to be high (59.3% in our study). Therefore, interpretation of the natremia value should also take into consideration the glycemia value.[32,35,36]

Numerous data published for rabbits report normal glycemia limits as 74 to 155 mg/dL and normal blood urea nitrogen limits as 5 to 30 mg/dL.[15–17,21,22,37,38] It is well known that stress and illness can cause plasma glucose levels to increase. Fear and stress from handling are frequently present in rabbits and may be responsible for glucose levels up to 270 mg/dL.[37–39]

Any pet rabbit presented to a veterinary clinic is subject to stress and possible mild dehydration during transportation. However, these changes seem to have no effect on the sodium levels and tonicity in healthy individuals in our study. This situation is most probably due to variations in sodium level in response to changes in glycemia and supports the fact that glucose acts as a permeant solute in the presence of normal insulin function.[36] However, in ill rabbits, a persistent high endogenous corticoid level can induce hyperglycemia, which leads to hyponatremia. To preserve electroneutrality, HCO_3 levels decrease. Corticoids also stimulate HCO_3 secretion in the kidneys and retention of chloride (this process is independent from Na). Stress can also produce respiratory alkalosis and subsequent increased HCO_3 excretion through the kidneys. Chronic stress leads to a decreased HCO_3 concentration and therefore can predispose the rabbit to metabolic acidosis. Furthermore, the muscular fatigue caused by hyperventilation and increased muscular tension derived from stress eventually leads to respiratory and metabolic acidosis. Loop diuretics induce lowering of sodium levels and chloride levels in rabbits (inducing high AnGap despite sodium loss).[30]

Hypernatremia is less common than hyponatremia. Intense thirst generally prevents it unless water is not available or a neurologic disorder that prevents access to water or interferes with recognition of thirst is present. A deficit of pure water, hypotonic fluid loss, or gain of impermeant solute can cause hypertonicity of the extracellular fluid and hypernatremia. Extrarenal causes of hypotonic fluid loss in rabbits include diarrhea, small intestinal obstruction, cutaneous burns, third-space loss (peritonitis or pancreatitis), and hypertonic fluid administration (hypertonic saline, sodium HCO_3). Renal causes are associated with chronic renal failure, nonoliguric acute renal failure, iatrogenic dieresis (mannitol administration, loop diuretics), persistent hyperglycemia, or postobstructive diuresis.

We observed slightly a higher concentration of venous sodium compared with arterial samples. We believe that this finding is a result of the dilution effect of heparin in smaller arterial samples. Equality of sodium levels has been reported previously in venous and arterial samples. This is the reason for obtaining at least 0.5 mL of blood during sampling with the technique described earlier. Smaller samples were proved to lead to artifactually decreased sodium results.

Chloride

Chloride levels in our experience are lower in rabbits compared with dogs and cats.[1–3,7] This finding can be explained by the significantly higher organic anion load in rabbits compared with that in carnivores or herbivores.[20] Normal lactate levels in rabbits can be up to 17 mmol/L higher than normal levels in carnivores and horses.[20] Despite this difference, the AnGap reference range in rabbits is similar to the typical values found in dogs and cats. Differences in the levels of sodium, unmeasured cations (in particular, calcium) or anions (phosphates, sulfates, ketoacids), albumin, and lactate in rabbits can be responsible for this finding.

Significant differences were found among hyponatremic, normonatremic, and hypernatremic samples. Chloremia seems to be directly proportional to natremia in rabbits, but it is less dependent of HCO_3 or AnGap levels.

Hypochloremic samples are commonly also hyponatremic, only one-third of them showing a compensatory HCO_3 increase. Although one-third of hypochloremic samples are alkalemic, pH is usually maintained within normal limits. This finding suggests that, in rabbits, hypochloremia does not elicit the increase in HCO_3 that would be expected, most probably because of the concurrent hyponatremia. The alkalinizing effect of hypochloremia is therefore less pronounced in this species.

Falsely increased chloride values were reported to be associated with increased uremia in human medicine using the i-STAT system.[40] Analysis performed on i-STAT results from pet rabbits in our center (ANOVA) did not show differences among samples with different uremia levels.

Potassium

Potassium is homeostatically important because it is essential for the maintenance of membrane potential. It also has a minor effect on the AnGap. However, significant changes in potassium levels, to the life-incompatible limit, are needed to induce changes in AnGap.[1]

Causes for hyperkalemia include acute renal failure, urine flow obstruction, severe tissue damage, hemolysis, metabolic acidosis, clotting, and incorrect sampling technique (delayed processing, excessive agitation, or use of ammonium heparin or K3EDTA anticoagulant). Hypokalemia can be caused by dietary insufficiency, loss of fluids from the gastrointestinal apparatus (mucoid diarrhea) or renal system (renal failure, loop diuretics), stress-induced (because of increased in catecholamine levels) alkalosis, and artifacts (hyperproteinemia and lipemia). Iatrogenic hypokalemia can be induced by insulin or glucose-containing fluids. Hypokalemia is associated with the floppy rabbit syndrome.[41–43]

Ionized Calcium

Calcium is found in the body in 3 forms: ionized (iCa), complexed (bound to phosphate, HCO_3, sulfate, citrate, and lactate) and protein-bound. iCa is the most important biologically active fraction and is responsible for the severe signs, symptoms, and alterations that may occur when calcium levels are abnormal. For accurate assessment of calcium status, iCa must be measured directly. Adjustment formulas to calculate iCa by means of total calcium (tCa) and protein or albumin concentration have not been recommended in dogs and cats.[44] The tCa concentration in rabbits is generally 30% to 50% higher than in other mammals and can vary widely depending on dietary intake.[45,46] iCa levels from 44 healthy rabbits in our center varied from 1.67 to 1.85 mmol/L, consistent with previously published data.[47–50] In the rabbit, the absorption of calcium from the gut is not regulated by 1,25-dihydroxyvitamin D.[51] The results of the injection of calcium gluconate and EDTA in an experimental study seemed to indicate that rabbits regulate their serum iCa concentration by rapid changes in parathyroid hormone (PTH) secretion and calcitonin in situations of hypercalcemia and hypocalcemia. However, the changes in PTH occur at high levels of calcium, suggesting that the parathyroid gland in this species is reset to respond to changes in iCa within their physiologic range.[47] Some of the most common causes of hypercalcemia are excessive dietary calcium, neoplasia, inflammatory disorders, and chronic renal failure.[43,44] Hypocalcemia has been associated with gastrointestinal disease, renal failure, acute pancreatitis, sepsis,[44] lactation[29] or some IV contrast media (especially sodium/meglumine diatrizoate),[52] and others. Conditions that cause acidosis can decrease the iCa levels because a higher level of protons increases the ratio of calcium ion binding by proteins.[53] This situation elicits progressive decalcification in acidosis during chronic renal insufficiency.

PACKED CELL VOLUME AND HB VALUES

It is common to find in the literature that packed cell volume (PCV) (hematocrit) and Hb results by the i-STAT method underestimate the real values (determined by reference methods) in humans and dogs.[11,12] When using the i-STAT system, the hematocrit is determined conductometrically, whereas Hb is calculated using the following formula: Hb (g/dL) = hematocrit (% PCV) $\times$ 0.34.

We performed the Passing and Bablok regression analysis of 148 samples from ill rabbits comparing simultaneous determination of PCV by the classic centrifugation method (3 minutes at 16000 $\times$ g) with that by the i-STAT system. The analysis provides the following regression line: $PCV_{centr} = 5 + PCV_{i\text{-}STAT}$. The 95% CI for the intercept value is 5% to 7.2%. The ± 1.96 residual standard deviation (RSD) for the predicted value is −4.5% to 4.5%, meaning that when an i-STAT-derived PCV result is used to predict the real PCV value, an underestimation or overestimation (up to 4.5%) is expected.

The same analysis was performed on 36 samples from ill rabbits comparing Hb determinations by Hemocue and i-STAT methods. The resulting regression line is $Hb_{Hemocue} = 0.1 + 0.98 \times Hb_{i\text{-}STAT}$. The Hb value by i-STAT analyzer seems to be almost identical to that determined by the Hemocue method. The ± 1.96 RSD for the predicted value is −1.3 to 1.3 g/dL, meaning that when an i-STAT- derived Hb result is used to predict the real Hb value, a mild underestimation or overestimation (up to 1.3 g/dL) is expected.

Both regression models show good linearity with R values for the PCV regression line and the Hb regression line of 0.91 and 0.96, respectively.

Example

$PCV_{i\text{-}STAT} = 30\%$
$Hb_{i\text{-}STAT} = 10.2$ mg/dL

According to the Passing and Bablok regression line, $PCV_{centr} = 35\%$ and $Hb_{Hemocue} = 10.1$ mg/dL.

The true PCV value lies between 30.5 and 39.5% and the true Hb value lies between 8.8 and 11.4 mg/dL with 95% confidence.

This example shows that, although the PCV and Hb misestimation by i-STAT might seem systematic and fits well with the linear model, the resulting intervals are too wide to be considered clinically irrelevant. Therefore, although the i-STAT method provides a good initial estimate, a determination by reference methods is still recommended to correctly evaluate the patient's PCV and Hb values.

REFERENCES

1. Bateman SW. Making sense of blood gas results. Vet Clin North Am Small Anim Pract 2008;38:543–57.
2. de Morais H, DiBartola S. Ventilatory and metabolic compensation in dogs with acid-base disturbances. J Vet Emerg Crit Care 1991;1:39–49.
3. Irizarry R, Reiss A. Arterial and venous blood gases: indications, interpretations, and clinical applications. Compend Contin Educ Vet 2009;31(10):E1–8.
4. Constable P. Clinical assessment of acid-base status: comparison of the Henderson-Hasselbalch and strong ion approaches. Vet Clin Pathol 2000; 29(4):115–28.
5. Corey H. Bench-to-bedside review: fundamental principles of acid-base physiology. Crit Care 2005;9(2):184–92.

6. Constable P. Clinical assessment of acid-base status: strong ion difference theory. Vet Clin North Am Food Anim Pract 1999;15(3):447–71.
7. Irizarry R, Reiss A. Beyond blood gases: making use of additional oxygenation parameters and plasma electrolytes in the emergency room. Compend Contin Educ Vet 2009;31(10):E1–8.
8. Severinghaus J, Astrup P. History of blood gas analysis. II. Ph and acid-base balance measurements. J Clin Monit 1985;1(4):259–77.
9. Severinghaus J. Acid-base balance controversy: case for standard-base excess as the measure of nonrespiratory acid-base imbalance. J Clin Monit 1991;7(3): 276–7.
10. DiBartola SP. Introduction to acid-base disorders. In: DiBartola SP, editor. Fluid, electrolyte and acid-base disorders in small animal practice. 3rd edition. St. Louis (MO): Elsevier; 2006. p. 229–51.
11. Schneider J, Dudziak R, Westphal K, et al. The i-STAT analyzer. A new, hand-held device for the bedside determination of hematocrit, blood gases, and electrolytes. Anaesthesist 1997;46(8):704–14.
12. Steinfelder-Visscher J, Teerenstra S, Gunnewiek JM, et al. Evaluation of the i-STAT point-of-care analyzer in critically ill adult patients. J Extra Corpor Technol 2008; 40(1):57–60.
13. Hopper K, Rezende M, Haskins S. Assessment of the effect of dilution of blood samples with sodium heparin on blood gas, electrolyte, and lactate measurements in dogs. Am J Vet Res 2005;66(4):656–60.
14. Benson KG, Paul-Murphy J. Clinical pathology of the domestic rabbit. Acquisition and interpretation of samples. Vet Clin North Am Exot Anim Pract 1999;2(3): 539–52.
15. Rezende M, Haskins S, Hopper K. The effects of ice-water storage on blood gas and acidbase measurements. J Vet Emerg Crit Care 2007;17(1):67–71.
16. Zhang J. Determination of the normal value blood routine and blood gas analysis of Japanese white rabbit. Journal of Anhui Agricultural Sciences 2008;36(5): 1887–8.
17. Topal A, Gül N. Comparison of the arterial blood gas, arterial oxyhaemoglobin saturation and end-tidal carbon dioxide tension during sevoflurane or isoflurane anaesthesia in rabbits. Ir Vet J 2006;59(5):278–81.
18. Hewitt CD, Innes DJ, Savory J, et al. Normal biochemical and hematological values in New Zealand white rabbits. Clin Chem 1989;35(8):1777–9.
19. Barzag MM, Bortolotti A, Omarini D, et al. Monitoring of blood gas parameters and acid-base balance of pregnant and non-pregnant rabbits (Oryctolagus cuniculus) in routine experimental conditions. Lab Anim 1992;26:73–9.
20. Vernay M. Origin and utilization of volatile fatty acids and lactate in the rabbit: influence of the faecal excretion pattern. Br J Nutr 1987;57:371–81.
21. Bar-Ilan A, Marder J, Samueloff S. In vivo and in vitro CO2 titration curves in the rabbit: adaptation to hypercapnic conditions. Comp Biochem Physiol A Comp Physiol 1984;78(2):217–20.
22. Krapf R. Mechanisms of adaptation to chronic respiratory acidosis in the rabbit proximal tubule. J Clin Invest 1989;83:890–6.
23. Akiba T, Rocco VK, Wamock DG. Parallel adaptation of the rabbit renal cortical sodium/proton antiporter and sodium/bicarbonate cotransporter in metabolic acidosis and alkalosis. J Clin Invest 1987;80(2):308–15.
24. Kiwull-Schöne H, Kalhoff H, Manz F, et al. Minimal-invasive approach to study pulmonary, metabolic and renal responses to alimentary acid-base changes in conscious rabbits. Eur J Nutr 2001;40:255–9.

25. Shafford HL, Schadt JC. Respiratory and cardiovascular effects of buprenorphine in conscious rabbits. Vet Anaesth Analg 2008;35(4):326–32.
26. Meinkoth JH, Cowell RL, Dorsey K. Metabolic acid-base abnormalities. In: Cowell RL, editor. Veterinary clinical pathology secrets. St. Louis (MO): Elsevier Mosby; 2004. p. 130–7.
27. Thrall MA, Weiser G, Allison RW, et al. Veterinary hematology and clinical chemistry. 2nd edition. Arnes (IO): Wiley-Blackwell; 2012.
28. Vaden SL, Knoll JS, Smith FW, et al. Blackwell's five minutes veterinary consult: laboratory tests and diagnostic procedures. Canine and feline. Arnes (IO): Wiley-Blackwell; 2009.
29. Harcourt-Brown F. Therapeutics. In: Harcourt-Brown F, editor. Textbook of rabbit medicine. Oxford (United Kingdom): Reed Educational and Professional; 2002. p. 94–120.
30. Bobowiec R, Wójcik M, Martelli F, et al. Changes in the anion gap induced by NH4Cl and furosemide in rabbits. Med Weter 2002;58(6):456–61.
31. Kiwull-Schone H, Kiwull P, Manz F, et al. Food composition and acid-base balance: alimentary alkali depletion and acid load in herbivores. J Nutr 2008; 138:431S–4S.
32. DiBartola SP. Disorders of sodium and water: hypernatremia and hyponatremia. In: DiBartola SP, editor. Fluid, electrolyte, and acid-base disorders in small animal practice. St Louis (MO): Elsevier Saunders; 2012. p. 45–79.
33. Bern M. Clinically significant pseudohyponatremia. Letters and correspondence. Am J Hematol 2006;81:558–61.
34. Illowsky BP, Laureno R. Encephalopathy and myelinolysis after rapid correction of hyponatremia. Brain 1987;110(Pt 4):855–67.
35. Nelson RW, Delaney SJ, Elliott DA. Electrolyte imbalances. In: Nelson RW, Couto CG, editors. Small animal internal medicine. 4th edition. St Louis (MO): Mosby Elsevier; 2009. p. 864–84.
36. Hillier TA, Abbott RD, Barrett EJ. Hyponatremia: evaluating the correction factor for hyperglycemia. Am J Med 1999;106(4):399–403.
37. Harcourt-Brown F. Textbook of rabbit medicine. Oxford: Butterworth-Heinemann; 2002. p. 141–64.
38. Mader DR. Basic approach to veterinary care. In: Quesenberry KE, Carpenter JW, editors. Ferrets, rabbits and rodents clinical medicine and surgery. 2nd edition. Philadelphia: WB Saunders; 2004. p. 147–54.
39. Harcourt-Brown FM, Harcourt-Brown NH. Blood glucose measurements in pet rabbits. In: Samour J, Montesinos A, editors. Proceedings of the 1st ECZM Meeting and 11th EAAV Conference. Madrid (Spain): European College of Zoological Medicine and European Association of Avian Veterinarians; 2011. p. 101–2.
40. Keith Pinckard J, Zahn J, Ashby L, et al. Falsely increased i-STAT® chloride results for blood samples with increased urea. Clin Chem 2001;47(11):2064–6.
41. Carpenter JW. Exotic animal formulary. 3rd edition. St. Louis (MO): Elsevier Saunders; 2005.
42. Melillo A. Rabbit clinical pathology. Journal of Exotic Pet Medicine 2007;16(3): 135–45.
43. Harcourt-Brown F. Clinical pathology. In: Harcourt-Brown F, editor. Oxford (United Kingdom): Reed Educational and Professional; 2002. p. 140–64.
44. Schenck PA, Chew DJ, Nagode LA, et al. Disorders of calcium: hypercalcemia and hypocalcemia. In: DiBartola SP, editor. Fluid, electrolyte and acid-base disorders in small animal practice. St. Louis (MO): Elsevier Saunders; 2012. p. 120–94.

45. Muñoz ME, Gonsales J, Esteller A. Bile pigment formation and excretion in the rabbit. Comp Biochem Physiol 1986;85(1):67–71.
46. Meredith A. General biology and husbandry. In: Meredith A, Flecknell PA, editors. Manual of rabbit medicine and surgery. 2nd edition. Gloucester (UK): BSAVA; 2006. p. 1–17.
47. Warren HB, Lausen NC, Segre GV, et al. Regulation of calciotropic hormones in vivo in the New Zealand white rabbit. Endocrinology 1989;125(5):2683–90.
48. Bas S, Bas A, Estepa JC, et al. Parathyroid gland function in the uremic rabbit. Domest Anim Endocrinol 2004;26(2):99–110.
49. Chang JM, Hwang SJ, Tsai JC, et al. In vivo effect of endothelin-1 on plasma calcium and parathyroid hormone concentrations. J Endocrinol 2000;165(2): 179–84.
50. Kamphues VJ, Carstensen P, Schroeder D, et al. Effect of increasing calcium and vitamin D supply on calcium metabolism in rabbits. J Anim Physiol Anim Nutr (Berl) 1986;56:191–208.
51. Jenkins JR. Gastrointestinal diseases. In: Quesenberry KE, Carpenter JW, editors. Ferrets, rabbits and rodents clinical medicine and surgery. 2nd edition. St Louis (MO): Elsevier Saunders; 2004. p. 161–71.
52. Hayakawa K, Maeda M, Mitsumori M, et al. Electrolyte disturbances caused by intravenous contrast media. Radiat Med 1992;10(5):171–5.
53. Toffaletti JG. Calcium, magnesium and phosphate. In: McClatchey KD, editor. Clinical laboratory medicine. Philadelphia: Lippincott Williams & Wilkins; 2002. p. 392–406.

Sexual Hormone Fluctuation in Chinchillas

Simone Celiberti, DVM[a], Alessia Gloria, DVM, PhD[b],*,
Alberto Contri, DVM, PhD[b], Augusto Carluccio, DVM, PhD[b],
Tanja Peric, DScA[c], Alessandro Melillo, DVM[a],
Domenico Robbe, DVM, PhD[b]

KEYWORDS

- Chinchillas • Hormones • Reproductive physiology • Estrus cycle

KEY POINTS

- The reproductive physiology of the chinchilla (*Chinchilla laniger*) is still subject to various studies because of the discordance of the data obtained from early work.
- The vaginal smear test is an indispensable aid in the monitoring of the various phases of the estrus cycle.
- Colpocytology has also been shown to be useful to determine the interestrus period during the spring.
- The chinchilla does not manifest an activity of a seasonal type but presents a continuous cycle where the diestrus phase varies.

INTRODUCTION

The reproductive physiology of the chinchilla (*Chinchilla laniger*) is subject to various studies because of the discordance of the data obtained from early work.[1] Its small size and the difficulty in carrying out repeated blood samples over prolonged periods have forced various authors to rely on alternative techniques to monitor the endocrine axis, giving important results but often in contrast with each other. Among these, the analysis of fecal progesterone has been used the most and has allowed a better understanding of the cyclical activity of this new animal.

This knowledge of this data could assist in the intensive breeding of this species and any eventual project for the conservation of chinchillas in the wild.

[a] OMNIAVET Veterinary Clinic, p.zza Omiccioli 5, Roma, Italy; [b] Department of Veterinary Clinical Sciences, University of Teramo, Viale Crispi 212, 64100 Teramo, Italy; [c] Department of Food Sciences, University of Udine, Udine, Italy
* Corresponding author.
E-mail address: gloriaalessia@libero.it

Vet Clin Exot Anim 16 (2013) 197–209
http://dx.doi.org/10.1016/j.cvex.2012.11.001
1094-9194/13/$ – see front matter © 2013 Elsevier Inc. All rights reserved.

vetexotic.theclinics.com

REPRODUCTIVE PHYSIOLOGY OF THE CHINCHILLA
Sexual Maturity

The female chinchilla manifests puberty after having reached its final adult weight, occurring around 240 days[2]; the male chinchilla acquires the capability to fecundate toward the eighth month. For reproduction purposes, it is better to use animals that have reached at least 1.5 years of age.[3] However, literature on the subject does not agree on when sexual maturity occurs in the female chinchilla; the accepted range varies from 8 weeks to 540 days.[4–9]

The Estrous Cycle

A fundamental characteristic of these hystricomorph rodents (chinchilla and guinea pig) that differentiates it considerably from myomorph rodents (rat and mouse) is the remarkable length of its estrous cycle. The adult female chinchilla develops a cyclic activity of the seasonal polyestrous positive photoperiod type,[10,11] even if in breeding continuous polyestrous–type cyclic activity can more frequently be observed.[12–15] In fact, in breeding conditions, births are frequently all year round. The estrous cycle lasts between 20 and 60 days,[16] with an average reproductive period of 35 days.[10] Ovulation occurs in a spontaneous manner coinciding with the estrus.[2] Sometimes the female chinchilla presents a "silent estrus," or rather, not accompanied by the opening of the vaginal slit, in particular during the unfavorable months of mating.[3] At the author's latitude (41°-54°N-12°–27°E), the mating season usually begins in January or February, although it is possible to observe female chinchillas in estrus during the latter half of October. The mating activity tends to decrease during the summer months, especially in July and August, when the fewest episodes are recorded. In wild chinchillas, which live in the southern hemisphere with seasons that are inverted with respect to the author's, 2 mating periods can be observed, midwinter (June to August) and mid-summer (December to February). These mating periods permit the maximum number of births during the less harsh seasons (spring to autumn). In particular, in the wild, the greatest number of deliveries is observed in spring (October to November); the less frequent deliveries are in autumn.[3]

The estrus of the chinchilla lasts between 12 and 48 hours and during this time the female chinchilla may accept the male chinchilla.[2] The most typical manifestation of the female chinchilla in estrus is the opening of the vaginal slit (**Fig. 1**), along with the discharge of a stringy, limpid, mucus secretion (**Fig. 2**), unaccompanied by any external genital edema.[17–20]

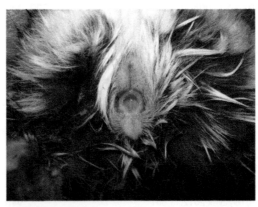

Fig. 1. The female chinchilla in estrus.

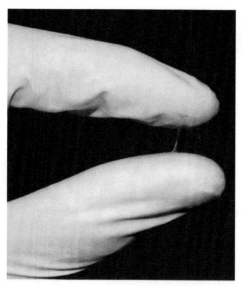

Fig. 2. Stringy, limpid, mucus secretion, typical of the chinchilla in estrus.

Mating

Because these animals are extremely timid and are active particularly at night, it is often difficult to observe the act of mating. Nevertheless, there are observations that can be made in the morning to prove mating occurred.

Certainly the most characteristic sign is the finding of the "copulating tap."[16,21–25] The sperm, after having been ejaculated into the vagina, coagulates, forming a "tap," which prevents the seminal liquid from leaving. A few hours after mating has occurred, contractions of the vagina push this tap out and the tap can be found in the cage. The form of this tap resembles a chrysalid and measures 2.5 cm in length by 6.7 mm in diameter, is yellow, and has the consistency of wax. If mating is suspected, an examination of the male chinchilla may supply further indications; an increase in the volume of the testicles will be noted in addition to finding a ring of fur around the penis, known as the "penile ring," which should be removed with extreme care (**Figs. 3** and **4**).

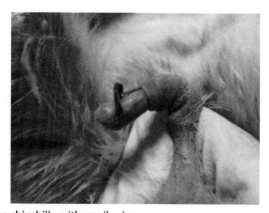

Fig. 3. Penis of the chinchilla with penile ring.

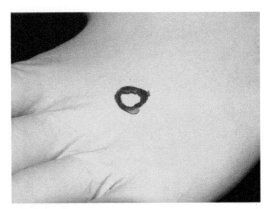

Fig. 4. Penile ring after removal.

Chinchillas, like other rodents (guinea pig), accept mating within 48 hours of delivery, with a high percentage of pregnancy.

Approximately 57.4 ± 2.6 days after delivery, the female chinchilla will manifest estrus and a further mating attempt will be possible.[2]

Pregnancy

In the early descriptions of the wild chinchilla, it was thought that these animals gave birth to a litter of between 5 and 7; today the numbers of chinchilla born in the wild and those bred in captivity are the same. The wild female chinchillas, captured during the last month of gestation, gave birth to 1.8 per pregnancy, a figure very similar to that obtained for bred ones, 2 to 3 per pregnancy,[2] with an average of 2 in the *C langer* and 1.4 in the *Chinchilla brevicaudata*.[3]

As far as the duration of the pregnancy is concerned, there are notable differences depending on the species of chinchilla in consideration. Indeed, the *C brevicaudata* has a gestation period of 128 days[26]; the *C laniger* has a gestation period of 111 days[26] and an intermediate time of approximately 115 days for the hybrid of the 2 species.[3]

Normally, the chinchilla, both domestic and wild, successfully completes 2 pregnancies per year, and even 3 a year may be possible with intensive breeding.

VALUES OF FECAL PROGESTERONE AND ESTROGENS IN THE INTENSIVE BREEDING OF CHINCHILLAS

For the present study, 24 nonpregnant chinchillas (*Claniger var La Plata*) were chosen at random and subdivided into 3 groups (group A; group B; group C). Group A (**Table 1**) and group B (**Table 2**), composed of 10 chinchillas each, respectively, were monitored during the autumn season (group A) and during the spring season (group B). Samples of fecal pellets of these animals were taken for the dosage of fecal metabolites of progesterone and vaginal smears to identify the phases of the estrus cycle. Group C (**Table 3**), composed of 4 subjects, was monitored during the autumn season and hematic samples were taken from these animals to quantify the dosage of progesterone and estrogen in addition to vaginal smear tests to individuate the phase of the estrus cycle. All the subjects varied in age from 1 to 4 years old, with a weight of approximately 547 ± 63 g. All the monitored animals showed no type of pathologic abnormality in the progress.

Table 1
Values of fecal progesterone obtained during the autumn season (group A)

	t0	t1	t2	t3	t4	t5	t6	t7	t8	t9
C.1	208.38	134.98	139.66	129.84	207.24	197.57	136.03	147.35	223.71	174.18
C.2	151.75	350.88	135.10	126.65	144.02	175.25	161.82	185.04	266.89	122.67
C.3	488.73	407.10	316.41	439.62	395.50	537.29	295.66	334.84	491.10	325.72
C.4	249.93	238.60	264.48	380.96	721.51	414.89	505.23	432.84	345.32	328.99
C.5	328.72	240.17	442.29	464.80	252.00	231.27	213.21	298.00	262.21	326.61
C.6	355.87	358.77	306.74	571.56	360.43	391.11	326.03	550.88	539.56	466.98
C.7	325.39	312.58	221.42	303.88	313.98	318.07	315.27	204.87	239.52	304.28
C.8	77.92	106.30	114.68	171.34	234.63	117.91	90.86	419.71	315.70	251.79
C.9	488.26	535.94	365.02	415.25	582.90	471.13	494.46	330.75	497.59	382.62
C.10	481.18	222.63	263.36	198.75	137.48	108.94	230.92	195.94	301.57	112.08
Media	315.61	290.79	256.92	320.26	334.97	296.34	276.95	310.02	348.32	279.59
DS±	144.62	129.35	106.59	157.04	189.84	151.92	140.46	130.16	117.34	114.35

Collection of Fecal Material and Execution of Vaginal Smear

During the study, 10 samples of feces were taken for each single animal (1 every 3 days) in the nonreproductive period (group A) and in the reproductive period (group B) and, contemporarily, vaginal smears were opportunely smeared onto slides and stained with Harris-Shorr coloring (**Fig. 5**).

Autumn Season

The values of fecal progesterone of all the animals in group A at different times, obtained during the autumn season, are reported in **Table 1**.

The average values of progesterone in all the animals at varying times are reported in **Fig. 6**. The graph shows the trend of progesterone during the period of collection with an average and deviation standard of 302.98 ± 28.13 ng/g and a range that varies from a minimum value of 256.92 ng/g to a maximum value of 348.32 ng/g. The lowest absolute value was 77.92 ng/g and the highest absolute value was 721.51 ng/g.

In these animals, it was not possible to recognize a common T0, which permitted the reporting of all the animals at a "similar" hormonal situation (similar to what occurred, instead, in those monitored during the spring season). In fact, during the entire period, none of them manifested the modifications that are typical of the estrus (the opening of the vaginal slit and the presence of stringy mucus) and in only 1 animal (C.8) was any change seen in the exfoliated vaginal cells, referable possibly to a "silent estrus"[3]; in

Table 2
Progesterone and estrogens during the autumn season

Animal	Progesterone (ng/mL)	Estrogen (pg/mL)
C.1	15.01	0.66
C.2	5.44	0.11
C.3	8.71	13.54
C.4	4.55	18.77
Media	8.42	8.27
DS	±4.73	±9.03

Table 3
Values of fecal progesterone obtained during the spring season (group B)

	t0	t1	t2	t3	t4	t5	t6	t7	t8	t9
C1	268.33	346.02	338.23	199.05	421.59	395.32	157.85	160.33	243.77	178.10
C2	508.40	794.21	729.91	910.52	656.64	630,54	454.33	797.25	643.81	632.92
C3	18.07	0.00	6.73	20.15	9.45	25.95	46.52	23.02	23.43	60.31
C4	0.00	59.12	18.14	44.96	46.42	68.28	66.80	32.83	0.00	21.87
C5	56.15	30.38	74.53	66.82	75.80	33.95	0.00	15.95	22.88	41.75
C6	48.34	88.89	63.95	40.67	94.12	48.65	42.94	78.47	47.60	53.26
C7	5.87	0.63	31.27	43.04	132.24	93.52	84.58	105.95	100.62	70.14
C8	114.69	95.25	128.06	60.81	52.84	70.65	8.98	0.00	24.80	24.43
C9	75.87	80.62	52.80	40.35	18.98	35.84	11.87	84.23	43.41	59.49
C10	13.85	46.31	53.81	33.80	33.44	58.05	17.00	49.00	40.55	29.34
Media	110.96	154.14	149.74	146.02	154.15	146.08	89.09	134.70	119.09	117.16
DS±	160.66	245.61	225.1	273.32	213.41	202.13	136.67	237.72	197.12	186.68

particular, the colpocytologic image showed an increase in the cellular and squama population, despite the high number of neutrophils and a modest presence of the other cellular types.

The results of the colpocytology obtained during the autumn period showed very similar images: the population of dominant cells was constant to that of neutrophils, accompanied by other cellular populations, in particular, parabasal cells and small intermediates (**Figs. 7** and **8**). This image is related to the "metaestrus" described by Bekyrürek and colleagues,[27,28] and to "diestrus" described by Gromadzka-Ostrowska and Szylarska-Gozdz.[10]

The high data obtained in the fecal progesterone of group A was confirmed by the following value of haematic progesterone of group C. The data obtained are reported in **Table 2**.

These data confirmed the presence of high concentrations of progesterone but this was not confirmed in the literature. Certain authors, indeed, maintain that the serum progesterone, during the autumn season, is attested to the value of 5.29 ± 0.70 ng/mL.[10]

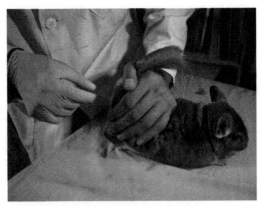

Fig. 5. Execution of the vaginal smear for colpocytology.

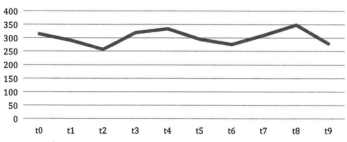

Fig. 6. The average fecal progesterone during the autumn season.

The low values of estrogen compared with the high values of progesterone confirm that the animals, at the moment the samples were taken, did not present anestrus but a phase of diestrus.

In addition to hematic samples, vaginal smears were taken to relate the hematic concentrations of progesterone to the colpocytology. From this, a similar image obtained from the previous sampling came to light. The exfoliated vaginal cells were characterized by the dominance of neutrophils and by the dominance of the presence of traces of the other cellular lines (cytologic diestrus).

Spring Season

The values of the fecal progesterone in all the animals in group B at various times, obtained during the spring season, are reported in **Table 3**.

The average values of progesterone in all animals at various times are reported in **Fig. 9**. The graph shows the trend of the progesterone, during the whole month of the collection period, with an average and deviation standard of 132.11 ± 22.03 ng/g, with a range between 89.09 ng/g and 154.15 ng/g. Then, if among these animals, animals C.1 and C.2 are not taken into consideration, whose values of progesterone are clearly higher than the other animals monitored at the same time, values of 46.80 ± 7.47 ng/g with a range between 34.84 ng/g and 57.91 ng/g are obtained. Clearly the lowest value was 0.00 ng/g, whereas the highest value was 910.53 ng/g (considering animals C.1 and C.2); if the above-mentioned animals are not taken into consideration, the highest value was 114.69 ng/g.

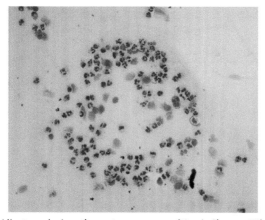

Fig. 7. Metaestrus/diestrus during the autumn season (Harris-Shorr ×20).

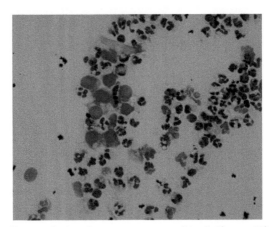

Fig. 8. Metaestrus/diestrus during the autumn season (Harris-Shorr ×40).

In the animals monitored during the spring season, it was possible to compare the values of the progesterone as if all of them were at the same hormonal moment. Indeed, thanks to the diagnostic help of the colpocytology, the author was able to report at time 0 all those preparations that showed a "cytologic" estrus. In 8 of 10 animals, it was possible to observe the typical changes of the exfoliated vaginal cells "characteristic" of the estrus: these, as described by Bekyürek and colleagues in 2002, are characteristic of the dominance of the superficial cells and squama (**Fig. 10**).

The results of the colpocytologic test showed that 2 subjects (C.3 and C.4) manifested more cytologic estruses over the spring period. In particular, chinchilla C.3 showed 2 estruses at a distance of 21 days; chinchilla C.4 showed 2 estruses 24 days apart.

The values of fecal progesterone compared at cytologic T0 are reported in **Table 4**. The values of fecal progesterone of the animals, which presented a "cytologic" estrus, are reported in red. As previously explained, animals C.3 and C.4 presented 2 cytologic estruses during the monitored period. From the values obtained during the

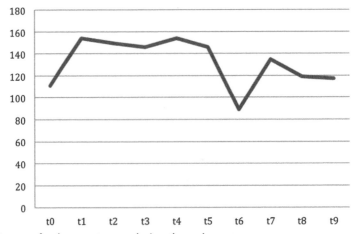

Fig. 9. Average fecal progesterone during the spring season.

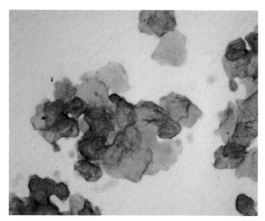

Fig. 10. "Cytologic" estrus during the spring period (Harris-Shorr ×40).

cytologic estrus, it can be deduced that not all subjects presented basal levels of progesterone.

By transferring these values onto a graph where T0 corresponds to the cytologic estrus, it was possible to represent the cyclic tendency of progesterone during the spring period (**Fig. 11**).

The values of progesterone in animals C.1 and C.2 are not included in the graph because the colpocytology obtained for these subjects revealed an image that refers to a situation of prolonged metaestrum/diestrum compatible with the high values of progesterone.

Table 4
Values of fecal progesterone reported at the cytologic estrus

	C.3	C.4	C.5	C.6	C.7	C.8	C.9	C.10	Media	±DS
−7			56.15			114.69			85.42	41.396
−6			30.38			95.25	75.87	13.85	53.84	38.078
−5			74.53	48.34		128.06	80.62	46.31	75.57	33.09
−4			66.82	88.89		60.81	52.80	53.81	64.62	14.708
−3			75.80	63.95		52.84	40.35	33.80	53.35	17.086
−2			33.95	40.67		70.65	18.98	33.44	39.54	19.105
−1	18.07		0.00	94.12	5.87	8.98	35.84	58.05	31.56	34.113
Estrus	0.00	0.00	15.95	48.65	0.63	0.00	11.87	17.00	11.76	16.669
1	6.73	59.12	22.88	42.94	31.27	24.80	84.23	49.00	40.12	24.256
2	20.15	18.14	41.75	78.47	43.04	24.43	43.41	40.55	38.74	19.295
3	9.45	44.96		47.60	132.24		59.49	29.34	53.85	42.114
4	25.95	46.42		53.26	93.52				54.79	28.309
5	46.52	68.28			84.58				66.46	19.092
6	23.02	66.80			105.95				65.26	41.489
7	23.43	32.83			100.62				52.29	42.112
8	60.31	0.00			70.14				43.48	37.977
9		21.87							21.87	

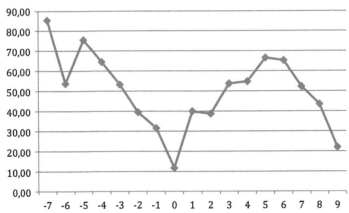

Fig. 11. Tendency of fecal progesterone during the cyclic activity in the chinchilla where time 0 corresponds to the cytologic estrus.

SUMMARY

Monitoring the reproductive cycle using colpocytology and fecal progesterone dosage represents a valid technique to understand the reproductive physiology of the species being considered.

Based on the evidence of the data found, the vaginal smear test is an indispensable aid in the monitoring of the various phases of the estrus cycle. In fact, by using the colpocytologic investigation, the author managed to identify the estrus phase that the animal presented at any certain moment in time. Not only did it enable to the confirmation of the variations in the fecal progesterone obtained in the different periods tested, but also using this method, it was possible to obtain the "cytologic" estrus in those animals that did not present the manifestations characteristic of these species. In fact, at the present time, it is not known whether the chinchilla may become pregnant following mating during a "silent" estrus. In particular, the cytologic estrus was observed in animals (chinchilla 8, autumn period; chinchilla 1 and 2 spring period) that presented high values of fecal progesterone and no anatomic modification referable to the estrus (opening of the vaginal slit and the presence of stringy mucus). In fact, as described by Grau,[3] chinchillas can manifest "silent" estruses, unaccompanied by the opening of the vaginal slit, especially in unfavorable mating months. The author thinks that the lack of the characteristic signs of the estrus is due to the high values of progesterone; however, this consideration must be investigated further.

The colpocytology has also been shown to be useful in determining the interestrus period during the spring; the author has in fact observed that 2 animals (chinchilla 3 and 4, reproductive season) had more cytologic estruses in the monitored period. In particular, chinchilla 3 manifested 2 cytologic estruses at a distance of 21 days from one another, whereas chinchilla 4 presented 2 cytologic estruses at a distance of 24 days. This finding confirms the data reported by Gromadzka-Ostrowska and Sylarska- Gozdz[10] that in the spring season the chinchilla has a variable cycle from 22 to 27 days.

Samples taken using feces offer numerous advantages: the feces are easy to collect and, more importantly in this type of animal the repeated sampling can be performed without disturbing the animal, because of the difficulty and complications in taking a hematic sample. Moreover, it would be impossible to monitor the endocrine axis for a long period of time using hematic sampling, because of the sheer volume of blood required.

Through this method, the animals have been monitored over a sufficiently long period during the autumn season and during the spring. During the autumn season, unexpected results were obtained. In fact, many authors report that the chinchilla is a seasonal animal that is photoperiod positive and during the summer to autumn season it is in anestrus.[16,21,22,28-32] In fact, the values of progesterone found were in sharp contrast with what was claimed in the earlier discussion. Indeed, from the author's data, the chinchilla presents very high values of progesterone during the autumn season (average, 302.98 ± 28.14 ng/g), inconsistent with anestrus. The author's results, on the other hand, validate the work of Gromadzka-Ostrowskka and Sylarska-Gozdz,[10] who maintain that during the autumn to winter period, the chinchilla presents a cycle of 70 to 90 days.

Because of the duration of the period tested, this last datum could not be confirmed and should be studied in depth through the prolonged monitoring (>90 days) of the reproductive axis of the animal. Based on the resulting data, however, it can be deduced that the chinchilla does not manifest an activity of a seasonal type but presents a continuous cycle where the diestrus phase varies. In fact, the obtained data proves that the chinchilla finds itself in a phase of prolonged diestrus, in the autumn period, in accordance with both the values of progesterone and the colpocytologic investigations. It would be extremely interesting to investigate the matter more in depth to understand which element determines the lengthening of the diestrus period.

In conclusion, it can be affirmed that the chinchilla manifests a reproductive activity of a continuous type and that the increase in mating during the spring season is due to a shorter diestrus period, and as a consequence, the animals present a shorter cycle with more frequent estruses.

REFERENCES

1. Weir BJ. Aspect of reproduction in the chinchilla. J Reprod Fertil 1966;12: 410–1.
2. Quesenberry KE, Carpenter JW. Ferrets, rabbits and rodents: clinical medicine and surgery. 2nd edition. St Louis (MO): Saunders; 2004. p. 243–59.
3. Grau J. La chinchilla, su crianza en todos los climas. El Ateneo; 1993.
4. Bonagura JD. Terapéutica veterinaria de pequeños animales. McGraw-Hill Interamericana; 2001.
5. Brookhyser KM, Aulerich RJ. Consumption of food, body weight, perineal colour and levels of progesterone in the serum of cyclic female chinchillas. J Endocrinol 1980;87:213–9.
6. Busso JM, Ponzio MF, Fiol De Cuneo M, et al. Noninvasive monitoring of ovarian endocrine activity in the chinchilla (Chinchilla lanigera). Gen Comp Endocrinol 2007;150(2):288–97.
7. Busso JM, Ponzio MF, Fiol De Cuneo M, et al. Reproduction in chinchilla (Chinchilla lanigera): current status of environmental control of gonadal activity and advances in reproductive techniques. Theriogenology 2012;78(1): 1–11.
8. Cabrera A. Catalogo de los mamíferos de America del sur. Parte II revista del museo argentino de ciencias naturales bernardino rivadavia. Zoologia 1961; 4(2):309–732.

9. Caliskaner S. Kurk hayvanlarinin beslenmesi. Ankara (Turkey): Ders kitabi: 376; 1993. p. 190–9.

10. Gromadzka – Ostrowska J, Szylarska – Gozdz E. Progesterone concentration and their seasonal changes during the estrus cycle of chinchilla. Acta Theriol 1984;29(20):251–8.

11. Wessel K. Does light affect reproduction in chinchillas too. Der Deutsche Pelztier-zuchter 1963;37:91–3.

12. Celiberti S, Robbe D, Tosi U, et al. Monitoraggio del ciclo riproduttivo nel cincillà (Chinchilla Lanigera) mediante colpocitologia e dosaggio del progesterone fecale. Atti SIRA 2010;8:205–8.

13. Czekala NM, Lasley BL. A technical note on sex determination in monomorphic birds using fecal steroid analysis. Int. Zoo Yearb 1977;17:209–11.

14. D'elia G, Teta P. Chinchilla lanigera. In: IUCN 2010. IUCN Red List of Threatened Species. 2008.

15. Fowler ME, Miller RE. Zoo and wild animal medicine. 5th edition. St Louis (MO): Saunders; 2003. p. 420–42.

16. Weir BJ. Chinchilla. In: Hafez ES, editor. Reproduction and breeding techniques for laboratory animals. Philadelphia: Lea and Febiger; 1970. p. 209.

17. Schwarzenberger F, Mostl E, Palme R, et al. Faecal steroid analysis for non-invasive monitoring of reproductive status in farm, wild and zoo animals. Anim Reprod Sci 1996;42:515–26.

18. Spontorno AE, Zuleta JP, Deane AL, et al. Chinchilla Laniger. Mamm Species 2004;758:1–9.

19. Tam WH. A comparative study of the production of progesterone by various hys-tricomorph rodents. J Endocrinol 1970;48:18–9.

20. Tappa B, Amao H, Takahashi KW. A simple method for intravenous injection and blood collection in the chinchilla (Chinchilla laniger). Lab Anim 1989;23:73–5.

21. Puzder M, Novikmec J. The principal reproductive indices in Chinchilla Laniger. Veterinarstvi 1992;42:258–9.

22. Thiede MR. Chinchillas als heimtiere, richting pflegen und verstehen. 3 Auflage. Munchen (Germany): Tyodata GmbH; 1994. p. 43–7.

23. Weir BJ. The induction of ovulation and oestrus in the chinchilla. J Reprod Fertil 1973;33:61–8.

24. Weir BJ. Reproductive characteristics of hystricomorph rodents. Symp Zool Soc Lond 1974;34:265–301.

25. Weir BJ, Rowlands IW. Functional anatomy of the hystricomorph ovary. Symp Zool Soc Lond 1974;34:302–32.

26. Gabrisch K, Zwart P. Medicina e chirurgia dei nuovi animali da compagnia, vol. II. Torino (Italy): UTET Ed; 2001. p. 173–96.

27. Adaro L, Orostegui C, Olivares R, et al. Variaciones morfométricas anuales del sistema reproductor masculino de la chinchilla en cautiverio (Chinchilla Laniger Grey [sic]). Avances en Producción Animal 1999;24:91–5.

28. Bekyürek T, Liman N, Bayram G. Diagnosis of sexual cycle by means of vaginal smear method in the chinchilla (chinchilla lanigera). Lab Anim 2002;36(1): 51–60.

29. Jakubow K, Gromadzka – Ostrowska J, Zalewska B. Seasonal changes in the haematological indices in peripheral blood of chinchilla (Chinchilla laniger L.). Journal of Small Exotic Animal Medicine 1984;78(4):845–53.

30. Jimenez JE. The extirpation and current status of Chinchilla lanigera and C. brevicauda. Biol Conserv 1996;77:1–6.

31. Kuroiwa J, Imamichi T. Growth and reproduction of the chinchilla-age at vaginal opening, oestrus cycle, gestation period, litter size, sex ratio and diseases frequently encountered. Jikken Dobutsu 1977;26:213–22 [in Japanese].

32. Munoz-Pedreros A. Orden rodentia. In: Munoz-Pedreros A, Yanez J, editors. Mamiferos de Chile. Valdivia (Chile): Ediciones Centro de Estudios Ambientales; 2000. p. 73–126.

Applications of Serum Protein Electrophoresis in Exotic Pet Medicine

Alessandro Melillo, DVM

KEYWORDS

- Electrophoresis • Exotic pets • Protein

KEY POINTS

- With exotic species, progress in the interpretation of the alteration of plasma proteins has been discontinuous and irregular.
- In several exotic species, especially those of small size, the need to work with small volumes of blood requires the clinician to collect the blood with an anticoagulant.
- In clinical practice, the normal plasma protein concentration is measured very simply by a refractometer.

Hundreds of proteins, having several different functions, circulate in the plasma that are, with the exception of immunoglobulins, largely synthesized in the liver. Plasma proteins in the complex are responsible for the colloidal osmotic effect necessary to maintain blood volume. Other important functions of plasma proteins are the buffer function of the blood pH (15%–20% of the total buffering capacity), transport of hormones, transport of drugs, and blood clotting. Different types of proteins are indispensable for the inflammatory reaction, the immune reaction, and for the process of healing and tissue repair. So, it is easily understood that the measurement of plasma proteins and the determination of their alterations may constitute an important method for assessing the health condition of a patient. Human medicine, such as the dog and cat's, has taken advantage for decades of this valuable diagnostic tool. With exotic species, progress in the interpretation of the alteration of plasma proteins has been more discontinuous and irregular. Despite this, the usefulness of this test is indisputable. This article analyzes the different applications of plasma protein electrophoresis in small mammals, birds, and reptiles.

METHOD OF ASSESSING PROTEINS

Traditionally in the medicine of dogs and cats, the measurement of protein is performed on the serum, the fluid that is obtained by centrifugation of a blood sample

Clinica Veterinaria OMNIAVET, Piazza G. Omiccioli 5, Roma 00125, Italy
E-mail address: birdalec@gmail.com

Vet Clin Exot Anim 16 (2013) 211–225
http://dx.doi.org/10.1016/j.cvex.2012.11.002
1094-9194/13/$ – see front matter © 2013 Elsevier Inc. All rights reserved.

allowed to clot in a test tube for 15 to 20 minutes, the time needed for fibrinogen to be used in the coagulation cascade. In several exotic species, especially of small size, the need to work with small volumes of blood requires the clinician to collect the blood with an anticoagulant (frequently natrium heparin or lithium heparin, sometimes heparinizing the syringe to avoid the coagulation of the sample during collection); therefore, centrifugation is achieved in plasma. The main difference between the 2 products is the absence in the serum of fribrinogen, the protein involved in the processes of coagulation; the concentration of total solids of the plasma is thus slightly higher than that of serum (about 5%) and the electrophoretic pattern from it will result in a higher incidence of β-globulin fraction where the fibrinogen normally migrates. In clinical practice, the normal plasma protein concentration is measured very simply by using a refractometer: a few drops of blood are collected in a heparin-ized capillary whose centrifugation gives the value of the microhematocrit (percentage of blood occupied by cells compared with plasma) and a small amount of plasma. Refractometry of that plasma allows easy estimation of the concentration of total solids. This method is simple and intuitive; however, it is not reliable if the sample quality is poor. Among the factors that interfere with the measurement of total solids by refractometer include hemolysis, lipemia, hyperbilirubinemia, azotemia, severe hyperglycemia, hypernatremia, hyperchloremia, and administration of colloids, including synthetic hemoglobin–based oxygen carriers. In the absence of these factors, the amount of nonprotein solids present in plasma is relatively constant, there-fore by subtracting the nonprotein component (1.5 g/dL) the value of total plasma proteins is obtained.

An increase in the concentration of total solids (hyperproteinemia) must always be evaluated in correlation with the microhematocrit value and reflects mainly dehydra-tion or increased synthesis of globulins for various pathologic conditions. The decrease in total solids (hypoproteinemia), vice versa, may reflect overhydration, decreased synthesis of albumin or immunoglobulin, or protein loss associated with hemorrhage, vasculitis, nephropathy, or enteropathy. With the exception of bleeding, which causes a loss of balanced albumins and globulins, in all pathologies involving protein loss albumin concentration falls to a greater extent than that of the globulins because of lower dimensions of the molecule, which allow easier migration through vascular endothelia. The measurement of total protein is certainly very useful, but for the purposes of a diagnosis that is as accurate as possible, it becomes essential to know the alterations of each protein fraction. For this purpose is used the charac-teristic of plasma proteins to be separated based on their charge and the consequent mobility in an electric field specially created. This method defines electrophoresis of proteins. The distribution of protein migrants on strips of cellulose acetate or agarose gel is represented graphically by a curve in which the extension and the height of each peak is corresponding to the breadth and the density of each protein fraction on the substrate migration.

Normally, 5 protein fractions are identified in the mammalian plasma, ordered according to the electric charge: albumin (high negative charge and low molecular weight, migrates to the anode and conventionally to the left of the track), α1-globulin, α2-globulin, and β-globulins and γ-globulins that present the greatest molecular weight and the lowest negative charge and then migrate to the right end of the curve. A different protein fraction is present in most birds and reptiles, with an even more negative charge than albumin that is positioned at the left in the same electrophoretic pattern and is therefore referred to as prealbumin. Conventionally, you find a point halfway between the beginning and end of the curve as the limit between the α2-globulin and β-globulins, and a point halfway to the start of β-globulins and the end of the track as the start of γ-globulin. With the exception of albumin, each peak represents a large number of different proteins that can be further separated by more complex examinations.

THE DIFFERENT FRACTIONS IN CIRCULATING PLASMA PROTEIN

Prealbumin is the protein fraction that migrates more rapidly and is positioned on the track before albumin. In species that have it, this is calculated with albumin in the ratio A/G. It is not normally detectable in mammals, except occasionally in cats, and it is normally found in human patients where it has the function of direct transport of thyroid hormones and indirectly of vitamin A by acting as a carrier protein that binds retinol. In the various avian species, it is present in variable amounts. For example, in the budgerigar (*Melopsittacus undulatus*) or in the cockatiel (*Nymphicus hollandicus*) it can constitute 75% of the total prealbumin + albumin, whereas in African gray parrots (*Psittacus erythacus*), it represents no more than 10% of total albumin and can also be completely absent.[1] In reptiles, the study of plasma proteins is still sporadic and fragmentary data exist, but migrating prealbumin has been reported in some species of chelonians: *Caretta caretta*,[2] *Geochelone radiata*,[3] *Chelonia mydas*,[4] and sauria (*Gallotia* spp),[5] as well as crocodiles (*Caiman* spp), but only with subsequent migration on polyacrylamide gels[6] apparently have similar transport functions, as in other orders.

Albumin constitutes the main fraction of the plasma proteins (in general between 35% and 50% of total protein and up to 60% to 65% in primates, including humans) and represents the main and more homogeneous peak in the electropherograms of all species. The main functions of albumin are to carry many molecules and maintain the oncotic pressure of the blood.[7]

The group of globulins include the acute phase proteins (APPs; α-globulins and β-globulins) and immunoglobulins (γ-globulins).

APPs are the body's response to trauma, inflammation, or infection. The local activation of granulocytes and macrophages causes the release of cytokines (mainly interleukin-6) that stimulate the liver to produce a series of glycoproteins. Alpha-1-antitrypsin, α-1-acid glycoprotein, α2-macroglobulin, C-reactive protein, haptoglobin, and fibrinogen are positive APPs, because their concentration increases in response to inflammation; albumin is considered a negative APP, as its synthesis decreases during inflammation, diverting liver protein synthesis to the proteins mentioned previously. The electrophoretic pattern of the APPs migrates to the peak of the α (α-1-acid glycoprotein, α2-macroglobulin, haptoglobin, protein C) and β (C-reactive protein, fibrinogen, complement, ferritin)-globulins, but with huge specific differences.

The group of γ-globulins is mainly composed of immunoglobulins, although some APPs, such as degradation products of the complement, can migrate into this area as well, especially in avian species. Immunoglobulins are quite impressive in size, consisting of 4 amino acid chains, 2 so-called "heavy" and 2 "light." Depending on the composition of the heavy chains, immunoglobulins are divided into classes named by letters of the Greek alphabet: gamma (IgG), mu (IgM), alpha (IgA), and epsilon (IgE). The IgG antibodies are produced in response to various bacterial, viral, or toxic stimuli; IgE (not present in all species) is mainly involved in allergic reactions; IgA is primarily responsible for the defense processes located at the mucosal level; and IgM has the characteristic of being active in pentameric form (ie, joining in groups of 5), thereby forming a protein complex of imposing size. IgM is secreted by B-lymphocytes and early plasma cells and its main function is to activate complement, whereas IgG is produced later and then plays a predominant action of opsonization, binding to the pathogen and allowing phagocytosis by macrophages. It is normally not possible to differentiate IgM from IgG through normal electrophoresis, but distinguishing the ones by the others is very important because it allows us to date the pathologic process in acute (IgM only) or chronic (IgG with or without IgM) and to differentiate an active process (IgM) by a seropositivity alone (IgG).

ELECTROPHORESIS OF PROTEINS IN THE RABBIT

Electrophoresis serum is used as a "screening" of interpretation of the humoral response and during not specific processes. Recent studies in rabbits have tried to bring to the surface the true diagnostic value of this report, in particular we tried to find a link between hypergammaglobulinemia and one of the diseases most commonly encountered in clinical practice veterinary medicine in lagomorphs: *Encephalitozoon cuniculi*.

The blood for sampling is collected in plain tubes (the use of tubes with accelerant is not possible because of the reduced volume of collectable blood in this species) and left to rest for about 30 minutes. The serum obtained is isolated and frozen at a temperature of $-18°C$ to be examined in the shortest possible time. Laboratory data have shown that a single cycle of freezing does not alter the electrophoretic pattern, whereas prolonged freezing determines a variation in the albumin/globulin ratio in favor of the latter. The serum of the rabbit contains, as in other mammals, various protein fractions: albumin, α-globulins, β-globulins, and γ-globulins. The α-globulins and β-globulins are generally divided into subunits of $\alpha1$ and $\alpha2$, and $\beta1$ and $\beta2$ (**Fig. 1**). Albumin constitutes the main fraction responsible for the oncotic pressure of body fluids, whereas the $\alpha1$-globulin, $\alpha2$-globulin, β-globulins, and γ-globulins are a smaller fraction responsible for the humoral response of the organism. Unlike the guinea pig, however, the area occupied by β-globulins is wider than that of the α-globulins. In rabbits, the normal Serum Protein Electrophoresis (SPE) pattern lacks a clear distinction between $\beta1$-globulins and $\beta2$-globulins, as present in dogs and cats, but when gammopathies in the β region occur, usually an extension of the electrophoretic band is seen, with consequent demarcation of the 2 peaks. The $\alpha1$-globulins, together with the $\alpha2$-globulins and β-globulins, increase in case of acute inflammation, expressing a more rapid response compared with that cell mediated. The γ fraction includes circulating immunoglobulins, complement, the degradation products of complement, and to a lesser extent some proteins that characterize the acute phase.[8]

Rabbit: normal pattern

ID: 02129010

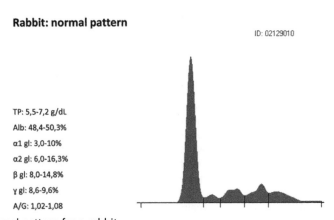

TP: 5,5-7,2 g/dL

Alb: 48,4-50,3%

α1 gl: 3,0-10%

α2 gl: 6,0-16,3%

β gl: 8,0-14,8%

γ gl: 8,6-9,6%

A/G: 1,02-1,08

Fig. 1. Normal pattern for a rabbit.

C-reactive protein is one of the first proteins produced by the body following an insult to any tissue. Despite being defined as an APP, it is also found in the course of chronic processes.[9] Placed inside a magnetic field (principle of electrophoresis of proteins), because of its shape, weight, and molecular electrostatic charge, such protein migrates to the right (toward the anode or negative electrode) in the area of β-globulins and γ-globulins to influence the path. Other APPs, such as aptoglobulina, α1 acid glycoprotein, and ceruloplasmin are normally found in the α and β fractions. In course of encephalitozoonosis we have seen a decrease of albumin, primarily because of the increased synthesis by hepatocytes of numerous immunoproteins (especially Ig) with consequent widening of the electrophoretic band in the region of β and γ. The β-globulin and γ-globulin can be found in course of chronic inflammatory processes (like bacterial, viral, or fungal infections), parasitism (*E cuniculi*), cancer, or immune-mediated diseases. In the specific case of protozoal infection by *E cuniculi*, healthy animals and seropositive animal SPE patterns only differ significantly in the γ fraction.[10] Results are very similar to those obtained by Didier in 1995, in a study of dogs showing clinical signs of encephalitozoon infection.[11] The hypergammaglobulinemia during encephalitozoonosis is usually mild to moderate; this value may be altered when rabbits with impaired immune response come in contact with the parasite, which may react with a decrease of circulating IgG and a possible increase in IgM.[12] The titration of IgM and IgG allows us to clarify the response against the parasite carried by the body at the time of collection. IgM increases usually in the early stages when the parasite exerts its action, decreasing up to be absent on the 38th day, whereas IgG increases more slowly in the course of infection but remains detectable for years.[13] The changes of γ-globulin have been shown to not be significantly different in animals with IgM titratable compared with animals with IgG increased. This shows that the hypergammaglobulinemia is an artifact resulting in a chronic inflammatory process. In support of this theory, it is believed that the organism remains latent in the body until it occurs in a suppression of the immune system, a phase in which the body eliminates spores in the urine.[14]

Contrary to what occurs in avian species, and in accordance with what occurs in dogs, hemolysis increases the β fraction, not the γ fraction.

ELECTROPHORESIS OF PROTEINS IN THE FERRET

In the otherwise rich literature on diseases of the ferret, electrophoresis is quite neglected, mainly because the main source of information on ferret diseases is US research, where electrophoresis is relatively unknown: the only application is described as an aid in diagnosis of Aleutian disease. Actually, it is a useful diagnostic tool in ferret species and its interpretation is not very different from that of the dog and cat. Being that the ferret is an animal of sufficient size, allowing access to the veins of good gauge as the cranial cava, it is recommended to draw blood without anticoagulant (heparin needle) to obtain serum instead of plasma and thus avoid the deposition of fibrinogen, which will inevitably alter the peak of β-globulins.

In a healthy ferret, as in dogs, the proteins migrate in the electric field in dividing fractions: albumin, α1-globulin, α2-globulin, β1-globulin, β2-globulin, and γ-globulin. Albumins represent approximately half of circulating proteins, for which the A/G ratio is about 1. IgA migrates in the field of α2 and β1 globulins, IgM in the field of β2 globulin or "fast" γ globulin, whereas the IgG in the field of slow γ-globulin (the far end of the track) (**Fig. 2**).

In ferrets, dehydration progresses very quickly in case of insufficient intake or increased losses, so hyperproteinemia is a frequently encountered clinical sign

Ferret: normal pattern

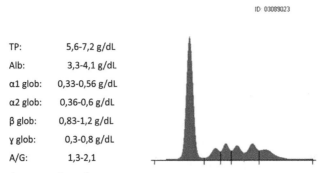

ID 03089023

TP:	5,6-7,2 g/dL
Alb:	3,3-4,1 g/dL
α1 glob:	0,33-0,56 g/dL
α2 glob:	0,36-0,6 g/dL
β glob:	0,83-1,2 g/dL
γ glob:	0,3-0,8 g/dL
A/G:	1,3-2,1

Fig. 2. Normal pattern for a ferret.

(for example in diarrhea, intestinal obstruction, acute gastritis, or renal failure) but in the case of noninfectious diseases, proteins raise in their entirety for hemoconcentration, so the pattern will result basically normal; in the case of inflammatory diseases, globulins increase, altering the electrophoretic curve. The most characteristic alteration is described in patients suffering from Aleutian disease. This disease, fortunately is infrequent (but certainly underdiagnosed) in Italy, is caused by a parvovirus (ADV) that affects the Mustelidae family, including mink and ferret. It is transmitted by feces and all body secretions and is particularly insidious because it evolves as a chronic disease, debilitating the ferret to the invariably fatal outcome. Aleutian disease causes lymphoplasmacytic infiltration and precipitation of immune complexes in various tissues from which a variety of symptoms is shown by sick animals. Blood tests are often vague, showing nonregenerative anemia, abnormal liver enzymes, and uremia; however, electrophoresis is revealing. Patients with ADV in fact have a marked hyperproteinemia with values up to 10 to 12 g/dL or more, but at the same time an important hypoalbuminemia: γ-globulins rise instead to constitute 20% to 60% of total protein, drawing a characteristic "horned" path and seriously altering the A/G ratio. Other diseases can cause hypergammaglobulinemia, although not as marked as ADV: other viruses such as influenza or distemper, pyoderma, kidney diseases with no protein loss, certain tumors, and systemic mycoses (*Blastomycosis, Coccidioides* spp). Another, more frequent, viral disease is catarrhal enteritis (ECE) caused by a coronavirus: kits are often asymptomatic carriers for adults who become instead gravely ill. In case of ECE, electrophoresis is characterized at the beginning by moderate hypoalbuminemia, which becomes more and more severe during the following weeks. Following the evolution of the disease, an increase in α2 or β1 may be noticed, meaning the production of IgA in the acute phase, then a peak of gammaglobulines even if significantly below that of ADV. After the second or third week, there is often hypogammaglobulinemia, evidence of the failure of the immune response.

It is also interesting to note the changes in the electrophoretic pattern in the case of liver disease. In the case of hepatic neoplasia, often the protein curve does not differ much from that of a healthy animal, except for a modest elevation of α2-globulins. More marked is the alteration in case of hepatic lipidosis and acute cholangitis-cholangiohepatitis, when the increase of α2-globulins is greater and reflects an intense inflammation. Chronic hepatitis and cholestasis phenomena, intrahepatic or extrahepatic, are reflected instead in a β-globulin peak, where transferrin, C-reactive protein, and generally the IgM migrate.

The decrease in the percentage of globulin is uncommon and is usually associated with renal failure or lymphoma. The hypoproteinemia usually indicates a defect in protein synthesis and has a negative prognostic value.[15]

ELECTROPHORESIS OF PROTEINS IN HYSTRICOMORPH RODENTS

The electrophoretic pattern of the guinea pig (*Cavia porcellus*) has been thoroughly studied in the experimental for which we know either paths in different normal farming conditions and adjustment of the normal bacterial flora (Specific pathogen free subjects and the like) and the reaction to various pathologies experimentally induced; however, very little is described in the field of clinical practice about the response of animals living in uncontrolled conditions that get sick spontaneously. Clinically healthy guinea pig serum proteins are separated into 7 sections: albumin, α1-globulin, α2-globulin, β1-globulin, β2-globulin (often divided into 2 peaks), and γ-globulins, and in some subjects prealbumins have been occasionally signaled (**Fig. 3**). The area occupied by β-globulins and γ-globulins in the complex is restricted in comparison with the well-developed area of the α-globulins and A/G ratio is high. By immunoelectrophoresis, up to 30 different protein migrants in those areas can be individuated, although not all were necessarily present in the same sample. An interesting study describes the changes in the electrophoretic pattern during the evolution of experimentally induced tuberculosis infection in a group of guinea pigs.[16] At the end of the first week, the electrophoretic pattern was still virtually unchanged, whereas at the fulfillment of the second, a large majority of individuals showed a marked increase in α2-globulins and the appearance of a new peak in the same region, characteristic of sick individuals and never found in healthy ones, named α2-T. At the third week, the α1 started to decrease whereas α2 increased further with increasing importance of α2-T peak, which persisted until the death of the subjects. More detailed studies have identified this protein as a glycoprotein, not macroglobulin. It is interesting to note that the response to tubercular infection occurs in the region of α2 in several species, including humans. Guinea pig lipoproteins tend instead to migrate in the β-globulin peak. The

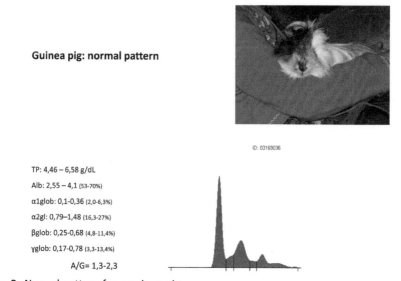

Guinea pig: normal pattern

ID: 03169036

TP: 4,46 – 6,58 g/dL

Alb: 2,55 – 4,1 (53-70%)

α1glob: 0,1-0,36 (2,0-6,3%)

α2gl: 0,79–1,48 (16,3-27%)

βglob: 0,25-0,68 (4,8-11,4%)

γglob: 0,17-0,78 (3,3-13,4%)

A/G= 1,3-2,3

Fig. 3. Normal pattern for a guinea pig.

same study also analyzed the serum of guinea pigs inoculated with killed mycobacteria: the electrophoresis of these subjects showed no increase of α2-globulins nor the appearance of α2-T, which can then be considered the sign of an organic reaction to the pathogen, but all the samples at the third week after inoculation showed a marked hypergammaglobulinemia. In another study, reaction to infection by *Entamoeba histolytica* was investigated, which consisted of hypoalbuminemia and increase of α-globulins and β-globulins.[17]

The importance of electrophoresis in the diagnosis of spontaneous disease in the guinea pig and chinchilla is currently studied: patterns from clinically healthy individuals are shown as a starting point for further observations (**Fig. 4**).

ELECTROPHORESIS OF PROTEINS IN PSITTACIFORMES

The first studies of serum proteins in birds were performed on domestic chickens, showing many similarities with the layout of mammals (eg, the production of APPs[18,19]), but also several differences: the widespread presence of prealbumin, for example, the lowest concentration of γ-globulin, and conversely the more marked response to inflammatory stimuli in the β-globulin field. Unfortunately for the needs of clinical practice, however, not only may the electrophoretic patterns of parrots differ from those of chickens,[20] but significant differences are found also among the different species of Psittaciformes (**Figs. 5–10**). This variability has led some investigators to doubt the possibility of obtaining reliable results by electrophoresis in avian species, especially with regard to the differentiation between the various globulin fractions.[21] The answer to this question is probably a better standardization of the techniques of electrophoresis and graphical representation, as well as a better understanding of the normal values of the different species. Normally, electrophoresis of birds is run on plasma samples obtained from heparinized blood: the percentages are derived from densitometric analysis of each protein fraction deposited on the gel and absolute values (g/dL) calculated by multiplying the percentage of each fraction for the value of total protein obtained from the refractometer.

Chinchilla: normal pattern

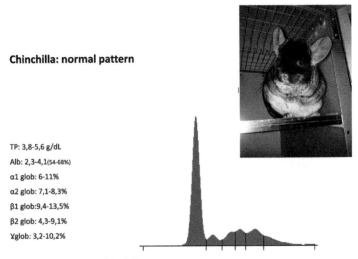

TP: 3,8-5,6 g/dL
Alb: 2,3-4,1(54-68%)
α1 glob: 6-11%
α2 glob: 7,1-8,3%
β1 glob:9,4-13,5%
β2 glob: 4,3-9,1%
Ɣglob: 3,2-10,2%

Fig. 4. Normal pattern for a chinchilla.

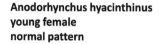

**Anodorhynchus hyacinthinus
young female
normal pattern**

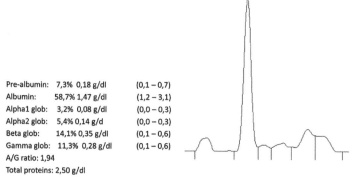

Pre-albumin:	7,3% 0,18 g/dl	(0,1 – 0,7)
Albumin:	58,7% 1,47 g/dl	(1,2 – 3,1)
Alpha1 glob:	3,2% 0,08 g/dl	(0,0 – 0,3)
Alpha2 glob:	5,4% 0,14 g/d	(0,0 – 0,3)
Beta glob:	14,1% 0,35 g/dl	(0,1 – 0,6)
Gamma glob:	11,3% 0,28 g/dl	(0,1 – 0,6)
A/G ratio: 1,94		
Total proteins: 2,50 g/dl		

Fig. 5. Normal pattern for *Anodorhynchus hyacinthinus*, young female.

The pattern of the normal chicken shows a marked peak of albumin, and globulins are divided between the β-globulin (IgM, IgA) and γ-globulin (IgG): transferrin, APP, migrates mainly in the β-globulins. In birds, the albumin protein fraction is undoubtedly preeminent; an interspecific important difference is noted in the group of prealbumin. Whereas in some species, such as the African gray, prealbumin is nearly or totally absent, similar to chickens, other species, such as the budgerigar or the monk parakeet (*Myopsitta monachus*), may have even more prealbumin than albumin. Conventionally, the A/G ratio is calculated by dividing the sum of prealbumin + albumin for the sum of the globulins. According to some investigators, however, it may be more correct to subtract the prealbumin, because it is not properly albumin and even a globulin. The opinion of the author is that this precaution not only is of little practical value but also potentially counterproductive, being that prealbumin, as albumin, has a negative APP and therefore its quantification, when present, has validity in the diagnosis of acute inflammation.

**Amazona ochrocephala:
young female getting
ready to lay an egg**

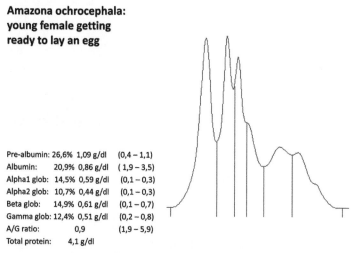

Pre-albumin:	26,6% 1,09 g/dl	(0,4 – 1,1)
Albumin:	20,9% 0,86 g/dl	(1,9 – 3,5)
Alpha1 glob:	14,5% 0,59 g/dl	(0,1 – 0,3)
Alpha2 glob:	10,7% 0,44 g/dl	(0,1 – 0,3)
Beta glob:	14,9% 0,61 g/dl	(0,1 – 0,7)
Gamma glob:	12,4% 0,51 g/dl	(0,2 – 0,8)
A/G ratio:	0,9	(1,9 – 5,9)
Total protein:	4,1 g/dl	

Fig. 6. An *Amazona ochrocephala* (young female) getting ready to lay an egg.

**Myopsitta monachus
male, 13 yo**

Adult specimen showing
Alpha globulins increase
Linked to acute inflammation

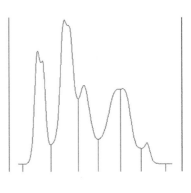

Pre-albumin:	19,8% 0,67 g/dl	(0,5 – 1,1)
Albumin:	33,0% 1,12 g/dl	(1,3 – 2,5)
Alpha-1 glob:	15,3% 0,52 g/dl	(0,0 – 0,3)
Alpha-2 glob:	25,8% 0,54 g/dl	(0,1 – 0,3)
Beta glob:	13,1% 0,45 g/dl	(0,2 – 0,6)
Gamma glob:	3,0% 0,1 g/dl	(0,1 – 0,5)

Fig. 7. *Myopsitta monachus* (male, 13 years old). Adult specimen showing α-globulin increase. It is linked to acute inflammation.

The β-globulins are the predominant group of globulins in all Psittaciformes: some species, such as the African gray, appear regularly divided into 2 subfractions, but the clinical value of this feature is still unclear.[22] The β-globulins increase from 15% to more than 35% in the Psittaciformes with chlamydiosis, aspergillosis, or sarcocystosis.[23,24] An increase of β-globulins has also been described in chickens experimentally inoculated with turpentine and other irritants,[18,19] demonstrating that most APPs (transferrin, fibrinogen, β lipoprotein, complement) in avian species migrate in this sector.[25] The transferrin appears to be the major APP in avian species (in contrast to what happens in mammals) and, although it is not specific to a particular disease,

**Cacatua moluccensis,
adult male**

Chronic FDB and self mutilation
worsening in late winter/spring
suggesting hormonal involvement

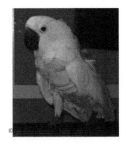

Prealbumin	8,9 %	* 12,0 - 28,0
Albumin	42,4 %	38,0 - 56,0
Alpha 1 globulin	11,3 %	*2,0 - 5,0
Alpha 2 globulin	6,8 %	2,0 - 7,0
Beta globulin	17,1 %	12,0 - 24,0
Gamma globulin	13,5 %	4,0 - 14,0
A/G Ratio	0,73 %	*0,50 - 0,64

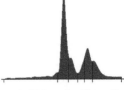

Fig. 8. *Cacatua moluccensis* (adult male). Chronic FDB and self-mutilation worsening in late winter/spring suggesting hormonal involvement.

Amazona aestiva

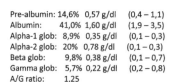 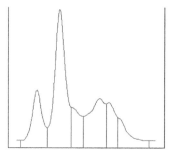

Elderly specimen showing increase of
alpha2 globulins linked to nephropathy

Pre-albumin:	14,6%	0,57 g/dl	(0,4 – 1,1)
Albumin:	41,0%	1,60 g/dl	(1,9 – 3,5)
Alpha-1 glob:	8,9%	0,35 g/dl	(0,1 – 0,3)
Alpha-2 glob:	20%	0,78 g/dl	(0,1 – 0,3)
Beta glob:	9,8%	0,38 g/dl	(0,1 – 0,7)
Gamma glob:	5,7%	0,22 g/dl	(0,2 – 0,8)
A/G ratio:	1,25		
Total proteins: 3,90 g/dl			

Fig. 9. *Amazona aestiva.* Elderly specimen showing increase of α2-globulins linked to nephropathy.

has an important prognostic value: its short half-life (24–48 hours) makes the monitoring of β-globulins an excellent indicator of the effectiveness of a therapy.

The α-globulins instead represent the group less defined and the whose measurement determines the highest margin of error.[22] Altogether they represent only 4% to 8% of total protein, and already this modest quantity (in comparison with that of mammals and also of other avian orders, such as Falconiformes) makes it difficult to precisely separate it from the 2 contiguous predominant peaks, albumins and β-globulins. They are divided into 2 fractions: the area of α1-globulins hosts mainly the α1 antitrypsin and in normal paths is not detectable as a well-defined peak; even in sick parrots an increase of this fraction has almost never been described, unlike what was observed in mammals. In some cases has been noted a selective increase dell'alfa1 antitrypsin, with or without moderate hypoalbuminemia, in Psittaciformes with heavy parasitism.[25] The main protein in the α2 area is instead α2 macroglobulin.

**Bubo bubo: the pattern from this
specimen looks normal, but the
bird is hypoproteinemic, possibly
as a consequence of a too severe
food restriction for training**

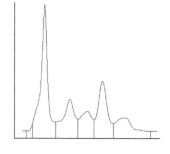

Pre – albumin:	0,3%	0,01 g/dl	(0,0 – 0,0)
Albumin:	42,5%	1,06 g/dl	(1,7 – 2,1)
Alpha1 glob:	16,4%	0,41 g/dl	(0,5 – 0,9)
Alpha2 glob:	11,0%	0,28 g/dl	(0,4 – 0,6)
Beta glob:	20,3%	0,51 g/dl	(0,7 – 1,5)
Gamma glob:	9,5%	0,23 g/dl	(0,2 – 0,6)
A – G ratio:	0,75		(0,50 – 0,90)
Total protein:		2,50 g/dl	(3,0 – 3,5)

Fig. 10. *Bubo bubo.* The pattern from this specimen looks normal, but the bird is hypoproteinemic, possibly as a consequence of a too severe food restriction for training.

The characteristic of this protein is its large size (molecular weight > 400,000) for which it is still retained by the filter even in the presence of serious renal damage. One of the few cases when significant elevations of $\alpha2$ are described is precisely acute nephritis, in which most of the proteins are lost through the kidneys and the percentage of macro-globulin increases accordingly: in response to other phlogistic stimuli, instead, incre-ments much more moderate and inconstant are noticed. Modest alterations of α-globulins have also been described in relation to the activation of the ovary, similarly as described in the human species. The increase of transferrin that occurs during this stage, however, also induces a concomitant peak of β-globulins.

The γ-globulins are a minor fraction in the electrophoretic pattern of the Psittaci-formes, on average 10% to 15% of the total protein. In the area of γ-globulin migrate mainly IgG so we see increments in this area only at a later stage of the pathology. Diseases in which we expect massive increases in γ-globulin are chronic diseases such as chlamydiosis or mycobacteriosis. Aspergillosis also belongs to the group of chronic diseases but, because of its immunosuppressing activity, often patients suffering from chronic fungal forms have apparently normal electrophoresis, as the humoral response is inhibited. Approximately 30% of patients suffering from aspergi-llosis show cyclical peaks in the β-globulins area, and only a small percentage show hypergammaglobulinemia. The normal response to a chronic inflammatory process is the production of a wide variety of antibodies that are expressed in a series of γ-globulin peaks or, more commonly, in a single peak with a large base: this phenomenon is named polyclonal gammopathy. In some cases, however, a single or very few immunoglobulins are massively produced, a phenomenon that is expressed in a peak-to-narrow base similar to that of albumin and is defined oligoclonal or monoclonal gammopathy. Normally behind this phenomenon there is a neoplastic proliferation of one or a few lines of B lymphocytes, even if in some cases, monoclonal gammopathies may occur in response to non-neoplastic stimuli as well, but anyway very serious.

It is worth considering that the low reliability reported by some investigators about the avian electrophoresis is to be traced back to improper collection, retention, and selection of the sample. Cray and colleagues[22] showed that serum refrigeration causes a discrete change in the albumin/globulin ratio, causing a progressive difficulty in defining and quantifying the α-globulins. Conversely, a freezing of the sample did not show adverse effects. Hemolysis is a phenomenon unfortunately present when sampling blood from small patients and difficult to control. In the dog, the products of hemolysis tend to migrate in the β-globulin region; conversely, those of birds seem to migrate primarily in the region of γ-globulin. This may be attributable to a structural difference of the protein or by a different technique analysis.[22] Lipemia is another frequent alteration especially in the serum of some South American species (*Amazona* spp, *Miopsitta*, *Pionus* spp): the electropherogram of a lipemic sample shows an artificial elevation in the region of β-globulins. In contrast, the β-globulins would be below the normal values related in the literature, in which serum would be used in place of plasma because the fibrinogen (absent in serum) migrates essentially in the β region.[26] This is, however, the only significant difference between the tracks from the 2 different spin cycles.

ELECTROPHORESIS OF FALCONIFORMES

Electrophoresis of birds of prey basically follows the same general considerations of Psittaciformes: common use of plasma instead of serum, need to standardize tech-niques, and to study the parameters of normality among the different species (**Figs. 11** and **12**). Compared with Psittaciformes, most Falconiformes do not present

Falco jugger, adult female
acute hypocalcemia related
to reproductive problems

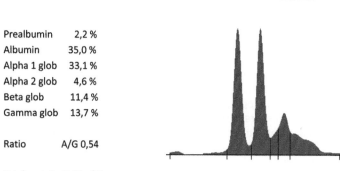

ID: 09129073

Prealbumin	2,2 %
Albumin	35,0 %
Alpha 1 glob	33,1 %
Alpha 2 glob	4,6 %
Beta glob	11,4 %
Gamma glob	13,7 %
Ratio	A/G 0,54

Total protein: 2,40 g/dl

Fig. 11. *Falco jugger* (adult female). Acute hypocalcemia related to reproductive problems.

prealbumin or present it in a minimal amount: vice versa, apparently healthy Falconi-formes have levels of α1-globulins and α2-globulins, markedly higher than the parrots. Major differences regarding the β-globulins and γ-globulins are not described. Elec-trophoresis is an important tool for the diagnosis of chlamydiosis and aspergillosis in Falconiformes. A text antibody positive for *Chlamydia* spp acquires a very different meaning in the presence of electrophoretic curve indicative of acute or chronic inflam-mation than in absence of any alteration; a marked alteration of electropherogram with

Reptiles: pogona vitticeps

Two seemingly healthy specimens,
well-housed and cared for, from a
successful breeding group

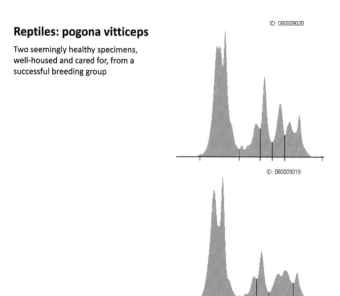

ID: 080009020

ID: 080009019

Fig. 12. *Pogona vitticeps.* Two seemingly healthy specimens, well housed and cared for, from a successful breeding group.

prevailing in the region of the β-globulins can support a presumptive diagnosis of aspergillosis also in case of a negative antibody test.[27] The electrophoresis has proved useful as a diagnostic and prognostic tool in Falconiformes even in the case of diseases such as mycobacteriosis, abscesses, and osteomyelitis.

ELECTROPHORESIS OF REPTILES

The use of electrophoresis in reptiles is still sporadic and most of the available data are anecdotal; nevertheless, they are interesting as a first element for future study. Serum proteins of reptiles migrate in a manner quite similar to those of birds and are divided on the track in the fractions of albumin, α1-globulin, α2-globulin, β-globulins, and γ-globulins. Prealbumin appears in some species (eg, *Geochelone radiata* and some turtles), in which it presumably has the same function of transport as in other animals. Albumins are also the preponderant portion of the curve in reptiles, whereas the globulins as a complex, like in birds, are in minimal concentration in healthy subjects.[28] In the fraction of α-globulins and β-globulins migrate mainly APPs and complement, whereas the γ-globulins are circulating antibodies; both β-globulin and γ-globulin can configure a single peak or two. Even in the absence of standardization, it can be seen how the electrophoretic pattern changes in subjects markedly ill compared with healthy subjects in reptiles as well. In an iguana (*Iguana iguana*) with evidence of osteometabolic disease, for example, is frequently observed the decrease of albumins and the marked increase in β globulins (APPs) that indicates suffering hepatic and renal function as a cause or consequence of the metabolic problem.[28] The alteration of the ratio A/G is one of the most interesting parameters to observe and evaluate, as it can reveal a dysproteinemia even in the presence of a normal value of total protein, thus inducing the clinician to further investigation. An important obstacle to the use of electrophoresis, as well as the biochemistry as an assessment of the health status of a reptile, is the marked variability linked not only to the species but also to temperature, ambient humidity, photoperiod, and in general to the season, that for heterothermic animals has much more influence on homeostasis than in homeothermic animals. Only the collection of an adequate volume of data will clarify the actual diagnostic value of this test in reptiles.

REFERENCES

1. Cray C, Tatum LM. Applications of protein electrophoresis in avian diagnostics. J Avian Med Surg 1998;12(1):4–10.
2. Gicking JC, Allen MF, Kendal EH, et al. Plasma protein electrophoresis of the Atlantic Loggerhead Sea Turtle *Caretta caretta*. J Herpetol Med Surg 2004; 14(3):13–8.
3. Zaias J, Norton T, Fickel A, et al. Biochemical and hematologic values for 18 clinically healthy radiated tortoises (*Geochelone radiata*) on St Catherines Island, Georgia. Vet Clin Pathol 2006;35(3):321–32.
4. Work TM, Rameyer RA, Balazs GH, et al. Immune status of free-ranging green turtles with fibropapillomatosis from Hawaii. J Wildl Dis 2001;37(3):574–81.
5. Martinez S, Rodriguez Dominguez MA, Mateo JA, et al. Comparative haematology and blood chemistry of endangered lizards (*Gallotia* species) in the Canary Islands. Vet Rec 2004;155(9):266–9.
6. Coppo JA, Mussart NB, Barboza NN, et al. Electrophoretic proteinogram reference interval from Argentina Northeastern captive caimans (crocodylia: Alligatoridae). InVet 2006;8(1):129–37.

7. Kaneko JJ, Harvey JW, Bruss ML, et al. Clinical biochemistry of domestic animals. Academic Press Elsevier; 2008.
8. Ceron JJ, Eckersall PD, Martinez-Subiela S, et al. Acute phase proteins in dogs and cats: current knowledge and future perspectives. Vet Clin Pathol 2005;34(2): 85–99.
9. Martinez Subiela S, Tecles F, Eckersall PD, et al. 2002 Serum concentration of acute phase proteins in dogs with leishmaniasis. Vet Rec 2002;150(8):241–4.
10. Cray C. New testing options for the diagnosis of *Encephalitozoon cuniculi* in rabbits. Exotic DVM 2009;11(2):27–8.
11. Didier ES, Vossbrinck CR, Baker M, et al. Identification and characterization of three *Encephalitozoon cuniculi* strains. Parasitology 1995;111:411–22.
12. Cox JC. Altered immune responsiveness associated with *Encephalitozoon cuniculi* infection in Rabbits. Infect Immun 1977;15(2):392–5.
13. Sobottka I, Iglauer F, Schuler T, et al. Acute and long term humoral immunity following active immunization of rabbits with inactivated spores of various *Encephalitozoon* species. Parasitol Res 2001;87(1):1–6.
14. Harcourt-Brown FM, Holloway HK. *Encephalitozoon cuniculi* in pet rabbits. Vet Rec 2003;152:427–31.
15. Boussarie PD. L'electrophorese des proteins seriques en pathologie du furet (*Mustela putorius* furo). Bull Acad Vet Fr 2007;160. n4.
16. Dardas TJ, Mallmann VH. Electrophoretic and immunoelectrophoretic studies of sera from normal, tuberculous and non infected tuberculin sensitive guinea pigs. J Bacteriol 1966;92(1).
17. Atchley FO, Auernheimer AH, Wasley MA. Electrophoretic studies of blood serum proteins in Guinea pigs inoculated with *Entoameba histolytica*. Parasitology 1961; 47(2).
18. Xie H, Huff GR, Huff WE, et al. Identification of ovotransferrin as an acute phase protein in chickens. Poult Sci 2002;81(1):112–20.
19. Tohjo H, Miyoshi F, Uchida E, et al. Polyacrylamide gel electrophoretic patterns of chicken serum in acute inflammation induced by intramuscular injection of turpentine. Poult Sci 1995;74(4):648–55.
20. Archer FJ, Battison AL. Differences in electrophoresis patterns between plasma albumins of the cockatiel (*Nymphicus hollandicus*) and the chicken (*Gallus gallus domesticus*). Avian Pathol 1997;26:865–70.
21. Rosenthal KL, Johnston MS, Shofer FS. Assessment of the reliability of plasma electrophoresis in birds. Am J Vet Res 2005;66(3):375–8.
22. Cray C, Rodriguez M, Zajas J. Protein electrophoresis of psittacine plasma. Vet Clin Pathol 2007;36(1):64–72.
23. Ivey ES. Serologic and plasma protein eletrophoretic findings in 7 psittacine birds with aspergillosis. J Avian Med Surg 2000;14(2):103–6.
24. Cray C, Zielezienski-Roberts K, Bonda M, et al. Serologic diagnosis of Sarcocystosis in Psittacine birds: 16 cases. J Avian Med Surg 2005;19(3):208–15.
25. Cray C. Plasma protein electrophoresis: an update. Proc Annu Conf Assoc Avian Vet 1997;209–12.
26. Lumeij JT, Maclean B. Total protein determination in pigeon plasma and serum: comparison of refractometric methods with the Biuret method. J Avian Med Surg 1996;10(3):150–2.
27. Tatum LM, Zajas J, Mealey BK, et al. Protein electrophoresis as a diagnostic and prognostic tool in raptor medicine. J Zoo Wildl Med 2000;31(4):497–502.
28. Zaias J, Cray C. Protein electrophoresis: a tool for the reptilian and amphibian practitioner. J Hum Mov Stud 2002;12:30–2.

Index

Note: Page numbers of article titles are in **boldface** type.

A

Vet Clin Exot Anim 16 (2013) 227–260
http://dx.doi.org/10.1016/S1094-9194(12)00101-6

vetexotic.theclinics.com

Moving?

Make sure your subscription moves with you!

To notify us of your new address, find your **Clinics Account Number** (located on your mailing label above your name), and contact customer service at:

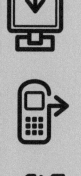

Email: journalscustomerservice-usa@elsevier.com

800-654-2452 (subscribers in the U.S. & Canada)
314-447-8871 (subscribers outside of the U.S. & Canada)

Fax number: 314-447-8029

Elsevier Health Sciences Division
Subscription Customer Service
3251 Riverport Lane
Maryland Heights, MO 63043

*To ensure uninterrupted delivery of your subscription, please notify us at least 4 weeks in advance of move.

Printed and bound by CPI Group (UK) Ltd, Croydon, CR0 4YY

03/10/2024

01040440-0010